a LANGE medical book

CURRENT
Practice Guidelines
In Primary Care
2012

Joseph S. Esherick, MD, FAAFP

Medical Director of Critical Care Services
Associate Director of Medicine
Ventura County Medical Center
Associate Clinical Professor of Family Medicine
David Geffen School of Medicine
Los Angeles, California

Daniel S. Clark, MD, FACC, FAHA

Director of Medicine and Cardiology
Ventura County Medical Center
Assistant Clinical Professor of Family Medicine
David Geffen School of Medicine
Los Angeles, California

Evan D. Slater, MD

Director, Hematology and Medical Oncology
Ventura County Medical Center
Assistant Clinical Professor of Medicine
David Geffen School of Medicine
Los Angeles, California

Mc Graw Hill **Medical**

New York   Chicago   San Francisco   L.   .   London
Madrid   Mexico City   Milan   New Delhi   San Juan   Seoul
Singapore   Sydney   Toronto

CURRENT Practice Guidelines in Primary Care, 2012

Copyright © 2012 by The McGraw-Hill Companies, Inc. Copyright © 2000 through 2009 by The McGraw-Hill Companies, Inc. All rights reserved. Printed in the United States of America. Except as permitted under the United States Copyright Act of 1976, no part of this publication may be reproduced or distributed in any form or by any means, or stored in a data base or retrieval system, without the prior written permission of the publisher.

1 2 3 4 5 6 7 8 9 0 DOC/DOC 17 16 15 14 13 12

ISBN 978-0-07-170194-5
MHID 0-07-170194-X
ISSN 1528-1612

Notice

Medicine is an ever-changing science. As new research and clinical experience broaden our knowledge, changes in treatment and drug therapy are required. The authors and the publisher of this work have checked with sources believed to be reliable in their efforts to provide information that is complete and generally in accord with the standards accepted at the time of publication. However, in view of the possibility of human error or changes in medical sciences, neither the authors nor the publisher nor any other party who has been involved in the preparation or publication of this work warrants that the information contained herein is in every respect accurate or complete, and they disclaim all responsibility for any errors or omissions or for the results obtained from use of the information contained in this work. Readers are encouraged to confirm the information contained herein with other sources. For example and in particular, readers are advised to check the product information sheet included in the package of each drug they plan to administer to be certain that the information contained in this work is accurate and that changes have not been made in the recommended dose or in the contraindications for administration. This recommendation is of particular importance in connection with new or infrequently used drugs.

This book was set in Times Roman by Cenveo Publisher Services.
The editors were James F. Shanahan and Karen G. Edmonson.
The production supervisor was Jeffrey Herzich.
Project management was provided by Cenveo Publisher Services.
RR Donnelley was printer and binder.

This book is printed on acid-free paper.

McGraw-Hill books are available at special quantity discounts to use as premiums and sales promotions, or for use in corporate training programs. To contact a representative please e-mail us at bulksales@mcgraw-hill.com.

This book is dedicated to all of our current and former residents at the Ventura County Medical Center.

Contents

Preface   *xiii*

1. DISEASE SCREENING

√   Abdominal Aortic Aneurysm 2
√   Alcohol Abuse & Dependence 3
√   Anemia 4
    Attention-Deficit/Hyperactivity Disorder 5
+   Bacteriuria, Asymptomatic 6
+   Bacterial Vaginosis 7
    Cancer
√   Bladder 8
√   Breast 10
√   Cervical 17
√   Colorectal 22
√   Endometrial 28
√   Gastric 31
√   Liver 32
√   Lung 33
√   Oral 35
√   Ovarian 36
√   Pancreatic 38
√   Prostate 39
√   Skin 42
√   Testicular 43
√   Thyroid 44
√   Carotid Artery Stenosis 45
+   Celiac Disease 46
√   Chlamydia 47
√   Cholesterol & Lipid Disorders
       Children 48
       Adults 49

√ denotes major 2009 updates.
+ denotes new topic for 2009.

√   Coronary Artery Disease 51
√   Dementia 54
√   Depression 55
√   Developmental Dysplasia of the Hip 56
√   Diabetes Mellitus
       Gestational 57
       Type 2 58
     Falls in the Elderly 60
√   Family Violence and Abuse 61
√   Gonorrhea 62
+   Group B Streptococcal Disease 63
+   Growth Abnormalities, Infant 64
√   Hearing Impairment 65
√   Hemochromatosis 66
+   Hemoglobinopathies 67
√   Hepatitis B Virus Infection, Chronic 68
√   Hepatitis C Virus Infection, Chronic 69
√   Herpes Simplex Virus, Genital 71
√   Human Immunodeficiency Virus 72
√   Hypertension
       Children & Adolescents 74
       Adults 75
+   Illicit Drug Use 77
√   Kidney Disease, Chronic 78
√   Lead Poisoning 79
+   Motor Vehicle Safety 81
√   Obesity
       Children 82
       Adults 83
√   Osteoporosis 84
+   Phenylketonuria 85
+   RH (D) Incompatibility 86
+   Scoliosis 87
     Speech & Language Delay 88
√   Syphilis 89
√   Thyroid Disease 90

√ denotes major 2009 updates.
+ denotes new topic for 2009.

√   Tobacco Use 91
√   Tuberculosis, Latent 93
√   Visual Impairment, Glaucoma, or Cataract 94

2. DISEASE PREVENTION

√   Primary Prevention of Cancer: NCI Evidence Summary 96
+   Dental Caries 104
√   Diabetes Mellitus, Type 2 105
+   Domestic Violence 106
+   Driving Risk 107
√   Endocarditis 108
√   Falls in the Elderly 109
+   Gonorrhea, Ophthalmia Neonatorum 110
+   Group B Streptococcal Infection 111
+   Human Immunodeficiency Virus, Opportunistic Infections 112
  Prevention Among HIV-Infected Adults 113
  Prevention Among HIV-Exposed and HIV-Infected Infants
   and Children 117
√   Hypertension 121
  Lifestyle Modifications 122
+   Immunizations
  Adults 123
  Infants and Children 124
  Children and Adolescents 125
+   Influenza
  Chemoprophylaxis 126
  Vaccination 127
+   Motor Vehicle Injury, Prevention 128
√   Myocardial Infarction 129
+   Neural Tube Defects 136
+   Obesity 137
√   Osteoporotic Hip Fractures 138
+   Pressure Ulcers 139
+   Sexually Transmitted Infections 141
√   Stroke 142

√ denotes major 2009 updates.
+ denotes new topic for 2009.

+   Sudden Infant Death Syndrome 147
+   Tobacco Use 148

3. DISEASE MANAGEMENT

+   Adrenal Incidentalomas 150
√   Alcohol Use Disorders 151
+   Androgen Deficiency Syndrome 152
+   Anxiety 153
√   Asthma 154
√   Atrial Fibrillation
     Management 156
+   Benign Prostatic Hyperplasia 163
+   Bronchitis, Acute 165
√   CA Survivorship
     Late Effects of CA Treatments 166
√   Carotid Artery Stenosis 171
    Cataract in Adults
     Evaluation & Management 172
√   Cerumen Impaction 174
    Cholesterol & Lipid Management
     Adults 175
     Children 177
    Constipation 178
    Contraceptive Use 179
√   Chronic Obstructive Pulmonary Disease
     COPD Exacerbations 182
     Stable COPD 183
     Changes in Classifications 184
     Recommendations 188
     Additional Changes 192
+   Coronary Artery Stent Therapy
     Use of Triple Anticoagulation Treatment 193
√   Delirium 195
√   Dementia 196
√   Depression 197

√ denotes major 2009 updates.
+ denotes new topic for 2009.

Diabetes Mellitus
Type 1 198
+   Type 2 200
+ Erectile Dysfunction 204
+ Glaucoma, Chronic Open Angle 205
+ Headache 206
Heart Failure 214
+ Hepatitis B Virus 215
+ Hepatitis C Virus 216
+ Hoarseness 217
+ Human Immunodeficiency Virus
Adults and Children 218
Pregnancy 220
Antiretroviral Therapy 222
Hypertension
Initiating Treatment 223
Lifestyle Modifications 224
Recommended Medications for Compelling Indications 225
Refractory Hypertension 226
+ Influenza 228
+ Kidney Disease
Chronic 229
Chronic-Mineral and Bone Disorders 231
+ Kidney Stones 232
+ Back Pain
Low 233
Evaluation and Management 234
Metabolic Syndrome
Identification & Management 235
+ Methicillin-Resistant Staphylococcus Aureus 236
+ Obesity Management 238
√ Osteoporosis 240
Glucocorticoid-Induced 242
Otitis Media, Acute 244
√ Palliative & End-of-Life Care
Pain Management 246
+ Abnormal Pap Smear 247

√ denotes major 2009 updates.
+ denotes new topic for 2009.

√   Perioperative Cardiovascular Evaluation 248
   Pneumonia, Community-Acquired
     Evaluation 250
     Suspected Pathogens 251
   Pregnancy
     Routine Prenatal Care 252
     Perinatal & Postnatal Guidelines 255
   Psoriasis, Plaque-Type 256
   Rheumatoid Arthritis
     Biologic Disease-Modifying Antirheumatic Drugs 257
     Nonbiologic Disease-Modifying Antirheumatic Drugs 258
+   Noninfectious Rhinitis Management 259
+   Sexually Transmitted Diseases 260
+   Management of Thyroid Nodules 267
   Tobacco Cessation 268
+   Acute Pharyngitis 271
+   Urinary Incontinence
     Stress 272
     Men 273
     Women 274
√   Urinary Tract Infections (UTIS) 275
+   Lower Urinary Tract Symptoms (LUTS) 277
+   Vertigo, Benign Paroxysmal Positional (BPPV) 278

4. APPENDICES

Appendix I: Screening Instruments
   Alcohol Abuse 280
   Depression 283
   Geriatric Depression Scale 287
Appendix II: Functional Assessment Screening in the Elderly 288
Appendix III: Screening and Prevention
 Guidelines in Perspective 290
Appendix IV: 95th Percentile of Blood Pressure
   Boys 292
   Girls 293
Appendix V: Body Mass Index Conversion Table 294

√ denotes major 2009 updates.
+ denotes new topic for 2009.

Appendix VI: Cardiac Risk-Farmingham Study
  Men 295
  Women 297
Appendix VII: Estimate of 10-Year Stroke Risk
  Men 299
  Women 300
√ Appendix VIII: Immunizations Schedules 302
Appendix IX: Professional Societies and Governmental
  Agencies 313

Index 317

Preface

Current Practice Guidelines in Primary Care, 2012 is intended for all clinicians interested in updated, evidence-based guidelines for primary care topics. This pocket-sized reference consolidates information from nationally recognized medical associations and government agencies into concise recommendations and guidelines of virtually all ambulatory care topics. This book is organized into topics related to disease screening, disease prevention, and disease management for quick reference to the evaluation and treatment of the most common primary care disorders.

The 2012 edition of Current Practice Guidelines in Primary Care contains fifty five new chapters and updates virtually every other primary care topic. It is a great resource for residents, medical students, midlevel providers, and practicing physicians in family medicine, internal medicine, pediatrics, and obstetrics and gynecology.

Although painstaking efforts have been made to find all errors and omissions, some errors may remain. If you find and error or wish to make a suggestion, please email us at pbg.ecommerce_custserv@mcgraw-hill.com.

Evan Slater, MD
Joseph Esherick, MD, FAAFP
Daniel S. Clark, MD, FACC, FAHA

1
Disease Screening

ABDOMINAL AORTIC ANEURYSM

Disease Screening	Organization	Date	Population	Recommendations	Comments	Source
Abdominal Aortic Aneurysm (AAA)	USPSTF ACC/AHA	2005 2006	Men aged 65–75 years who have ever smoked	One-time screening for AAA by ultrasonography. No recommendation for or against screening for AAA in men aged 65–75 years who have never smoked.	1. Cochrane review (2007): Significant decrease in AAA-specific mortality in men (OR, 0.60, 95% CI 0.47–0.99) but not for women. (*Cochrane Database of Syst Rev.* 2007;2:CD002945; http://www.thecochranelibrary.com) 2. Early mortality benefit of screening (men aged 65–74 years) maintained at 7-year follow-up. Cost-effectiveness of screening improves over time. (*Ann Intern Med.* 2007;146:699) 3. Surgical repair of AAA should be considered if diameter ≥ 5.5 cm or if AAA expands ≥ 0.5 cm over 6 months to reduce higher risk of rupture. Meta-analysis: endovascular repair associated with fewer postoperative adverse events and lower 30-day and aneurysm-related mortality but not all-cause mortality compared to open repair. [*Br J Surg.* 2008;95(6):677]	http://www.ahrq.gov/clinic/uspstf/uspsaneu.htm *Circulation.* 2006;113(11): e463–e654 *J Vasc Surg.* 2007;45:1268–1276
	USPSTF	2005	Women	Routine screening is not recommended.		
	CMS	2007	Men aged 65–75 years who have smoked at least 100 cigarettes in their lifetime or who have a family history of AAA.	Recommend one-time ultrasound screening for AAA.	4. Asymptomatic AAA between 4.4 and 5.5 cm. should have regular ultrasound surveillance with surgical intervention when AAA expands > 1 cm per year or diameter reaches 5.5 cm. (*Cochrane Database of Sys Rev.* 2008, CD001835) http://www.thecochranelibrary.com) 5. Medicare covers one-time limited screening.	http://www.medicare.gov/navigation/manage-your-health/preventive-services/abdominal aortic-aneurysm.aspx

ALCOHOL ABUSE & DEPENDENCE						
Disease Screening	Organization	Date	Population	Recommendations	Comments	Source
Alcohol Abuse & Dependence	AAFP USPSTF VA/DOD ICSI	2010 2004 2009 2010	Adults	Screen all adults in primary care settings, including pregnant women, for alcohol misuse.	1. Screen annually using validated tool. 2. AUDIT score ≥ 4 for men and ≥ 3 for women and SASQ reporting of ≥ 5 drinks in a day (men) or ≥ 4 drinks in a day (women) in the past year are valid and reliable screening instruments for identifying unhealthy alcohol use. 3. The TWEAK and the T-ACE are designed to screen pregnant women for alcohol misuse.	http://www.guidelines.gov/content.aspx?id=34005 http://www.ahrq.gov/clinic/pocketgd1011/pocketgd1011.pdf http://www.icsi.org/preventive_services_for_adults/preventive_services_for_adults_4.html
	VA/DOD	2009	Adults	Provide brief intervention to those who have a positive alcohol misuse screen. Brief interventions during future visits.		http://www.guidelines.gov/content.aspx?id=15676
	AAFP USPSTF ICSI	2010 2004 2010	Adolescents Children and adolescents	Insufficient evidence to recommend for or against screening or counseling interventions to prevent or reduce alcohol misuse by adolescents.	1. AUDIT and CAGE questionnaires have not been validated in children or adolescents. 2. Reinforce not drinking and driving or riding with any driver under the influence. 3. Reinforce to women the harmful effects of alcohol on fetuses.	http://www.guidelines.gov/content.aspx?id=34005 http://www.icsi.org/preventive_services_for_children_guideline_/preventive_services_for_children_and_adolescents_2531.html

Disease Screening	Organization	Date	Population	Recommendations	Comments	Source
Anemia	AAFP	2006	Infants aged 6–12 months	Perform selective, single hemoglobin or hematocrit screening for high-risk infants.[a]	Reticulocyte hemoglobin content is a more sensitive and specific marker than is serum hemoglobin level for iron deficiency. One-third of patients with iron deficiency will have a hemoglobin level > 11 g/dL.	http://www.aafp.org/online/en/home/clinical/exam.html
	USPSTF	2006	Infants aged 6–12 months	Evidence is insufficient to recommend for or against routine screening, but risk assessment based on diet, socioeconomic status, prematurity, and low birth weight should be done.	Recommends routine iron supplementation in high-risk children aged 6–12 months.	
	USPSTF	2006	Pregnant women	Screen all women with hemoglobin or hematocrit at first prenatal visit.	1. Insufficient evidence to recommend for or against routine use of iron supplements for nonanemic pregnant women (USPSTF). 2. When acute stress or inflammatory disorders are not present, a serum ferritin level is the most accurate test for evaluating iron deficiency anemia. Among women of childbearing age, a cut-off of 30 ng/mL has sensitivity of 92%, specificity of 98% (*Blood.* 1997;89:1052–1057). 3. Severe anemia (hemoglobin < 6) associated with abnormal fetal oxygenation and transfusion should be considered. In iron-deficient women intolerant of oral iron, intravenous iron sucrose or iron dextran should be given.	http://www.ahrq.gov/clinic/cpgsix.htm

[a]Includes infants living in poverty, blacks, Native Americans and Alaska Natives, immigrants from developing countries, preterm and low-birth-weight infants, and infants whose principal dietary intake is unfortified cow's milk or soy milk. Less than two servings per day of iron-rich foods (iron-fortified breakfast cereals or meats).

ATTENTION-DEFICIT/HYPERACTIVITY DISORDER

Disease Screening	Organization	Date	Population	Recommendations	Comments	Source
Attention Deficit/ Hyperactivity Disorder (ADHD)	AAFP AAP	2000	Children aged 6–12 years with inattention, hyperactivity, impulsivity, academic underachievement, or behavioral problems	Initiate an evaluation for ADHD. Diagnosis requires the child meet DSM-IV criteria[a] and direct supporting evidence from parents or caregivers and classroom teacher. Evaluation of a child with ADHD should include assessment for coexisting disorders.	1. The rise in stimulant prescriptions since 1990 plateaued in 2002. *(Am J Psychiatr.* 2006;163:579) 2. Current estimates are that 8.7% of U.S. children/adolescents and 5% of adults meet criteria for ADHD *(Arch Pediatr Adolesc Med.* 2007;161:857; *Am J Psychiatr.* 2006;163:716). Worldwide prevalence is estimated at 5.3%. *(Am J Psychiatr.* 2007;164:942) 3. The U.S. Food and Drug Administration (FDA) approved a "black box" warning regarding the potential for cardiovascular side effects of ADHD stimulant drugs. *(NEJM.* 2006;354:1445)	*Pediatrics.* 2000; 105: 1158

[a]DSM-IV Criteria for ADHD:

I: Either A or B.

A: *Six or more of the following symptoms of inattention have been present for at least 6 months to a point that is disruptive and inappropriate for developmental level.*

Inattention: (1) Often does not give close attention to details or makes careless mistakes in schoolwork, work, or other activities. (2) Often has trouble keeping attention on tasks or play activities. (3) Often does not seem to listen when spoken to directly. (4) Often does not follow instructions and fails to finish schoolwork, chores, or duties in the workplace (not due to oppositional behavior or failure to understand instructions). (5) Often has trouble organizing activities. (6) Often avoids, dislikes, or does not want to do things that take a lot of mental effort for a long period of time (such as schoolwork or homework). (7) Often loses things needed for tasks and activities (eg, toys, school assignments, pencils, books, or tools). (8) Is often easily distracted. (9) Is often forgetful in daily activities.

B: *Six or more of the following symptoms of hyperactivity-impulsivity have been present for at least 6 months to an extent that is disruptive and inappropriate for developmental level.*

Hyperactivity: (1) Often fidgets with hands or feet or squirms in seat. (2) Often gets up from seat when remaining in seat is expected. (3) Often runs about or climbs when and where it is not appropriate (adolescents or adults may feel very restless). (4) Often has trouble playing or enjoying leisure activities quietly. (5) Is often "on the go" or often acts as if "driven by a motor." (6) Often talks excessively.

Impulsivity: (1) Often blurts out answers before questions have been finished. (2) Often has trouble waiting one's turn. (3) Often interrupts or intrudes on others (eg, butts into conversations or games).

II: Some symptoms that cause impairment were present before age 7 years.

III: Some impairment from the symptoms is present in two or more settings (eg, at school/work and at home).

IV: There must be clear evidence of significant impairment in social, school, or work functioning.

V: The symptoms do not happen only during the course of a pervasive developmental disorder, schizophrenia, or other psychotic disorder. The symptoms are not better accounted for by another mental disorder (eg, mood disorder, anxiety disorder, dissociative disorder, or a personality disorder).

BACTERIURIA, ASYMPTOMATIC

Disease Screening	Organization	Date	Population	Recommendations	Comments	Source
Bacteriuria, Asymptomatic	AAFP USPSTF	2010 2008	Pregnant women	Recommend screening for bacteriuria at first prenatal visit or at 12–16 weeks gestation.	http://www.guidelines.gov/content. aspx?id=34005 http://www.uspreventiveservicestaskforce. org/uspstf08/asymptbact/asbactrs.htm	
	AAFP USPSTF	2010 2008	Men and nonpregnant women	Recommends against routine screening for bacteriuria.		

Disease Screening	Organization	Date	Population	Recommendations	Comments	Source
BACTERIAL VAGINOSIS						
Bacterial Vaginosis	AAFP USPSTF	2010 2008	Pregnant women at high risk for preterm delivery	Insufficient evidence to recommend for or against routine screening.	http://www.guidelines.gov/content.aspx?id=34005 http://www.uspreventiveservicestaskforce.org/uspstf08/bv/bvrs.htm	
	AAFP USPSTF	2010 2008	Low-risk pregnant women	Recommend against routine screening.		

CANCER, BLADDER

Disease Screening	Organization	Date	Population	Recommendations	Comments	Source
Cancer, Bladder	AAFP	2008	Asymptomatic persons	Recommends against routine screening for bladder cancer (CA) in adults.	1. *Benefits:* There is inadequate evidence to determine whether screening for bladder CA would have any impact on mortality. *Harms:* Based on fair evidence, screening for bladder CA would result in unnecessary diagnostic procedures with attendant morbidity. (NCI, 2008).	http://www.aafp.org/online/en/home/clinical/exam.html
	USPSTF	2004			2. A high index of suspicion should be maintained in anyone with a history of smoking (4–7-fold increased risk),[a] exposure to industrial toxins (aromatic amines, benzene) or therapeutic pelvic radiation, cyclophosphamide chemotherapy, history of *Schistosoma haematobium* cystitis, hereditary nonpolyposis colon CA (Lynch syndrome) and history of transitional cell carcinoma of ureter (50% risk of subsequent bladder CA). Large screening studies in these high-risk populations have not been performed.	http://www.ahrq.gov/clinic/uspstf/uspsblad.htm

CANCER, BLADDER

Disease Screening	Organization	Date	Population	Recommendations	Comments	Source
Cancer, Bladder (continued)					3. Urine cytology with only 10% positive predictive value, urinary biomarkers (nuclear matrix protein 22, telomerase) with suboptimal sensitivity and specificity.	http://www.cancer.gov/cancer_information/testing

[a]Individuals who smoke are four to seven times more likely to develop bladder CA than are individuals who have never smoked. Additional environmental risk factors: exposure to aminobiphenyls; aromatic amines; azo dyes; combustion gases and soot from coal; chlorination byproducts in heated water; aldehydes used in chemical dyes and in the rubber and textile industries; organic chemicals used in dry cleaning, paper manufacturing, rope and twine making, and apparel manufacturing; contaminated Chinese herbs; arsenic in well water. Additional risk factors: prolonged exposure to urinary *Schistosoma haematobium* bladder infections, cyclophosphamide, or pelvic radiation therapy for other malignancies.

Disease Screening	Organization	Date	Population	Recommendations[a,b]	Comments	Source
CANCER, BREAST						
Cancer, Breast	ACS	2008	Women aged 20–39 years	Inform women of benefits and limitations of breast self-exam (BSE). Educate concerning reporting a lump or breast symptoms. Clinical breast exam (CBE) every 2–3 years. Breast imaging not indicated for average-risk women.	1. *Benefits of mammography screening:* Based on fair evidence, screening mammography in women aged 40–70 years decreases breast CA mortality. The benefit is higher in older women (reduction in risk of death in women aged 40–49 years = 15%–20%, 25%–30% in women aged ≥ 50 years. *Harms:* Based on solid evidence, screening mammography may lead to potential harm by overdiagnosis (indolent tumors that are not life-threatening) and unnecessary biopsies for benign disease. (NCI, 2008)	http://www.cancer.org
	ACP	2007	Women aged 40–49 years	Perform individualized assessment of breast CA risk; base screening decision on benefits and harms of screening (see Comment 1) as well as on a woman's preferences and CA risk profile.	2. BSE does not improve breast CA mortality (*Br J Cancer.* 2003;88:1047) and increases the rate of false-positive biopsies. (*J Natl Cancer Inst.* 2002;94:1445) 3. Twenty-five percent of breast CAs diagnosed before age 40 years are attributable to *BRCA1* or 2 mutations.	*Ann Intern Med.* 2007;146:511

Disease Screening	Organization	Date	Population	Recommendations[a,b]	Comments	Source
CANCER, BREAST						
Cancer, Breast (continued)	UK-NHS	2006	Women aged 40–49 years	Based on current evidence, routine screening is not recommended.	4. The sensitivity of annual screening of young (aged 35–49 years) high-risk women with magnetic resonance imaging (MRI) and mammography is superior to either alone, but MRI is associated with a significant increase in false-positives. (*Lancet.* 2005;365:1769) 5. Computer-aided detection in screening mammography appears to reduce overall accuracy (by increasing false-positive rate), although it is more sensitive in women aged < 50 years with dense breasts. (*NEJM.* 2007;356:1399)	http://www.cancerscreening.nhs.uk
	AAFP	2008	Women aged ≥ 40 years	Mammography, with or without CBE, every 1–2 years after counseling about potential risks and benefits.	Evidence is insufficient to recommend for or against routine CBE alone, or teaching or performing a routine BSE.	http://www.aafp.org/online/en/home/clinical/exam.html

Disease Screening	Organization	Date	Population	Recommendations[a,b]	Comments	Source
CANCER, BREAST						
Cancer, Breast (continued)	ACS	2008	Women aged ≥40 years	Mammography and CBE yearly; if > 20% lifetime risk of breast CA, annual mammogram + MRI. *BRCA-1* and 2 mutation-positive women should begin MRI and mammogram screening at age 30 years or younger depending on family history. Lymphoma survivors with a history of mediastinal radiation should begin mammography and MRI yearly 10 years after radiation.	1. In high-risk women, probability of breast CA when mammogram is negative = 1.4% (1.2%–1.6%) versus when mammogram plus MRI are negative = 0.3% (0.1%–0.8%) (*Ann Intern Med.* 2008;148:671) MRI two to three times as sensitive as mammogram, but 2-fold increase in false-positives—use in selected high-risk population (*J Clin Onc.* 2005;23:8469. *J Clin Onc.* 2009;27:6124) 2. If lifetime risk of breast CA is between 15% and 20%, women should discuss risks/benefits of adding annual MRI to mammography screening. Sensitivity of MRI superior to mammography, especially in higher-risk women aged < 50 years with dense breasts (increasing breast density increases risk of breast CA and lowers sensitivity of mammogram). A > 75% breast density increases risk of breast CA 5-fold. (*J Clin Onc.* 2010; 28:3830)	http://www.cancer.org *CA Cancer J Clin.* 2007;57:75

Disease Screening	Organization	Date	Population	Recommendations[a,b]	Comments	Source
CANCER, BREAST						
Cancer, Breast (continued)	UK-NHS	2006	Women aged 50–70 years Women aged >70 years	Program-initiated mammography screening of all women every 3 years. Patient-initiated screening covered by National Health Service (NHS).	Annual versus 3-year screening interval showed no significant difference in predicted breast CA mortality, although relative risk reduction among annually screened women had nonsignificant reduction of 5%–11%. (*Eur J Cancer.* 2002;38:1458)	http://www.cancerscreening.nhs.uk
	AGS	2005	Women aged 70–85 years	If estimated life expectancy ≥ 5 years, then offer screening mammography ± CBE every 1–2 years.	Incidence of breast CA highest in this age range but significant comorbidities and competing causes of death compared with that of younger women.	http://www.americangeriatrics.org/products/positionpapers/breast_cancer_position_statement.pdf
	AAFP	2008	Women with family history associated with increased risk (breast CA aged < 50 years or ovarian CA at any age) for deleterious mutations in *BRCA1* or *BRCA2* genes[c]	Refer for genetic counseling and evaluation for *BRCA* testing.	1. In one study, nearly half of *BRCA*-positive women developed malignant disease detected by mammography < 1 year after a normal screening mammogram. (*Cancer.* 2004;100:2079). 2. Consider mammography plus MRI screening in high-risk women. (*CA Cancer J Clin.* 2011;61:8–30) 3. Management of an inherited predisposition to breast CA is controversial. (*NEJM.* 2007;357:154) Risk-reducing surgery versus enhanced surveillance with yearly magnetic resonance imaging (MRI) and mammography.	http://www.aafp.org/online/en/home/clinical/exam.html http://www.ahrq.gov/clinic/uspstf/uspstfbrgen.html

					CANCER, BREAST	
Disease Screening	Organization	Date	Population	Recommendations[a,b]	Comments	Source
Cancer, Breast (continued)	USPSTF	2009	Women aged 50–74 years	—biennial screening mammography —BSE teaching not recommended —inconclusive data for screening women aged >75 years	These recommendations for women aged 40–50 years have been widely criticized and largely ignored by other advisory organizations as inconsistent with available data. Subsequent trial from Norway showed significant benefit in mortality reduction (28%) in the aged 40–49 years subset. Analysis of data sets continues but there has been no major change in practice patterns (*Am J Roentgenol.* 2011;196:112. *Am J Coll Rad.* 2010;7:18. *Cancer.* 2011;117:7). (*Eur J Cancer.* 2010;46:3137)	http://www.ahrqior/clinic/uspstf
			Women aged 40–50 years	—Decision to begin screening mammography before age 50 years should be individualized according to benefit versus harm for each patient.		
	NCCN	2011	Aged 20–40 years (average risk)	CBE every 1–3 years—breast awareness education	A woman with mediastinal radiation at age 20–25 years will have a 75-fold increased risk of breast CA at age 35 years versus age-matched controls.	www.nccn.org
			Aged > 40 years (average risk)	Annual CBE, annual mammogram. MRI not recommended in average-risk patients.		
			Acquired increased risk—prior thoracic radiation therapy	CBE q6–12 months, annual mammogram and annual MRI beginning 8–10 years after radiation therapy or age 25 years, whichever occurs last	Salpingo-oophorectomy will decrease risk of breast CA in *BRCA1* and 2 carriers by 50% and decrease risk of ovarian CA by 90%–95%.	

					CANCER, BREAST		
Disease Screening	Organization	Date	Population	Recommendations[a,b]	Comments		Source
Cancer, Breast (continued)	USPSTF	2009	Lifetime risk of breast CA > 20% based on family history, genetic predisposition (*BRCA1* or 2).	Aged < 25 years annual CBE, breast awareness education, and referral to genetic counselor	Tamoxifen or raloxifene not studied as de novo chemo prevention in *BRCA1* or 2 patients, but tamoxifen will decrease risk of contralateral breast CA by 50% in *BRCA*-mutated breast CA patients. (*Int J Cancer.* 2006;118:2281).		http://www.ahrqigor/clinic/uspstf
	NCCN	2011	History of lobular carcinoma in situ atypical hyperplasia or history of breast CA	Aged > 25 years, annual mammogram and MRI, CBE q6–12 months, consider risk-reducing strategies (surgery, chemo prevention)	Risk-reducing bilateral mastectomy in *BRCA1* and 2 mutation carriers results in a 90% risk reduction in incidence of breast CA and a 90% rate of satisfaction with risk-reducing surgery (*NEJM.* 2001;345:159. *JAMA.* 2010;304:967)		www.NCCN.org

[a]Debate about the value of screening mammograms was triggered by a Cochrane review published on October 20, 2001 (*Lancet.* 2001;358:1340–1342). This review cited a number of methodologic and analytic flaws in the large long-term mammography trials. The USPSTF and NCI concluded that the flaws were problematic but unlikely to negate the consistent and significant mortality reductions observed in the trials.

[b]Summary of current evidence: *CA Cancer J Clin.* 2011;61:8–30.

[c]1. Women not of Ashkenazi Jewish heritage:

Two first-degree relatives with breast CA, one of whom received the diagnosis at age ≤50 years.

A combination of ≥3 first- or second-degree relatives with breast CA.

A combination of both breast and ovarian CA among first- and second-degree relatives.

A first-degree relative with bilateral breast CA.

A combination of ≥2 first- or second-degree relatives with ovarian CA.

A first- or second-degree relative with both breast and ovarian CA.

A history of breast CA in a male relative.

2. Women of Ashkenazi Jewish heritage: Any first-degree relative (or second-degree relatives on the same side of the family) with breast or ovarian CA.

CANCER, BREAST				
TABLE A: HARMS OF SCREENING MAMMOGRAPHY				
Harm	**Internal Validity**	**Consistency**	**Magnitude of Effects**	**External Validity**
Treatment of insignificant CAs (overdiagnosis, true-positives) can result in breast deformity, lymphedema, thromboembolic events, new CAs, or chemotherapy-induced toxicities.	Good	Good	Approximately 20%–30% of breast CAs detected by screening mammograms represent overdiagnosis. (*BMJ.* 2009;339:2587) Oncotype DX (a predictive panel of 15 breast CA genes) can reduce the use of chemotherapy by 50% in node-negative hormone receptor-positive patients.	Good
Additional testing (false-positives)	Good	Good	Estimated to occur in 30% of women screened annually for 10 years, 7%–10% of whom will have biopsies. This creates anxiety and negative quality of life impact. (*Ann Int Med.* 2009;151:738)	Good
False sense of security, delay in CA diagnosis (false-negatives)	Good	Good	About 10%–30% of women with invasive CA will have negative mammogram results, especially if young with dense breasts or with lobular or high-grade CAs (*Radiology.* 2005;235:775).	Good
Radiation-induced mutation can cause breast CA, especially if exposed before age 30 years. Latency is more than 10 years, and the increased risk persists lifelong.	Good	Good	In women beginning screening at age 40 years, benefits far outweigh risks of radiation inducing breast CA. Women should avoid unnecessary CT scanning. (*BJC.* 2005;93:590)	Good

Source: NCI. 2010—http://www.cancer.gov

Disease Screening	Organization	Date	Population	Recommendations	Comments	Source
CANCER, CERVICAL						
Cancer, Cervical	ACS	2008	Women within 3 years after first sexual intercourse or by age 21 years, whichever comes first[a]	Annual Pap smear until age 30 years (every 2 years if liquid-based Pap test) (ACS).[b] Human papillomavirus (HPV) DNA testing not recommended if aged < 30 years (majority of young patients will clear the infection). At age ≥ 30 years, if three consecutive normal Pap smear results, may screen with Pap smears every 2–3 years; or screen every 3 years with Pap smear plus HPV DNA test. Continue to screen annually if risk factors present.[c]	1. Cervical CA is causally related to infection with HPV (> 70% associated with either HPV-18 or HPV-16 genotype) (See new ACIP HPV recommendations, Appendix VIII). 2. Immunocompromised women (organ transplantation, chemotherapy, chronic steroid therapy, or human immunodeficiency virus [HIV]) should be tested twice during the first year after initiating of screening and annually thereafter (*CA Cancer J Clin.* 2011;61:8). 3. Women with a history of cervical CA or in utero exposure to diethylstilbestrol (DES) should continue average risk protocol for women aged < 30 years indefinitely. 4. HPV vaccination of young women is now recommended by ACIP, UK-NHS, and others. Cervical CA screening recommendations have not changed for women receiving the vaccine because the vaccine covers only 70% of HPV serotypes that cause cervical CA (*MMWR.* 2007;56(RR-2):1–24).	http://www.cancer.org http://www.survivorshipguidelines.org

	CANCER, CERVICAL					
Disease Screening	Organization	Date	Population	Recommendations	Comments	Source
Cancer, Cervical (continued)	AAFP	2007	Women who have ever had sex and have a cervix[a]	Strongly recommends Pap smear at least every 3 years.[d]	5. Long-term use of oral contraceptives may increase risk of cervical CA in women who test positive for cervical HPV DNA (*Lancet.* 2002;359:1085). Smoking increases risk of cervical CA 4-fold. (*AJ Epidemiology.* 1990;131:945).	http://www.aafp.org/online/en/home/clinical/exam.html
	USPSTF	2003			6. A vaccine against HPV-16 and 18 significantly reduces the risk of acquiring transient and persistent infection. [*NEJM.* 2002;347:1645. *Obstet Gynecol.* 2006;107(1):4]. 7. *Benefits:* Based on solid evidence, regular screening of appropriate women with the Pap test reduces mortality from cervical CA. Screening is effective when started within 3 years after first vaginal intercourse. *Harms:* Based on solid evidence, regular screening with the Pap test leads to additional diagnostic procedures and treatment for low-grade squamous intraepithelial lesions (LSILs), with uncertain long-term consequences on fertility and pregnancy. Harms are greatest for younger women, who have a higher prevalence of LSILs. LSILs often regress without treatment. False-positives in postmenopausal women are due to mucosal atrophy. (NCI, 2008)	http://www.ahrq.gov/clinic/uspstf/uspscerv.htm

Disease Screening	Organization	Date	Population	Recommendations	Comments	Source
Cancer, Cervical (continued)	IARC	2005	Women aged < 25 years	Routine screening is not recommended.	UK-NHS initiated an HPV immunization program for girls aged 12–13 years in September 2008.	http://screening.iarc.fr
	UK-NHS	2004				http://www.cancerscreening.nhs.uk
	IARC	2005	Women aged 25–49 years	Routinely screen every 3 years (IARC: if country has sufficient resources; otherwise, every 5 years).	UK-NHS contacts all eligible women who are registered with a primary care doctor.	http://screening.iarc.fr
	UK-NHS	2004	Women aged 50–64 years	Routinely screen every 5 years with conventional cytology.		http://www.cancerscreening.nhs.uk
	IARC	2005	Women aged ≥ 65 years	Women who have always tested negative in an organized screening program should cease screening once they attain the age of 65 years.		http://screening.iarc.fr

CANCER, CERVICAL

Disease Screening	Organization	Date	Population	Recommendations	Comments	Source
Cancer, Cervical (continued)	UK-NHS	2004	Women aged ≥ 65 years	Screen women who have not been screened since age 50 years or who have had recent abnormal test results.	Stop screening after age 65 years if there are three consecutive normal test results.	http://www.cancerscreening.nhs.uk
	ACOG	2009	Begin at age 21 years independent of sexual history	Every 2 years from ages 21–29.	Women aged ≥ 30 years can extend interval to every 2–3 years if: three consecutive negative screens, no history of cervical intraepithelial neoplasia 2 or 3, not immunocompromised, no HIV, and not exposed to DES. No more often than 3 years if cervical cytology and HPV testing combined.	ACOG Practice bulletin *Obstet Gynecol.* 2009; 114:1409.
	USPSTF	2003	Women aged > 65 years	Recommends against routine screening if woman has had adequate recent screening and normal Pap smear results and is not otherwise at high risk for cervical CA.[c]	Beyond age 70 years, there is little evidence for or against screening women who have been regularly screened in previous years. Individual circumstances, such as the patient's life expectancy, ability to undergo treatment if CA is detected, and ability to cooperate with and tolerate the Pap smear procedure, may obviate the need for cervical CA screening.	http://www.ahrq.gov/clinic/uspstf/uspscerv.htm
	ACS	2008	Women aged ≥ 70 years	Discontinue screening if ≥ three normal Pap smear results in a row and no abnormal Pap smear results in the last 10 years.[e]		http://www.cancer.org

Disease Screening	Organization	Date	Population	Recommendations	Comments	Source
CANCER, CERVICAL						
Cancer, Cervical (continued)	ACS ACOG USPSTF	2008 2009 2003	Women without a cervix	Recommends against routine Pap smear screening in women who have had a total hysterectomy or removal of the cervix for benign disease and no history of abnormal cell growth.		http://www.cancer.org http://www.ahrq.gov/clinic/uspstf/uspscerv.htm ACOG Committee Opinion, No. 357, Dec 2006

[a] If sexual history is unknown or considered unreliable, screening should begin at age 18 years.

[b] New tests to improve CA detection include liquid-based/thin-layer preparations, computer-assisted screening methods, and HPV testing (*Am Fam Phys.* 2001;64:729. *N Engl J Med.* 2007;357:1579. *JAMA.* 2009;302:1757).

[c] High-risk factors include DES exposure before birth, HIV infection, or other forms of immunosuppression, including chronic steroid use.

[d] Most of the benefit can be obtained by beginning screening within 3 years of onset of sexual activity or at age 21 years, whichever comes first.

[e] Women with a history of cervical CA, DES exposure, HIV infection, or a weakened immune system should continue to have screenings as long as they are in more than 5-year life expectancy.

Disease Screening	Organization	Date	Population	Recommendations	Comments	Source
					CANCER, COLORECTAL	
Cancer, Colorectal	ACS USMTFCC[a] ACR	2008		See Table on page 26. Tests that find polyps and CA are preferred.	Although colonoscopy is the *de facto* gold standard for colon CA screening, choice of screening technique depends on risk, co morbidities, insurance coverage, patient preference, and availability. Above all, do something to screen for colon CA.	*CA Cancer J Clin.* 2008;58:130 *de facto*
	AAFP USPSTF	2008 2002	Aged ≥ 50 years at average risk[b]	Screen with one of the following strategies[c,d,e]. 1. Fecal occult blood test (FOBT) annually[f] 2. Flexible sigmoidoscopy every 5 years	1. The USPSTF "strongly recommends" colorectal cancer (CRC) screening in this group. 2. Flexible sigmoidoscopy and one-time FOBT mandating a colonoscopy if either yields positive results will miss 25% of significant proximal neoplasia. This strategy should include yearly FOBT. (*N Engl J Med.* 2001;345:555) 3. FOBT alone decreased CRC mortality by 33% compared with those who were not screened. (*Gastroenterology.* 2004;126)	http://www.aafp.org/online/en/home/clinical/exam.html http://www.cancer.org *Gastrointestinal Endoscopy.* 2006;63:546

Disease Screening	Organization	Date	Population	Recommendations	Comments	Source
CANCER, COLORECTAL						
Cancer, Colorectal (continued)				3. FOBT annually plus flexible sigmoidoscopy every 5 years	4. Accuracy of colonoscopy is operator dependent—rapid withdrawal time, poor prep, and lack of experience will increase false-negatives. (*N Engl J Med.* 2006;355:2533)	*Gastroenterology.* 2003;124:544
				4. Colonoscopy every 10 years[g] 5. CT colonoscopy		http://www.ahrq.gov/clinic/uspstf/uspscolo.htm
	ACOG	2007	Women at average risk aged ≥ 50 years	Preferred Method: • Colonoscopy every 10 years Other Appropriate Methods: • FOBT annually • Flexible sigmoidoscopy every 5 years • FOBT annually plus flexible sigmoidoscopy every 5 years • Double-contrast barium enema every 5 years	5. Percentage of U.S. adults receiving some form of CRC screening has increased from 44% in 1999 to 63% in 2008 (*Arch Int Med.* 2011; 171:647).	ACOG Committee Opinion, No. 357, Nov 2007
	UK-NHS	2007	Adults aged 60–69 years Adults aged ≥ 70 years	Program screened every 2 years with FOBT[c] Patient-initiated screening covered by NHS		http://www.cancerscreening.nhs.uk/bowel/index.html

Disease Screening	Organization	Date	Population	Recommendations	Comments	Source
	CANCER, COLORECTAL					
Cancer, Colorectal (continued)	ACS USMTFCC[a]	2008	Persons at increased risk based on family history but without a definable genetic syndrome[b]	*Group I:* Screening colonoscopy at age 40 years, or 10 years younger than the earliest diagnosis in the immediate family, and repeated every 5 years.[h]		*CA Cancer J Clin.* 2008;58:130
	ACR ASGE	2008	Very high-risk hereditary nonpolyposis colorectal cancer (HNPCC) (3%–4% of all CRCs) proven gene carrier—evaluate if Bethesda criteria is met	*Group II:* Follow average risk recommendations, but begin at age 40 years. Colonoscopy every 2 years beginning at age 20–25 years then yearly at age 40 years.[h]	Increased risk of non-CRC (endometrial, ovary, upper gastrointestinal, renal pelvis, ureter) requires systematic screening. Extra-intestinal tumors include hepatoblastoma (AFP screening recommended in families with this tumor), adrenal tumors, osteomas, brain tumors, skin CA, and thyroid CA.	*Am J Gastroenterol.* 2009;104:739 *J Clin Onc.* 2003;21:2397. *Gut.* 2008;57:704.

CANCER, COLORECTAL

Disease Screening	Organiza-tion	Date	Population	Recommendations	Comments	Source
Cancer, Colorectal (continued)			Classic familial adenomatous polyposis (FAP)	At-risk children should be offered genetic testing at age 10–12 years. Flexible sigmoidoscopy or colonoscopy every 12 months starting at age 10–12 years. Elective colectomy based on number and histology of polyps—usually done by early 20s; upper endoscopy every 5 years if no gastric or duodenal polyps starting in early 20s.		*JAMA.* 2006;296:1507

[a]U.S. Multisociety Task Force on Colorectal Cancer. (ACG, ACP, AGA, ASGE)

[b]Risk factors indicating need for earlier/more frequent screening: personal history of CRC or adenomatous polyps or hepatoblastoma, CRC or polyps in a first-degree relative aged < 60 years or in 2 first-degree relatives of any age, personal history of chronic inflammatory bowel disease, and family with hereditary CRC syndromes [*Ann Intern Med.* 1998;128(1):900. *A J Gastroenterol.* 2009;104:739. *NEJM.* 1994;331(25):1669. *NEJM.* 1995;332(13):861]. Additional high-risk group: history of ≥ 30 Gy radiation to whole abdomen; all upper abdominal fields; pelvic, thoracic, lumbar, or sacral spine. Begin monitoring 10 years after radiation or at age 35 years, whichever occurs last. (http://www. survivorshipguidelines.org). Screening colonoscopy in those aged ≥ 80 years results in only 15% of the expected gain in life expectancy seen in younger patients (*JAMA.* 2006;295:2357). ACG treats African Americans as high-risk group. See separate recommendation above.

[c]A positive result on an FOBT should be followed by colonoscopy. An alternative is flexible sigmoidoscopy and air-contrast barium enema.

[d]FOBT should be performed on 2 samples from 3 consecutive specimens obtained at home. A single stool guaiac during annual physical exam is not adequate.

[e]USPSTF did not find direct evidence that a screening colonoscopy is effective in reducing CRC mortality rates.

[f]Use the guaiac-based test with dietary restriction, or an immunochemical test without dietary restriction. Two samples from each of 3 consecutive stools should be examined without rehydration. Rehydration increases the false-positive rate.

[g]Population-based retrospective analysis: risk of developing CRC remains decreased for > 10 years following negative colonoscopy findings (*JAMA.* 2006;295:2366).

[h]*Group I:* First-degree relative with colon CA or adenomatous polyps at age < 60 years, or 2 first-degree relatives with CRC or adenomatous polyps at any time. *Group II:* First-degree relative with CRC or adenomatous polyps at age ≥ 60 years or 2 second-degree relatives with CRC.

Revised Bethesda criteria for testing for HNPCC (Lynch syndrome)—screen for tumor microsatellite instability if CRC diagnosed in a patient aged <50 years, presence of synchronous, metachronous CRC or other HNPCC defining tumor at any age. CRC with microsatellite unstable type histology (mucinous, signet ring, infiltrating lymphocytes) in patients aged < 60 years. CRC diagnosed in one or more first-degree relatives with HNPCC-related tumor with one of the cancers diagnosed at age < 50 years. CRC diagnosed under age 50. CRC diagnosed in 2 or more first-degree or second-degree relatives with HNPCC-related tumors regardless of age. Confirmation of HNPCC is made by genetic evaluation of the involved genes (*J Natl Cancer Inst.* 2004;96:261).

CANCER, COLORECTAL

The following options are acceptable choices for CRC screening in average-risk adults beginning at age 50 years. Since each of the following tests has inherent characteristics related to prevention potential, accuracy, costs, and potential harms, individuals should have an opportunity to make an informed decision when choosing one of the following options.

In the opinion of the guidelines development committee, *colon CA prevention* should be the primary goal of CRC screening. Tests that are designed to detect both early CA and adenomatous polyps should be encouraged if resources are available and patients are willing to undergo an invasive test.

Tests That Detect Adenomatous Polyps and Cancer

Test	Interval	Key Issues for Informed Decisions
FSIG with insertion to 40 cm or to the splenic flexure	Every 5 years	Complete or partial bowel prep is required.
		Because sedation usually is not used, there may be some discomfort during the procedure.
		The protective effect of sigmoidoscopy is primarily limited to the portion of the colon examined.
		Patients should understand that positive findings on sigmoidoscopy usually result in a referral for colonoscopy.
Colonoscopy	Every 10 years	Complete bowel prep is required.
		Procedural sedation is used in most centers; patients will miss a day of work and will need a chaperone for transportation from the facility.
		Risks include perforation and bleeding, which are rare but potentially serious; most of the risk is associated with polypectomy (*Ann Intern Med.* 2009;150;1).
DCBE	Every 5 years	Complete bowel prep is required.
		If patients have one or more polyps ≥ 6 mm, colonoscopy will still be needed for biopsy or polyp removal; follow-up colonoscopy will require complete bowel prep.
		Risks of DCBE are low; rare cases of perforation have been reported—radiation exposure is a concern (*NEJM.* 2007;357;1403).
CTC	Every 5 years	Complete bowel prep is required.
		If patients have one or more polyps ≥ 6 mm, colonoscopy will be recommended; if same-day colonoscopy is not available, a second complete bowel prep will be required before colonoscopy.
		Risks of CTC are low; rare cases of perforation have been reported.
		Extracolonic abnormalities may be identified on CTC that could require further evaluation (7%–15% of CT exams). Not as sensitive as colonoscopy for polyps < 1 cm and especially for polyps ≤ 6 mm.

TESTS THAT PRIMARILY DETECT CANCER		
Test	**Interval**	**Key Issues for Informed Decisions**
gFOBT with high sensitivity for CA	Annual	Depending on manufacturer's recommendations, two to three stool samples collected at home are needed to complete testing; a single stool gathered during a digital exam in the clinical setting is not an acceptable stool test and should not be done.
FIT with high sensitivity for CA	Annual	
		Positive test results are associated with an increased risk of colon CA and advanced neoplasia; colonoscopy should be recommended if the test results are positive.
		If the test result is negative, it should be repeated annually.
		Patients should understand that one-time testing is likely to be ineffective.
sDNA with high sensitivity for CA	Interval uncertain	An adequate stool sample must be obtained and packaged with appropriate preservative agents for shipping to the laboratory.
		The unit cost of the currently available test is significantly higher than are other forms of stool testing.
		If the test result is positive, colonoscopy will be recommended.
		If the test result is negative, the appropriate interval for a repeat test is uncertain. sDNA testing is not widely used at this time (*Ann Intern Med*. 2008;149:441).

Note: CRC, colorectal cancer; CA, cancer; FSIG, flexible sigmoidoscopy; DCBE, double-contrast barium enema; CTC, computed tomography colonography; CT, computed tomography; gFOBT, guaiac-based fecal occult blood test; FIT, fecal immunochemical test; sDNA, stool DNA

CANCER, ENDOMETRIAL

Disease Screening	Organization	Date	Population	Recommendations	Comments	Source
Cancer, Endometrial	ACS	2008	All postmenopausal women	Inform women about risks and symptoms of endometrial CA, and strongly encourage them to report any unexpected bleeding or spotting. This is especially important for women with an increased risk of endometrial CA (history of unopposed estrogen therapy, tamoxifen therapy, late menopause, nulliparity, infertility or failure to ovulate, obesity, diabetes, or hypertension).	1. *Benefits:* There is inadequate evidence that screening with endometrial sampling or transvaginal ultrasound (TVU) decreases mortality. *Harms:* Based on solid evidence, screening with TVU will result in unnecessary additional exams because of low specificity. Based on solid evidence, endometrial biopsy may result in discomfort, bleeding, infection, and, rarely, uterine perforation. (NCI, 2008) 2. Presence of atypical glandular cells on Pap test from postmenopausal (aged > 40 years) women not taking exogenous hormones is abnormal and requires further evaluation (TVU and endometrial biopsy). Pap test is insensitive for endometrial screening.	http://www.cancer.org

CANCER, ENDOMETRIAL

Disease Screening	Organization	Date	Population	Recommendations	Comments	Source
Cancer, Endometrial (continued)					3. Endometrial thickness of <4 mm on TVU is associated with low risk of endometrial CA. (*Am J of Obstet Gynecol.* 2001;184:70) 4. Most cases of endometrial CA are diagnosed as a result of symptoms reported by patients (uterine bleeding), and a high proportion of these cases are diagnosed at an early stage and have high rates of cure. (NCI, 2008) 5. Tamoxifen use for 5 years raises the risk of endometrial CA 2–3-fold, but CAs are low stage, low grade, with high cure rates. (*J Natl Cancer Inst.* 1998;90:1371)	
	ACS	2008	All women at high risk for endometrial CA[a]	Annual screening beginning at age 35 years with endometrial biopsy.	1. Variable screening with ultrasound among women (aged 25–65 years; $n = 292$) at high risk for HNPCC mutation detected no CAs from ultrasound. Two endometrial cases occurred in the cohort that presented with symptoms. (*Cancer.* 2002;94:1708)	http://www.cancer.org

| | CANCER, ENDOMETRIAL | | | | |

Disease Screening	Organization	Date	Population	Recommendations	Comments	Source
Cancer, Endometrial (continued)					2. The Women's Health Initiative (WHI) demonstrated that combined estrogen and progestin did not increase the risk of endometrial CA but did increase the rate of endometrial biopsies and ultrasound exams prompted by abnormal uterine bleeding. (*JAMA*. 2003:290)	

[a]High-risk women are those known to carry HNPCC-associated genetic mutations, or at high risk to carry a mutation, or who are from families with a suspected autosomal dominant predisposition to colon CA (45%–50% lifetime risk of endometrial CA).

Disease Screening	Organization	Date	Population	Recommendations	Comments	Source
CANCER, GASTRIC						
Cancer, Gastric			Average-risk population	There are currently no recommendations regarding screening for gastric CA.	1. Population endoscopic screening for gastric CA in moderate- to high-risk population subgroups is cost-effective (Japan, South America). (*Clin Gastroenterol Hepatol.* 2006;4:709).	
Adenocarcinoma of gastroesophageal junction	ASGE	2006	Diagnosis—Barrett's esophagus with or without gastroesophageal reflux disease	—No dysplasia— scope every 3 years —Mild dysplasia— scope in 6 months, then yearly High-grade dysplasia— surgery or endoscopic therapy	2. Patients at increased risk for gastric CA should be educated about risk and symptoms. (*Helicobacter pylori*, pernicious anemia, HNPCC, post-partial gastrectomy) 3. *Benefits:* There is fair evidence that screening would result in no decrease in gastric CA mortality in the United States. *Harms:* There is good evidence that esophagogastroduodenoscopy screening would result in rare but serious side effects, such as perforation, cardiopulmonary events, aspiration pneumonia, and bleeding. (NCI, 2008)	*Gastrointest Endosc.* 2006;63:570

	CANCER, LIVER				
Disease Screening	Organization	Date	Population	Recommendations	Comments	Source
Cancer, Liver (Hepatocellular Carcinoma [HCC])	AASLD	2010 update	Adults at high risk for HCC;[a] especially those awaiting liver transplantation should be entered into surveillance programs.	Surveillance with ultrasound at 6-month intervals.	1. Alpha Fetoprotien (AFP) alone should not be used for screening unless ultrasound is not available (low sensitivity).	Hepatology. 2005;42:1208
					2. *Benefits:* Based on fair evidence, screening would not result in a decrease in HCC-related mortality. *Harms:* Based on fair evidence, screening would result in rare but serious side effects associated with needle biopsy, such as needle-track seeding, hemorrhage, bile peritonitis, and pneumothorax (NCI, 2008).	
	British Society of Gastroenterology	2003	Adults	Surveillance with abdominal ultrasound and AFP every 6 months should be considered for high-risk groups.[a]		*Gut.* 2003;52(suppl III):iii
						http://www.bsg.org.uk/

[a]*HBsAg+ persons (carriers):* Asian males aged ≥ 40 years; Asian females aged ≥ 40 years, Africans aged > 20 years. *Non-hepatitis B carriers:* family history of HCC; all cirrhotics; alcoholic cirrhosis; genetic hemochromatosis; primary biliary cirrhosis, alpha-1-antitrypsin deficiency with cirrhosis, hepatitis C with cirrhosis, hemochromatosis with cirrhosis.

CANCER, LUNG

Disease Screening	Organization	Date	Population	Recommendations	Comments	Source
Cancer, Lung	AAFP USPSTF	2008 2004	Asymptomatic persons	Evidence is insufficient to recommend for or against lung CA screening.	1. Counsel all patients against tobacco use, even when aged > 50 years. Smokers who quit gain ~10 years of increased life expectancy. (*BMJ.* 2004;328)	http://www.aafp.org/online/en/home/clinical/exam.html http://www.ahrq.gov/clinic/uspstf/uspslung.htm
	ACCP	2008	Asymptomatic persons	Based on good evidence, routine screening for lung CA with chest x-ray (CXR), sputum cytology is not recommended.	2. *Benefits:* Based on fair evidence, screening with sputum cytology or CXR does not reduce mortality from lung CA. Evidence is inadequate to assess mortality benefit of low-dose CT (LDCT). *Harms:* Based on solid evidence, screening would lead to false-positive test results and unnecessary invasive procedures. (NCI, 2008) 3. Spiral CT screening can detect greater number of lung CAs in smokers with a > 10 pack/year exposure. (*NEJM.* 2006;355:1763–1771)	http://www.chestnet.org/education/guidelines/index.php

CANCER, LUNG

Disease Screening	Organization	Date	Population	Recommendations	Comments	Source
Cancer, Lung (continued)				Routine screening with LDCT is not recommended except in the context of a clinical trial.	4. Although screening increases the rate of lung CA diagnosis and treatment, it may not reduce the risk of advanced lung CA or death from lung CA. (*JAMA.* 2007;297:995)	*Chest.* 2003;123:835–885 *CA Cancer J Clin.* 2004;54:41 http://www.ctfphc.org
	ACS	2001	Asymptomatic persons	Guidance in shared decision making regarding screening of high-risk persons.	5. The NCI has reported initial data from the National Lung Screening Trial (NLST), a randomized controlled trial comparing LDCT and CXR yearly × 3 with 8-year follow-up. 53,500 men and women aged 50–74 years, 30 pack/year smokers were randomized. A 20.3% reduction in deaths from lung CA was reported for the LDCT group. Problems with false-positives and cost of workup were noted, but benefits may lead to a change in guidelines.	http://www.cancer.org http://www.cancer.gov/nlst

	CANCER, ORAL					

Disease Screening	Organization	Date	Population	Recommendations	Comments	Source
Cancer, Oral	AAFP USPSTF	2008 2004	Asymptomatic persons	Evidence is insufficient to recommend for or against routinely screening adults for oral CA.	1. Risk factors: regular alcohol or tobacco use. 2. A randomized controlled trial of visual screening for oral CA (at 3-year intervals) showed decreased oral CA mortality among screened males (but not females) who were tobacco and/or alcohol users over an 8-year period. (*Lancet.* 2005;365:1927)	http://www.aafp.org/online/en/home/clinical/exam.html http://www.ahrq.gov/clinic/uspstf/uspsoral.htm
	COG	2006	History of radiation to head, oropharynx, neck, or total body Acute/chronic graft-versus-host disease	Annual oral cavity exam	Significant increase in HPV (subtypes 16 and 18)-related squamous cell cancer of the oropharynx (base of tongue and tonsil) in nonsmokers. 20%–30% improvement in cure rate versus that for smoking-related cancers. (*N Engl J Med.* 2010;363:24)	http://www.survivorshipguidelines.org

Disease Screening	Organization	Date	Population	Recommendations	Comments	Source
Cancer, Ovarian	AAFP USPSTF	2008 2004	Asymptomatic women at average risk[a]	Recommends against routine screening. Beware of symptoms of ovarian CA that can be present in early-stage disease (abdominal, pelvic, and back pain; bloating and change in bowel habits; urinary symptoms).	1. Risk factors: age > 60 years; low parity; personal history of endometrial, colon, or breast CA; family history of ovarian CA; and hereditary breast/ovarian CA syndrome. Use of oral contraceptives for 5 years decreases the risk of ovarian CA by 50%. (*JAMA.* 2004;291:2705) 2. *Benefit:* There is inadequate evidence to determine whether routine screening for ovarian CA with serum markers such as CA-125 levels,	http://www.aafp.org/online/en/home/clinical/exam.html http://www.ahrq.gov/clinic/uspstf/uspsovar.htm
	AAFP USPSTF	2008 2005	Women whose family history is associated with an increased risk for deleterious mutations in *BRCA1* or *BRCA2* genes[b]	Recommends referral for genetic counseling and evaluation for *BRCA* testing. Does not recommend routine screening in this group. Screening with CA-125, TVU, and pelvic exam can be considered but there is no evidence in this population that screening reduces risk of death from ovarian CA.	TVU, or pelvic exam would result in a decrease in mortality from ovarian CA. *Harm:* Problems have been lack of specificity (positive predictive value) and need for invasive procedures to make a diagnosis. Based on solid evidence, routine screening for ovarian CA would result in many diagnostic laparoscopies and laparotomies for each ovarian CA found. (NCI, 2008) (*JAMA.* 2011;305:2295). 3. Additionally, CAs found by screening have not consistently been found to be lower stage. (*Lancet Oncol.* 2009;10:327)	http://www.aafp.org/online/en/home/clinical/exam.html http://www.ahrq.gov/clinic/uspstf/uspsbrgen.htm

CANCER, OVARIAN

CANCER, OVARIAN

Disease Screening	Organization	Date	Population	Recommendations	Comments	Source
Cancer, Ovarian (continued)	ACOG NCCN	2009 2011		Recommends screening with CA-125 and TVUs at age 30–35 years or 5–10 years earlier than earliest onset of ovarian CA in family members.	4. Preliminary results from the Prostate, Lung, Colorectal and Ovarian (PLCO) Cancer Screening Trial: At the time of baseline exam, positive predictive value for invasive cancer was 3.7% for abnormal CA-125 levels, 1% for an abnormal TVU results, and 23.5% if both tests showed abnormal results. (*Am J Obstet Gynecol.* 2005;193:1630)	

[a]Lifetime risk of ovarian CA in a woman with no affected relatives is 1 in 70. If 1 first-degree relative has ovarian CA, lifetime risk is 5%. If 2 or more first-degree relatives have ovarian CA, lifetime risk is 7%. Women with 2 or more family members affected by ovarian cancer have a 3% chance of having a hereditary ovarian cancer syndrome. If *BRCA1* mutation lifetime risk of ovarian CA is 45%–50%, if *BRCA2* mutation lifetime risk is 15%–20%, Lynch syndrome = 8%–10% lifetime risk of ovarian CA.

[b]USPSTF recommends against routine counseling or routine BRCA testing of women whose family history is not associated with increased risk for deleterious mutation in *BRCA1* or *BRCA2* genes.

CANCER, PANCREATIC

Disease Screening	Organization	Date	Population	Recommendations	Comments	Source
Cancer, Pancreatic	AAFP USPSTF	2008 2004	Asymptomatic persons	Recommends against routine screening.	1. Cigarette smoking has consistently been associated with increased risk of pancreatic CA. *BRCA2* mutation is associated with a 5% lifetime risk of pancreatic CA. Blood group O with lower risk and diabetes with a 2-fold higher risk of pancreatic CA. (*J Nat Cancer Inst.* 2009;101:424. *J Clin Onc.* 2009;27:433) 2. USPSTF concluded that the harms of screening for pancreatic CA due to the very low prevalence, limited accuracy of available screening tests, invasive nature of diagnostic tests, and poor outcomes of treatment exceed any potential benefits.	http://www.aafp.org/online/en/home/ clinical/exam.html http://www.ahrq.gov/clinic/uspstf/ uspspanc.htm

Disease Screening	Organization	Date	Population	Recommendations	Comments	Source
CANCER, PROSTATE						
Cancer, Prostate	ACS	2008	Men aged ≥ 50 years[a]	Offer annual prostate-specific antigen (PSA) and digital rectal exam (DRE) if ≥ 10-year life expectancy.[b] Discuss risks and benefits of screening strategy.	1. Discouraging tests or not offering tests is not appropriate. 2. Men who ask their doctors to make the decision on their behalf should be tested.	http://www.cancer.org
	AAFP USPSTF	2008 2008	Asymptomatic men	Evidence insufficient to recommend for or against routine screening using PSA or DRE. In men aged ≥ 75 years, USPSTF recommends against screening.	1. There is good evidence that PSA can detect early-stage prostate CA (2-fold increase in organ-confined disease at presentation with PSA screening), but mixed and inconclusive evidence that early detection improves health outcomes or mortality. 2. Two long-awaited studies add to the confusion. A U.S. study of 76,000 men with increased prostate CA found in screened group, but no reduction in risk of death from prostate CA. A European study of 80,000 men showed a decrease rate of death from prostate CA by 20% but significant overdiagnosis. 1410 men needed to be screened and 48 cases of prostate CA found to prevent one death from prostate CA. Patients older than age 70 years had an increased death rate in the screened group. (*N Engl J Med.* 2009;360:1310, 1320)	http://www.aafp.org/online/en/home/clinical/exam.html http://www.ahrq.gov/clinic/uspstf/uspsprca.htm

Disease Screening	Organization	Date	Population	Recommendations	Comments	Source
CANCER, PROSTATE						
Cancer, Prostate (continued)					3. *Benefit:* Insufficient evidence to establish whether a decrease in mortality from prostate CA occurs with screening by DRE or serum PSA. *Harm:* Based on solid evidence, screening with PSA and/or DRE detects some prostate CAs that would never have caused important clinical problems. Based on solid evidence, current prostate CA treatments result in permanent side effects in many men, including erectile dysfunction and urinary incontinence. (NCI, 2008) 4. Men with localized, low-grade prostate CAs (Gleason score 2–4) have a minimal risk of dying from prostate CA during 20 years of follow-up (6 deaths per 1000 person-years). (*JAMA.* 2005;293:2095)	

Disease Screening	Organization	Date	Population	Recommendations	Comments	Source
Cancer, Prostate (continued)					5. Radical prostatectomy (vs watchful waiting) reduces disease-specific and overall mortality in patients with early-stage prostate CA. (*N Engl J Med.* 2001; 364:1708). This benefit was seen only in men aged <65 years. Active surveillance for low-risk patients (*J Clin Onc.* 2010;28:126) is safe and increasingly used as an alternative to radical prostatectomy. A gene signature profile reflecting virulence and treatment responsiveness in prostate CA is needed. 6. PSA velocity (>0.5–0.75 ng/year rise) is predictive for the presence of prostate CA especially with a PSA of 4–10. (*Eur Urol.* 2009;56:573)	
	EAU	2007	Asymptomatic men	There is a lack of evidence to support or disregard widely adopted, population-based screening programs for early detection of prostate CA.		www.uroweb.org
	UK-NHS	2007	Asymptomatic men	Informed decision making	See informational leaflet at: http://www.cancerscreening.nhs.uk/prostate/prostate-patient-info-sheet.pdf	www.cancerscreening.nhs.uk

[a]Men in high-risk groups (one or more first-degree relatives diagnosed before age 65 years, African Americans) should begin screening at age 45 years. Men at higher risk due to multiple first-degree relatives affected at an early age could begin testing at age 40 years. (http://www.cancer.org/)
[b]Men who ask their doctor to make the decision should be tested. Discouraging testing or not offering testing is inappropriate.

CANCER, SKIN

Disease Screening	Organization	Date	Population	Recommendations	Comments	Source
Cancer, Skin (melanoma)	AAFP USPSTF	2008 2009	Asymptomatic persons	Evidence is insufficient to recommend for or against routine screening using a total-body skin exam for early detection of cutaneous melanoma, basal cell carcinoma, or squamous cell skin CA.[a,b]	*Benefits:* Evidence is inadequate to determine whether visual exam of the skin in asymptomatic individuals would lead to a reduction in mortality from melanomatous skin CA. *Harms:* Based on fair though unqualified evidence, visual exam of the skin in asymptomatic persons may lead to unavoidable increases in harmful consequences. (NCI, 2008)	http://www.aafp.org/online/en/home/clinical/exam.html http://www.ahrq.gov/clinic/uspstf/uspsskca.htm
	Sloan-Kettering	2006	Asymptomatic persons	Routine screening is not recommended.[c]		

[a]Clinicians should remain alert for skin lesions with malignant features when examining patients for other reasons, particularly patients with established risk factors. Risk factors for skin CA include: evidence of melanocytic precursors (atypical moles), large numbers of common moles (>50), immunosuppression, any history of radiation, family or personal history of skin CA, substantial cumulative lifetime sun exposure, intermittent intense sun exposure or severe sunburns in childhood, freckles, poor tanning ability, and light skin, hair, and eye color.

[b]Consider educating patients with established risk factors for skin CA (see above) concerning signs and symptoms suggesting skin CA and the possible benefits of periodic self-exam. Alert at-risk patients to significance of asymmetry, border irregularity, color variability, diameter > 6 mm, and evolving change in previous stable mole. All suspicious lesions should be biopsied (excisional or punch not a shave biopsy) (*Ann Int Med.* 2009;150:188) (USPSTF) (ACS) (COG).

[c]Consider dermatologic risk assessment if family history of melanoma in ≥ 2 blood relatives, presence of multiple atypical moles, or presence of numerous actinic keratoses.

CANCER, TESTICULAR						
Disease Screening	Organization	Date	Population	Recommendations	Comments	Source
Cancer, Testicular	AAFP USPSTF	2008 2011	Asymptomatic adolescent and adult males[a]	Recommend against routine screening. Be aware of risk factors for testicular CA—previous testis CA (2%–3% risk of 2nd cancer), cryptorchid testis, family history of testis CA, HIV (increased risk of seminoma), Klinefelter's syndrome.	*Benefits:* Based on fair evidence, screening would not result in appreciable decrease in mortality, in part because therapy at each stage is so effective. *Harm:* Based on fair evidence, screening would result in unnecessary diagnostic procedures (NCI, 2011).	http://www.aafp.org/online/en/home/clinical/exam.html http://www.ahrq.gov/clinic/uspstf/uspstest.htm
	ACS	2004	Asymptomatic men	Testicular exam by physician as part of routine cancer-related checkup.		http://www.cancer.org
	EAU	2008	High-risk males[a]	Self-physical exam is advisable.		www.uroweb.org

[a]Patients with history of cryptorchidism, orchiopexy, family history of testicular CA, or testicular atrophy should be informed of their increased risk for developing testicular CA and counseled about screening. Such patients may then elect to be screened or to perform testicular self-exam. Adolescent and young adult males should be advised to seek prompt medical attention if they notice a scrotal abnormality. (USPSTF)

	CANCER, THYROID					

Disease Screening	Organization	Date	Population	Recommendations	Comments	Source
Cancer, Thyroid	AAFP	2010	Asymptomatic persons	Recommends against the use of ultrasound screening in asymptomatic persons. Be aware of higher-risk patients: radiation administered in infancy and childhood for benign conditions (thymus enlargement, acne) have an increased risk beginning 5 years after radiation and may appear more than 20 years later; nuclear fallout exposure; history of goiter; family history of thyroid disease; female gender; Asian race. (*Int J Cancer.* 2001;93:745)	Neck palpation for nodules in asymptomatic individuals has sensitivity of 15%–38%, specificity of 93%–100%. Only a small proportion of nodular thyroid glands are neoplastic, resulting in a high false-positive rate. (USPSTF)	http://www.aafp.org/online/en/home/clinical/exam.html http://www.cancer.org

	CAROTID ARTERY STENOSIS				
Disease Screening	Organization	Date	Population	Recommendations	Comments	Source
Carotid Artery Stenosis (CAS) (asymptomatic)	ASN USPSTF AHA/ASA	2007 2010	Asymptomatic adults	Screening of the general population or a selected population based on age, gender, or any other variable alone is not recommended.	1. The prevalence of internal CAS of ≥ 70% varies from 0.5%–8% based on population-based cohort utilizing carotid duplex ultrasound. General population > age 65 years estimated prevalence of 1%. No risk stratification tool further distinguishes the importance of CAS. No evidence suggests that screening for asymptomatic CAS reduces fatal or nonfatal strokes. 2. Carotid duplex ultrasonography to detect CAS ≥ 60%; sensitivity, 94%; specificity, 92%. [*Ann Intern Med.* 2007;147(12):860] 3. If true prevalence of CAS is 1%, number needed to screen to prevent 1 stroke over 5 years = 4368; to prevent 1 disabling stroke over 5 years = 8696. [*Ann Intern Med.* 2007;147(12):860]	*J Neuroimaging.* 2007;17:19–47 http://www.ahrq.gov/clinic/uspstf/uspsacas.htm USPFT 2007 (AHRQ # 08-05102-EF-1) *Stroke.* 2010:42

Disease Screening	Organization	Date	Population	Recommendations	Comments	Source
CELIAC DISEASE						
Celiac Disease	NICE	2009	Children and adults	Serologic testing to screen for celiac disease should be performed for any of the following signs, symptoms, or associated conditions: chronic diarrhea, failure to thrive, persistent or unexplained gastrointestinal symptoms, prolonged fatigue, recurrent abdominal pain, cramping or distension, unexplained weight loss, unexplained anemia, autoimmune thyroid disease, dermatitis herpetiformis, irritable bowel syndrome, type 1 diabetes, or first-degree relatives with celiac disease.	1. Patients must continue a gluten-containing diet during diagnostic testing. 2. IgA tissue transglutaminase (TTG) is the test of choice. 3. IgA endomysial antibody test is indicated if the TTG test is equivocal. 4. Avoid anti-gliadin antibody testing. 5. Consider serologic testing for any of the following: Addison disease, amenorrhea, autoimmune hepatitis, autoimmune myocarditis, chronic immune thrombocytopenic purpura (ITP), dental enamel defects, depression, bipolar disorder, Down syndrome, Turner's syndrome, epilepsy, lymphoma, metabolic bone disease, chronic constipation, polyneuropathy, sarcoidosis, Sjögren's syndrome, or unexplained alopecia.	http://www.nice.org.uk/nicemedia/pdf/CG86FullGuideline.pdf

Disease Screening	Organization	Date	Population	Recommendations	Comments	Source
CHLAMYDIA						
Chlamydia	CDC ICSI	2010 2010	Women aged ≤ 25 years who are sexually active	Annual screening	1. Chlamydia is a reportable infection to the Public Health Department in every state.	http://www.cdc.gov/mmwr/pdf/rr/rr5912.pdf http://www.icsi.org/preventive_services_for_adults/preventive_services_for_adults_4.html
	CDC	2010	Women aged ≤ 35 years who are sexually active and in juvenile detention or jail	At intake and then annual screening		http://www.cdc.gov/mmwr/pdf/rr/rr5912.pdf
	CDC	2010	Young heterosexual men	Insufficient evidence for or against routine screening		http://www.cdc.gov/mmwr/pdf/rr/rr5912.pdf
	CDC	2010	Homosexual men	Annual testing for men who have had insertive or receptive intercourse in the past year	1. Urine nucleic amplification acid test (NAAT) for chlamydia for men who have had insertive intercourse 2. NAAT of rectal swab for men who have had receptive anal intercourse	http://www.cdc.gov/mmwr/pdf/rr/rr5912.pdf

CHOLESTEROL & LIPID DISORDERS

Disease Screening	Organization	Date	Population	Recommendations	Comments	Source
Cholesterol & Lipid Disorders	USPSTF	2007	Infants, children, adolescents, or young adults (aged < 20 years)	Insufficient evidence to recommend for or against routine population lab screening.[a]	1. Childhood drug treatment of dyslipidemia lowers lipid levels but effect on childhood or adult outcomes pending. 2. Lifestyle approach is recommended starting after age 2 years.	http://www.ahrq.gov/clinic/uspstf/uspschlip.htm *Pediatrics.* 2007;120:e189–e214 *Circulation.* 2007;115: 1948–1967
	AHA	2007		Selective screening aged > 2 years with a parent aged < 55 years with coronary artery disease, peripheral artery disease, cerebrovascular disease, or hyperlipidemia should be screened with fasting panel.		*Pediatrics.* 2008;122:198–208
	Pediatrics	2008		Selective screening aged > 2 years if positive family history (FH) of dyslipidemia, presence of dyslipidemia, or the presence of overweight, obesity, hypertension, diabetes, or a smoking history.		

CHOLESTEROL & LIPID DISORDERS

Disease Screening	Organization	Date	Population	Recommendations	Comments	Source
Cholesterol & Lipid Disorders (continued)	NCEP III	2004	Adult men and women aged > 20 years	Check fasting lipoprotein panel (if testing opportunity is nonfasting, use nonfasting total cholesterol [TC] and high-density lipoprotein [HDL]) every 5 years if in desirable range; otherwise see management algorithm.[b]	3. There are no recommendation at which age screening should be discontinued. Screening should continue beyond age 65 years if the individual patient would benefit from long-term lipid management. [*Geriatrics*. 2000;55(8):48]	*Circulation.* 2002;106:3143–3421 *Circulation.* 2004;110: 227–239 http://www.nhlbi.nih.gov/ guidelines/cholesterol/ atp3upd04.htm
	USPSTF	2008	Men aged > 35 years	Grade A recommendation. Optimal screening interval uncertain	4. Treatment decisions should be based on at least two cholesterol levels.	http://www.ahrq.gov/ clinic/uspstf/uspschol. htm
			Men aged 20–35 years	Only if at increased risk for coronary heart disease (CHD) Grade B recommendation	5. Screen with fasting lipid panel to include TC, low-density-lipoprotein cholesterol (LDL-C), high-density-lipoprotein cholesterol (HDL-C), and triglycerides.	
			Women aged > 45 years	Screen if at increased risk of CHD Grade A recommendation		
			Women aged 20–45 years	Screen if at increased risk of CHD Grade B recommendation No recommendation for or against routine screening in men aged 20–35 years or in women aged ≥ 20 years who are not at increased risk of CHD.		

CHOLESTEROL & LIPID DISORDERS

Disease Screening	Organization	Date	Population	Recommendations	Comments	Source
Cholesterol & Lipid Disorders (continued)	AAFP	2008	Men aged ≥ 35 years	Strongly recommends routine screening for lipid disorders		http://www.aafp.org/exam/ http://www.ahrq.gov/clinic/uspstf/uspschol.htm
			Women aged ≥ 45 years	Strongly recommends screening only if at increased risk of CHD.[c]		
				Random total cholesterol and HDL-C or fasting lipid profile, periodicity based on risk factors for all patients.		

[a]AHA: Low efficacy of targeted screening of children based on family history. Sensitivity and specificity of screening complicated by variability in TC and HDL based on race, gender, and sexual maturation. (*Circulation.* 2007;115:1948–1967).

[b]Classify fasting TC < 200 mg/dL as desirable, 200–239 mg/dL as borderline, or ≥ 240 mg/dL as high. Classify HDL < 40 as low, and ≥ 60 as high. Classify LDL < 100 as optimal, 100–129 as near or above optimal, 130–159 as borderline high, 160–189 as high, and ≥ 190 as very high. If TC < 200 mg/dL and HDL ≥ 40 mg/dL, then repeat in 5 years; if nonfasting TC ≥ 200 mg/dL or HDL < 40 mg/dL, then check fasting lipids and risk-stratify based on LDL (see Management Algorithm). Advanced lipoprotein testing does not predict carotid intima-media thickness better than traditionally measured lipid values. (*Ann Intern Med.* 2005;142:742–750).

[c]Hypertension, smoking, diabetes, family history of CHD before age 50 years (male relatives) or age 60 years (female relatives), family history suggestive of familial hyperlipidemia.

CORONARY ARTERY DISEASE					
Disease Screening	**Organization**	**Date**	**Population**	**Recommendations**	**Comments**	**Source**

Disease Screening	Organization	Date	Population	Recommendations	Comments	Source
Coronary Artery Disease	AAFP USPSTF	2008 2004	Adults at low risk of CHD events[a]	Recommends *against* routine screening in men and women with resting electrocardiogram (ECG), exercise treadmill test (ETT), or electron-beam CT for coronary calcium at low risk for CHD risk.[b]	USPSTF recommends against screening asymptomatic individuals due to the high false-positive results, the low mortality with asymptomatic disease, and the iatrogenic diagnostic and treatment risks.	http://www.aafp.org/online/en/home/clinical/exam.html *Circulation.* 2005;111:682–696 http://www.ahrq.gov/clinic/uspstf/uspsacad.htm 2004 *Ann Intern Med.* 2004;140:569 *Circulation.* 2005;112:771–776
	AHA ESC	2010 2003	All asymptomatic adults aged ≥ 20 years	Framingham Risk Score, including blood pressure (BP) and cholesterol level, should be obtained. SCORE Risk System is an alternate choice. No benefit in genetic testing, advanced lipid testing, natriuretic-peptide testing, high-sensitivity C-reactive protein (CRP), ankle-brachial index, carotid intima-medial thickness, coronary artery score on electron-beam CT, homocysteine level, lipoprotein (a) level, CT angiogram, MRI, or stress echocardiography regardless of CHD risk.		*Circulation.* 2007;115:402–426 *J Am Coll Cardiol.* 2010;56(25):2182–2199 http://www.uspreventiveservicestaskforce.org/uspstf/uspscoronaryhd.htm 2009

Disease Screening	Organization	Date	Population	Recommendations	Comments	Source
CORONARY ARTERY DISEASE						
Coronary Artery Disease (continued)			Adults at intermediate risk of CHD events	May be reasonable to consider use of coronary artery calcium and high-sensitivity C-reactive protein (hsCRP) measurements in patients at intermediate risk according to Framingham Score[b] hsCRP is not recommended in low- or high-risk individuals.		
	AAFP	2008	Adults at high risk of CHD events[a]	Insufficient evidence to recommend for or against routine screening with ECG, ETT, or electron-beam CT for coronary calcium, ankle-brachial index, carotid intima-media thickness.[b]		*Arch Intern Med.* 2011;171(11): 977–982
	AHA	2007				http://www.aafp.org/online/en/home/clinical/exam.html
	USPSTF	2009				http://www.ahrq.gov/clinic/uspstf/uspsacad.htm *Annals Intern Med.* 2009;151:474–482

CORONARY ARTERY DISEASE

Disease Screening	Organization	Date	Population	Recommendations	Comments	Source
Coronary Artery Disease (continued)	ACCF/AHA	2010	Women	Cardiac risk stratification by the Framingham Risk Score should be used. High risk in women should be considered when the risk is $\geq$ 10% rather than $\geq$ 20%. An alternative 10-year risk score to consider is the Reynolds Risk Score, although it requires measurement of hsCRP.		AHA Guidelines. *J Am Coll Cardiol.* 2011;57(12): 1404–1423

[a]Increased risk for CHD events: older age, male gender, high BP, smoking, elevated lipid levels, diabetes, obesity, sedentary lifestyle. Risk assessment tool for estimating 10-year risk of developing CHD events available online, or *see Appendix VI* and *VII.* http://hp2010.nhlbihin.net/atpiii/calculator.asp?usertype=prof

[b]AHA scientific statement (2006): Asymptomatic persons should be assessed for CHD risk. Individuals found to be at low risk (< 10% 10-year risk) or at high risk (> 20% 10-year risk) do not benefit from coronary calcium assessment. High-risk individuals are already candidates for intensive risk-reducing therapies. In clinically selected, intermediate-risk patients, it may be reasonable to use electron-beam CT or multidetector computed tomography (MDCT) to refine clinical risk prediction and select patients for more aggressive target values for lipid-lowering therapies. (*Circulation.* 2006;114:1761–1791).

	DEMENTIA				
Disease Screening	**Organization**	**Date**	**Population**	**Recommendations**	**Comments**	**Source**
Dementia	ICSI	2010	Adults	Insufficient evidence to recommend for or against routine dementia screening.		http://www.icsi.org/preventive_services_for_adults/ preventive_services_for_adults_4.html

Disease Screening	Organization	Date	Population	Recommendations	Comments	Source
DEPRESSION						
Depression	USPSTF	2009	Children aged 7–11 years	Insufficient evidence to recommend for or against routine screening.		http://www.uspreventiveservicestaskforce.org/uspstf09/depression/chdeprart.pdf
	USPSTF	2009	Adolescents	Screen all adolescents aged 12–18 years for major depressive disorder (MDD) when systems are in place to ensure accurate diagnosis, appropriate psychotherapy, and adequate follow-up.	1. Screen in primary care clinics with the Patient Health Questionnaire for Adolescents (PHQ-A) (73% sensitivity; 94% specificity) or the Beck Depression Inventory-Primary Care (BDI-PC) (91% sensitivity; 91% specificity). See *Appendix 1.* 2. Treatment of adolescents with selective serotonin reuptake inhibitors (SSRIs), psychotherapy, or combined therapy decreases MDD symptoms. 3. SSRI may increase suicidality in some adolescents, emphasizing the need for close follow-up.	
	USPSTF ICSI	2009 2010	Adults	Recommend screening adults for depression when staff-assisted support systems are in place for accurate diagnosis, effective treatment, and follow-up.	1. Asking two simple questions may be as accurate as formal screening tools: a. "Over the past 2 weeks, have you felt down, depressed, or hopeless?" b. "Over the past 2 weeks, have you felt little or no interest or pleasure in doing things?" 2. Optimal screening interval is unknown.	http://www.uspreventiveservicestaskforce.org/uspstf09/adultdepression/addeprrs.pdf http://www.icsi.org/preventive_services_for_adults/preventive_services_for_adults_4.html

Disease Screening	Organization	Date	Population	Recommendations	Comments	Source
DEVELOPMENTAL DYSPLASIA OF THE HIP						
Developmental Dysplasia of the Hip (DDH)	ICSI AAFP	2010 2010	Infants	Evidence is insufficient to recommend routine screening for DDH in infants as a means to prevent adverse outcomes.	1. There is evidence that screening leads to earlier identification; however, 60%–80% of the hips of newborns identified as abnormal or suspicious for DDH by physical exam and > 90% of those identified by ultrasound in the newborn period resolve spontaneously, requiring no intervention.	http://www.icsi.org/preventive_services_for_children_guideline_/preventive_services_for_children_and_adolescents_2531.html http://www.guidelines.gov/content.aspx?id=34005
	USPSTF	2006	Infants	Same Recommendation As Above	The USPSTF was unable to assess the balance of benefits and harms of screening for developmental dysplasia of hip (DDH) but was concerned about the potential harms associated with treatment, both surgical and nonsurgical, of infants identified by routine screening.	

	GESTATIONAL DIABETES				
Disease Screening	Organization	Date	Population	Recommendations	Comments	Source
Diabetes Mellitus, Gestational (GDM)	AAFP	2010	Pregnant women	Evidence is insufficient to recommend for or against routine screening.	1. No high-quality evidence is available that shows that screening (vs testing women with symptoms) for GDM reduces important adverse health outcomes for mothers or their infants. Also, no high-quality evidence is available on the sensitivity or specificity of GDM screening [*Ann Intern Med.* 2008;148(10):766)]	http://www.guidelines.gov/content.aspx?id=34005

Disease Screening	Organization	Date	Population	Recommendations	Comments	Source
DIABETES, TYPE 2 ABUSE						
Diabetes Mellitus (DM), Type	ADA	2011	Pregnant women	1. Screen for undiagnosed DM type 2 at first prenatal visit if aged ≥ 45 years or if risk factors for DM are present.[a] 2. For all other women, screen at 24–28 weeks with a 75-gm 2-hour oral glucose tolerance test (OGTT).	1. Preexisting diabetes if: a. Fasting glucose ≥ 126 mg/dL b. 2-hour glucose ≥ 200 mg/dL after 75-gm glucose load c. Random glucose ≥ 200 mg/dL with classic hyperglycemic symptoms d. Hemoglobin A1c ≥ 6.5% 2. Criteria for GDM by 75-gm 2-hour OGTT if any of the following are abnormal: a. Fasting ≥ 92 mg/dL (5.1 mmol/L) b. 1 hour ≥ 180 mg/dL (10.0 mmol/L) c. 2 hour ≥ 153 mg/dl (8.5 mmol/L)	http://care.diabetesjournals.org/content/34/Supplement_1/S11.full.pdf+html
	ADA	2011	Children at start of puberty or aged ≥ 10 years	1. Screen all children at risk for DM type 2[b]		

DIABETES, TYPE 2 ABUSE

Disease Screening	Organization	Date	Population	Recommendations	Comments	Source
Diabetes Mellitus (DM), Type (continued)	ADA	2011	Adults	1. Screen asymptomatic adults aged ≥ 45 years or if risk factors for DM are present.[a]	1. Australian Carbohydrate Intolerance Study in Pregnant Women (ACHOIS): Treatment of a screening-detected population with mild gestational diabetes reduced serious neonatal and maternal outcomes [*Ann Intern Med.* 2008;148(10):766] 2. Fasting plasma glucose ≥ 126 mg/dL or a casual plasma glucose ≥ 200 mg/dL meets threshold for diabetes diagnosis, if confirmed on a subsequent day, *and precludes the need for glucose challenge.* (ADA)	http://www.guidelines.gov/content.aspx?id=34005 http://www.ahrq.gov/clinic/pocketgd1011/pocketgd1011.pdf
	AAFP USPSTF	2010 2010	Hypertensive adults	Screen asymptomatic adults with sustained BP (either treated or untreated) > 135/80 mm Hg.	Screen at least every 3 years in asymptomatic adults.	
	AAFP USPSTF	2010 2010	Adults	Evidence is insufficient to recommend for or against routinely screening asymptomatic adults with a BP < 135/80 mm Hg.		

[a]DM risk factors: overweight (BMI ≥ 25 kg/m²) AND an additional risk factor: physical inactivity; first-degree relative with DM; high-risk ethnicity (eg, African American, Latino, Native American, Asian American, Pacific Islander); history of GDM; prior baby with birth weight > 9 lb; hypertension (HTN) on therapy or with BP ≥ 140/90 mm Hg; HDL–C level < 35 mg/dL (0.90 mmol/L) and/or a triglyceride level > 250 mg/dL (2.82 mmol/L); polycystic ovary syndrome; history of impaired glucose tolerance or HgbA1c ≥ 5.7%; *Acanthosis nigricans*; or cardiovascular disease.

[b]Test asymptomatic children if BMI > 85% for age/sex, weight for height > 85th percentile, or weight > 120% of ideal for height PLUS ANY TWO of the following: family history of DM in first- or second-degree relative; high-risk ethnic group (eg, Native American, African American, Latino, Asian American, or Pacific Islander); Acanthosis nigricans; HTN; dyslipidemia, polycystic ovary syndrome; small-for-gestational-age birth weight; maternal history of DM or GDM during the child's gestation.

FALLS IN THE ELDERLY

Disease Screening	Organization	Date	Population	Recommendations	Comments	Source
Falls in the Elderly	NICE	2004	All older persons	Ask at least yearly about falls.[a,b,c]	1. Individuals are at increased risk if they report at least two falls in the previous year, or one fall with injury.	http://www.nice.org.uk
	AAOS	2001			2. Calcium and vitamin D supplementation reduces falls by 45% over 3 years in women, but no effect is seen in men. (*Arch Intern Med.* 2006;166:424)	*JAGS.* 2001;49:664–672
	AGS	2001			3. A fall prevention clinic appears to reduce the number of falls among the elderly. (*Am J Phys Med Rehabil.* 2006;85:882)	http://www.americangeriatrics.org/products/positionpapers/falls.pdf
	British Geriatrics Society	2001			4. See also page 109 for fall prevention and Appendix II.	http://www.bgs.org.uk/
	CTF	2005	All persons admitted to long-term care facilities	Recommend programs that target the broad range of environmental and resident-specific risk factors to prevent falls and hip fractures.[d]	5. 15.9% of U.S. adults aged ≥ 65 years fell in the preceding 3 months; of these, 31.3% sustained an injury that resulted in a doctor visit or restricted activity for at least 1 day. [*MMWR Morb Mortal Wkly Rep.* 2008;57(9):225]	http://www.ctfphc.org

[a]All who report a single fall should be observed as they stand up from a chair without using their arms, walk several paces, and return (see Appendix II). Those demonstrating no difficulty or unsteadiness need no further assessment. Those who have difficulty or demonstrate unsteadiness, have ≥ 1 fall, or present for medical attention after a fall should have a fall evaluation (see fall prevention, page 109).

[b]Risk factors: Intrinsic: lower extremity weakness, poor grip strength, balance disorders, functional and cognitive impairment, visual deficits. Extrinsic: polypharmacy (≥ 4 prescription medications), environment (poor lighting, loose carpets, lack of bathroom safety equipment).

[c]Free "Tip Sheet" for patients from AGS (http://www.healthinaging.org/public_education/falls_tips.php).

[d]Post-fall assessments may detect previously unrecognized health concerns.

	FAMILY VIOLENCE AND ABUSE				
Disease Screening	Organization	Date	Population	Recommendations	Comments	Source
Family Violence and Abuse	AAFP	2010	Children, women, and older adults	Insufficient evidence to recommend for or against routine screening of parents or guardians for the physical abuse or neglect of children, of women for intimate partner violence, or of older adults or their caregivers for elder abuse.	1. Recent studies show that screening for intimate partner violence in emergency departments and pediatric clinics shows high prevalence (10%–20%) and does not increase harm. (*Ann Emerg Med.* 2008;51:433. *Pediatrics.* 2008;121:e85) 2. In screening for intimate partner violence, women prefer self-completed approaches (written or computer-based) over face-to-face questioning. (*JAMA.* 2006;296:530) 3. All providers should be aware of physical and behavioral signs and symptoms associated with abuse and neglect, including burns, bruises, and repeated suspect trauma.	http://www.uspreventiveservicestaskforce.org/uspstf/uspsfamv.htm http://www.guidelines.gov/content.aspx?id=34005

GONORRHEA

Disease Screening	Organization	Date	Population	Recommendations	Comments	Source
Gonorrhea	CDC	2010	Sexually active women	Annually screen all women at risk for gonorrhea.[a]	Gonorrhea is a reportable illness to state Public Health Department.	http://www.cdc.gov/mmwr/pdf/rr/rr5912.pdf
	CDC	2010	Women aged ≤ 35 years who are sexually active and in juvenile detention or jail	Screen at intake and then annual screenings		http://www.cdc.gov/mmwr/pdf/rr/rr5912.pdf
	CDC	2010	Homosexual men	Annual testing for men who have had insertive or receptive intercourse in the past year		http://www.cdc.gov/mmwr/pdf/rr/rr5912.pdf

[a]Women aged < 25 years are at highest risk for gonorrhea infection. Other risk factors that place women at increased risk include a previous gonorrhea infection, the presence of other sexually transmitted diseases (STDs), new or multiple sex partners, inconsistent condom use, commercial sex work, and drug use.

GROUP B STREPTOCOCCAL DISEASE

Disease Screening	Organization	Date	Population	Recommendations	Comments	Source
Group B Streptococcal (GBS) Disease	CDC	2010	Pregnant women	Universal screening of all women at 35–37 gestational weeks for GBS colonization with a vaginal-rectal swab	Women who are colonized with GBS should receive intrapartum antibiotic prophylaxis to prevent neonatal GBS sepsis.	http://www.cdc.gov/mmwr/preview/mmwrhtml/rr5910a1.htm?s_cid=rr5910a1_w

GROWTH ABNORMALITIES, INFANT

Disease Screening	Organization	Date	Population	Recommendations	Comments	Source
Growth Abnormalities, Infant	CDC	2010	Children 0–59 months	Use the 2006 World Health Organization (WHO) international growth charts for children aged < 24 months.	1. The Centers for Disease Control and Prevention (CDC) and American Academy of Pediatricians (AAP) recommend the WHO as opposed to the CDC growth charts for children aged < 24 months 2. The CDC growth charts should still be used for children aged 2–19 years. 3. This recommendation recognizes that breast-feeding is the recommended standard of infant feeding and therefore the standard against which all other infants are compared.	http://www. uspreventiveservicestaskforce. org/uspstf09/adultdepression/ addeprrs.pdf

HEARING IMPAIRMENT

Disease Screening	Organization	Date	Population	Recommendations	Comments	Source
Hearing Impairment	AAFP USPSTF	2010 2008	Newborns	Routine screening of all newborn infants for hearing loss.	1. Screening involves either a one-step or a two-step process. 2. The two-step process includes otoacoustic emissions (OAEs) followed by auditory brainstem response (ABR) in those who fail the OAE test. 3. The one-step process uses either OAE or ABR testing.	http://www.guidelines.gov/content.aspx?id=34005 http://www.uspreventiveservicestaskforce.org/uspstf08/newbornhear/newbhears.htm
	ICSI	2010	Newborns	Universal screening of infants for congenital hearing loss should be performed during the first month of life.		http://www.icsi.org/preventive_services_for_children__guideline_/preventive_services_for_children_and_adolescents_2531.html
	AAFP ICSI USPSTF	2010 2010 2011	Adults aged >50 years	Question older adults periodically about hearing impairment, counsel about availability of hearing aid devices, and make referrals for abnormalities when appropriate. See also Appendix II: Functional Assessment Screening in the Elderly.	1. 20%–40% of adults aged >50 years and >80% of adults aged ≥80 years have some degree of hearing loss. 2. Additional research is required to determine if hearing loss screening can lead to improved health outcomes. 3. No harm from hearing loss screening. 4. No harm related to hearing aid use.	http://www.guidelines.gov/content.aspx?id=34005 http://www.icsi.org/preventive_services_for_adults/preventive_services_for_adults_4.html http://www.uspreventiveservicestaskforce.org/uspstf11/adulthearing/adulthearart.pdf

Disease Screening	Organization	Date	Population	Recommendations	Comments	Source
Hemochromatosis (hereditary)	AAFP USPSTF	2008 2006	Asymptomatic adults	Recommends against routine genetic screening for hemochromatosis. Patients with a family history should be counseled with further testing based on clinical considerations. (*Arch Int Med.* 2006;166:269. *Blood.* 2008;111:3373).	1. There is fair evidence that clinically significant disease due to hereditary hemochromatosis is uncommon in the general population. Male homozygotes for C282Y gene mutation have a 2-fold increase in the incidence of iron overload-related symptoms compared with females. 2. There is poor evidence that early therapeutic phlebotomy improves morbidity and mortality in screening-detected versus clinically detected individuals.	http://www.aafp.org/online/en/home/clinical/exam.html http://www.ahrq.gov/clinic/uspstf/uspshemoch.htm
	ACP	2005	Adults	Insufficient evidence to recommend for or against screening.[a] In case-finding for hereditary hemochromatosis, serum ferritin and transferrin saturation tests should be performed.	1. If testing is performed, cut-off values for serum ferritin levels > 200 μg/L in women and > 300 μg/L in men and transferrin saturation > 45% may be used as criteria for case-finding, but there is no general agreement about diagnostic criteria. 2. For clinicians who choose to screen, one-time screening of non-Hispanic white men with serum ferritin level and transferrin saturation has highest yield.	*Ann Intern Med.* 2005;143:517–521 http://www.acponline.org/clinical/guidelines/ *N Engl J Med.* 2004;350:2383

[a]Discuss the risks, benefits, and limitations of genetic testing in patients with a positive family history of hereditary hemochromatosis or those with elevated serum ferritin levels or transferrin saturation.

Disease Screening	Organization	Date	Population	Recommendations	Comments	Source
Hemoglobinopathies	AAFP USPSTF	2010 2007	Newborns	Recommend screening all newborns for hemoglobinopathies (including sickle cell disease).	Newborn screen tests for phenylketonuria (PKU), hemoglobinopathies, and hypothyroidism	http://www.guidelines.gov/content.aspx?id=34005 http://www.uspreventiveservicestaskforce.org/uspstf07/sicklecell/sicklers.htm

HEMOGLOBINOPATHIES

HEPATITIS B VIRUS INFECTION, CHRONIC

Disease Screening	Organization	Date	Population	Recommendations	Comments	Source
Hepatitis B Virus (HBV) Infection, Chronic	USPSTF ACOG AAP AAFP CDC	2009 2007 2006 2010 2010	Pregnant women	Screen all women with HBsAg at their first prenatal visit.	1. Breast-feeding is not contraindicated in women with chronic HBV infection if the infant has received hepatitis B immunoglobulin (HBIG)-passive prophylaxis and vaccine-active prophylaxis. 2. All pregnant women who are HBsAg-positive should be reported to the Local Health Department to ensure proper follow-up. 3. Immunoassays for HBsAg have sensitivity and specificity > 98% (*MMWR*. 1993;42:707).	http://www.annals.org/content/150/12/I-36.full http://publichealth.lacounty.gov/mch/ReproductiveHealth/PreconceptionHealth/PCHFiles/Hepatitis%20in%20Pregnancy%20ACOG.pdf http://www.guidelines.gov/content.aspx?id=34005 http://www.cdc.gov/mmwr/pdf/rr/rr5912.pdf
	NIH AASLD	2009 2009	Adults and children	1. Recommend routine screening for HBV infection of newly arrived immigrants from countries where the HBV prevalence rate is > 2%.[a] 2. Screen all patients with chronically elevated alanine transaminase (ALT), homosexual men, persons with multiple sexual partners, injection drug users, jail inmates, dialysis patients, household contacts of persons with chronic HBV infection, and persons infected with either hepatitis C virus (HCV) or HIV.		http://www.guidelines.gov/content.aspx?id=14240 http://www.guidelines.gov/content.aspx?id=15475

[a] Immigrants from Asia, Africa, South Pacific, Middle East (except Israel), Eastern Europe (except Hungary), the Caribbean, Malta, Spain, Guatemala, and Honduras.

Disease Screening	Organization	Date	Population	Recommendations	Comments	Source
HEPATITIS C VIRUS INFECTION, CHRONIC						
Hepatitis C Virus (HCV) Infection, Chronic	ACOG CDC	2007 2010	Pregnant women at increased risk[a]	Perform routine counseling and testing at the first prenatal visit.	1. Route of delivery has not been shown to influence rate of vertical transmission of HCV infection. Cesarean section should be reserved for obstetric indications only. 2. Breast-feeding is not contraindicated in women with chronic HCV infection.	http://publichealth.lacounty.gov/mch/ReproductiveHealth/PreconceptionHealth/PCHFiles/Hepatitis%20in%20Pregnancy%20ACOG.pdf http://www.cdc.gov/mmwr/pdf/rr/rr5912.pdf

	AASLD	2009	Persons at increased risk for HCV infection[a]	Recommend HCV antibody testing by enzyme immunoassay in all high-risk adults.	1. HCV RNA testing should be performed for:
					  a. Positive HCV antibody test result in a patient
					  b. When antiviral treatment is being considered
					  c. Unexplained liver disease in an immunocompromised patient with a negative HCV antibody test result
					  d. Suspicion of acute HCV infection
					2. HCV genotype should be determined in all HCV-infected persons prior to interferon treatment.
					3. Seroconversion may take up to 3 months.
					4. 15%–25% of persons with acute hepatitis C resolve their infection; of the remaining, 10%–20% develop cirrhosis within 20–30 years after infection, and 1%–5% develop hepatocellular carcinoma.
					5. Patients testing positive for HCV antibody should receive a nucleic acid test to confirm active infection. A quantitative HCV RNA test and genotype test can provide useful prognostic information prior to initiating antiviral therapy. (*JAMA.* 2007;297:724).
						http://www.aasld.org/practiceguidelines/Documents/Hepatitis%20C%20UPDATE.pdf

HEPATITIS C VIRUS INFECTION, CHRONIC

Disease Screening	Organization	Date	Population	Recommendations	Comments	Source
Hepatitis C Virus (HCV) Infection, Chronic (continued)	AAFP	2010	General asymptomatic adults	Recommends against routine screening for HCV infection in adults who are not at increased risk.[a]		http://www.guidelines.gov/content.aspx?id=34005

[a]HCV risk factors: HIV infection, sexual partners of HCV-infected persons, persons seeking evaluation or care for STDs, including HIV, history of injection drug use, persons who have ever been on hemodialysis, intranasal drug use, history of blood or blood component transfusion or organ transplant prior to 1992, hemophilia, multiple tatooes, children born to HCV-infected mothers, and healthcare providers who have sustained a needle stick injury.

HERPES SIMPLEX VIRUS, GENITAL

Disease Screening	Organization	Date	Population	Recommendations	Comments	Source
Herpes Simplex Virus (HSV), Genital	AAFP CDC	2010 2010	Adolescents and adults	Recommends against routine serological screening for HSV.		http://www.guidelines.gov/content.aspx?id=34005 http://www.cdc.gov/mmwr/pdf/rr/rr5912.pdf
	AAFP CDC	2010 2010	Pregnant women	Recommends against routine serological screening for HSV to prevent neonatal HSV infection.	1. In women with a history of genital herpes, routine serial cultures for HSV are not indicated in the absence of active lesions. 2. Women who develop primary HSV infection during pregnancy have the highest risk for transmitting HSV infection to their infants.	http://www.guidelines.gov/content.aspx?id=34005 http://www.cdc.gov/mmwr/pdf/rr/rr5912.pdf

HUMAN IMMUNODEFICIENCY VIRUS

Disease Screening	Organization	Date	Population	Recommendations	Comments	Source
Human Immunodeficiency Virus (HIV)	AAFP USPSTF	2010 2005	Pregnant women	Clinicians should screen all pregnant women for HIV.	Rapid HIV antibody testing during labor identified 34 HIV-positive women among 4849 women with no prior HIV testing documented (prevalence, 7 in 1000). Eighty-four percent of women consented to testing. Sensitivity was 100%, specificity was 99.9%, positive predictive value (PPV) was 90%. (*JAMA.* 2004;292:219).	http://www.guidelines.gov/content.aspx?id=34005 http://www.ahrq.gov/clinic/uspstf/uspshivi.htm
	CDC	2010	Pregnant women	Include HIV testing in panel of routine prenatal screening tests. Retest high-risk women at 36 weeks' gestation. Rapid HIV testing of women in labor who have not received prenatal HIV testing.		http://www.cdc.gov/mmwr/pdf/rr/rr5912.pdf
	CDC	2010	Adolescents and adults who seek evaluation and treatment for STDs	HIV screening should be offered to all people who seek evaluation for STDs and all adolescents who are sexually active or who engage in injection drug use.	1. HIV testing should be voluntary and must have a verbal consent to test. Patients may "opt out" of testing. 2. Educate and counsel all high-risk patients regarding HIV testing, transmission, risk-reduction behaviors, and implications of infection.	http://www.cdc.gov/mmwr/pdf/rr/rr5912.pdf

HUMAN IMMUNODEFICIENCY VIRUS

Disease Screening	Organization	Date	Population	Recommendations	Comments	Source
Human Immunodeficiency Virus (HIV) (continued)	AAFP	2010	Adolescents and adults at increased risk[a]	Strongly recommends screening.	1. If acute HIV is suspected, also use plasma RNA test. 2. False-positive results with electroimmunoassay (EIA): nonspecific reactions in persons with immunologic disturbances (eg, systemic lupus erythematosus or rheumatoid arthritis), multiple transfusions, recent influenza, or rabies vaccination. 3. Confirmatory testing is necessary using Western blot or indirect immunofluorescence assay. 4. Awareness of HIV positively reduces secondary HIV transmission risk and high-risk behavior and viral load if on highly active antiretroviral therapy HAART. (CDC, 2006)	http://www.guidelines.gov/content.aspx?id=34005
	AAFP USPSTF	2010 2005	Adolescents and adults who are not at increased risk	Insufficient evidence to recommend for or against routine screening.		http://www.guidelines.gov/content.aspx?id=34005 http://www.uspreventiveservicestaskforce.org/uspstf/uspshivi.htm

[a]Risk factors for HIV: men who have had sex with men after 1975; multiple sexual partners; history of IVDU; prostitution; history of sex with an HIV-infected person; history of sexually transmitted disease; history of blood transfusion between 1978–1985; or persons requesting an HIV test.

HYPERTENSION, CHILDREN & ADOLESCENTS

Disease Screening	Organization	Date	Population	Recommendations	Comments	Source
Hypertension (HTN), Children & Adolescents	AAFP Pediatrics	2006 2004	Age 3–20 years[a]	Children aged ≥ 3 years should have BP measured as part of routine evaluation.	1. Hypertension: average systolic blood pressure (SBP) or diastolic blood pressure (DBP) ≥ 95th percentile for gender, age, and height on ≥ 3 occasions. See *Appendices*. 2. Prehypertension: average SBP or DBP 90th–95th percentile. 3. Adolescents with BP ≥ 120/80 mm Hg are prehypertensive.	http://www.aafp.org/afp/2006/0501/p.1558.html *Pediatrics.* 2004;114:555–576 Amer Family Physician. 2006; 73 (9): 1558-1568.
	NHLBI	2004	Aged 3–20 years[a]		4. Evaluation of hypertensive children: assess for additional risk factors. Follow-up BP: if normal, repeat in 1 year; if prehypertensive, repeat BP in 6 months; if Stage 1, repeat in 2 weeks; if symptomatic or Stage 2, refer or repeat in 1 week. 5. Indications for antihypertensive drug therapy in children: symptomatic HTN, secondary HTN, target-organ damage, diabetes, persistent HTN despite nonpharmacologic measures.	http://www.nhlbi.nih.gov/ *Contemp Pediatr.* Oct 14, 2008
	Bright Futures	2008	Aged 3–21 years[a]	Annual screening	6. Accumulating evidence suggests that ambulatory BP monitoring is a more accurate method for diagnosis of HTN in children and allows better assessment for therapy.	http://www.brightfutures.org *Hypertension.* 2008;52:433–451

[a] In children aged < 3 years, conditions that warrant BP measurement: prematurity; very low birth weight, or neonatal complications; congenital heart disease; recurrent urinary tract infections (UTIs), hematuria, or proteinuria; renal disease or urologic malformations; family history of congenital renal disease; solid-organ transplant; malignancy or bone marrow transplant; drugs known to raise BP; systemic illnesses; increased intracranial pressure.

				HYPERTENSION, ADULTS		
Disease Screening	Organization	Date	Population	Recommendations	Comments	Source
Hypertension (HTN), Adults	USPSTF AAFP USPSTF	2009 2008 2007	Adults aged > 18 years	1. Screen for HTN 2. HTN > 140/90 mm Hg 3. Diagnosis after two or more BP readings obtained at least two visits over several weeks		*Am Fam Physician.* 2009;79(12):1087–1088 http://www.aafp.org/online/en/home/clinical/exam.html http://www.ahrq.gov/clinic/uspstf/uspshype.htm
	ESH ESC	2007	Adults	The diagnosis of HTN is usually based on at least two BP readings at least two visits, although in cases of *severe BP elevation*, especially if associated with end-organ damage, the diagnosis can be based on measurements taken at a single visit.		*J Hypertens.* 2007;25:1105 http://www.escardio.org/knowledge/guidelines/Guidelines_list.htm?hit=quick
	JNC VII (NHLBI)	2003	Aged > 18 years	Normal: recheck in 2 years (see Comments). Pre-HTN: recheck in 1 year. Stage 1 HTN: confirm within 2 months. Stage 2 HTN: evaluate or refer to source of care within 1 month (evaluate and treat immediately if BP > 180/110).	1. Pre-HTN: SBP 120–139 or DBP 80–89. 2. Stage 1 HTN: SBP 140–159 or DBP 90–99. 3. Stage 2 HTN: SBP ≥ 160 or DBP ≥ 100 (based on average of ≥ 2 measurements on ≥ 2 separate office visits). 4. Perform physical exam and routine labs.[a] 5. Pursue secondary causes of HTN.[b]	*JAMA.* 2003;289:2560. *Hypertension.* 2003;42:1206

HYPERTENSION, ADULTS						
Disease Screening	**Organization**	**Date**	**Population**	**Recommendations**	**Comments**	**Source**
Hypertension, Adults (continued)					6. Treatment goals are for BP < 140/90, unless patient has diabetes or renal disease (< 130/80). See JNC VII Management Algorithm, page 148.	
					7. Ambulatory BP monitoring is a better (and independent) predictor of cardiovascular outcomes compared with office visit monitoring and is covered by Medicare when evaluating white- coat HTN. (*NEJM.* 2006;354:2368). Increased frequency of systolic HTN compared with younger patients. HTN is more likely associated with end-organ damage and more often associated with other risk factors.	*J Am Coll Cardiol.* 2011;57(20):2037–2110.
	ACCF/AHA	2011	Aged > 65 years	Identification and treatment of systolic and diastolic HTN in the very elderly is beneficial in reduction in all-cause mortality and stroke death.		

a Physical exam should include: measurements of height, weight, and waist circumference; funduscopic exam (retinopathy); carotid auscultation (bruit); jugular venous pulsation; thyroid gland (enlargement); cardiac auscultation (left ventricular heave, S_3 or S_4, murmurs, clicks); chest auscultation (rales, evidence of chronic obstructive pulmonary disease); abdominal exam (bruits, masses, pulsations); exam of lower extremities (diminished arterial pulsations, bruits, edema); and neurologic exam (focal findings). Routine labs include urinalysis, complete blood count, electrolytes (potassium, calcium), creatinine, glucose, fasting lipids, and 12-lead electrocardiogram.
b Pursue secondary causes of HTN when evaluation is suggestive (clues in parentheses) of: (1) pheochromocytoma (labile or paroxysmal HTN accompanied by sweats, headaches, and palpitations); (2) renovascular disease (abdominal bruits); (3) autosomal dominant polycystic kidney disease (abdominal or flank masses); (4) Cushing's syndrome (truncal obesity with purple striae); (5) primary hyperaldosteronism (hypokalemia); (6) hyperparathyroidism (hypercalcemia); (7) renal parenchymal disease (elevated serum creatinine, abnormal urinalysis); (8) poor response to drug therapy; (9) well-controlled HTN with an abrupt increase in BP; (10) SBP > 180 or DBP > 110 mm Hg; or (11) sudden onset of HTN.

ILLICIT DRUG USE

Disease Screening	Organization	Date	Population	Recommendations	Comments	Source
Illicit Drug Use	AAFP USPSTF ICSI	2010 2008 2010	Adults, adolescents, and pregnant women	Insufficient evidence to recommend for or against routine screening for illicit drug use.		http://www.guidelines.gov/content.aspx?id=34005 http://www.uspreventiveservicestaskforce.org/uspstf08/druguse/drugrs.htm http://www.icsi.org/preventive_services_for_adults/preventive_services_for_adults_4.html

KIDNEY DISEASE, CHRONIC

Disease Screening	Organization	Date	Population	Recommendations	Comments	Source
Kidney Disease, Chronic (CKD)	NICE	2008	Adults	1. Monitor glomerular filtration rate (GFR) at least annually in people prescribed drugs known to be nephrotoxic.[a] 2. Screen renal function in people at risk for CKD.[b]		http://www.nice.org.uk/nicemedia/live/12069/42117/42117.pdf

[a]Examples: calcineurin inhibitors, lithium, or nonsteroidal anti-inflammatory drugs (NSAIDs)

[b]DM, HTN, cardiovascular disease, structural renal disease, nephrolithiasis, benign prostatic hyperplasia (BPH), multisystem diseases with potential kidney involvement (eg, systemic lupus erythematosus [SLE]), family history of Stage 5 CKD or hereditary kidney disease, or personal history of hematuria or proteinuria.

LEAD POISONING						

Disease Screening	Organization	Date	Population	Recommendations	Comments	Source
Lead Poisoning	AAFP	2010	Children aged 1–5 years	1. Insufficient evidence to recommend for or against routine screening in asymptomatic children at increased risk. 2. Recommends against screening in asymptomatic children at average risk.	1. Risk assessment should be performed during prenatal visits and continue until aged 6 years. 2. CDC personal risk questionnaire: a. Does your child live in or regularly visit a house (or other facility, eg, daycare) that was built before 1950? b. Does your child live in or regularly visit a house built before 1978 with recent or ongoing renovations or remodeling (within the last 6 months)? c. Does your child have a sibling or playmate who has or did have lead poisoning? (http://www.cdc.gov/nceh/lead/publications/screening.htm)	http://www.guidelines.gov/content.aspx?id=34005
	AAFP	2010	Pregnant women	Recommends against screening in asymptomatic pregnant women.		http://www.guidelines.gov/content.aspx?id=34005

LEAD POISONING

Disease Screening	Organization	Date	Population	Recommendations	Comments	Source
Lead Poisoning (continued)	CDC	2010	Pregnant women	Routine blood lead testing of pregnant women is recommended in clinical settings that serve populations with specific risk factors for lead exposure.[a]		http://www.cdc.gov/nceh/lead/publications/LeadandPregnancy2010.pdf
	CDC	2009	Children aged 1–5 years	Recommend blood lead screening in Medicaid-eligible children at increased risk for lead exposure.[b]	Screen at ages 1 and 2 years, or by age 3 years if a high-risk child has never been screened.	http://www.cdc.gov/mmwr/preview/mmwrhtml/rr5809a1.htm

[a]Important risk factors for lead exposure in pregnant women include recent immigration, pica practices, occupational exposure, nutritional status, culturally specific practices such as the use of traditional remedies or imported cosmetics, and the use of traditional lead-glazed pottery for cooking and storing food.
[b]Child suspected by parent, healthcare provider, or Health Department to be at risk for lead exposure; sibling or playmate with elevated blood lead level; recent immigrant, refugee, or foreign adoptee; child's parent or caregiver works with lead; household member uses traditional folk or ethnic remedies or cosmetics or who routinely eats food imported informally from abroad; residence near a source of high lead levels.

MOTOR VEHICLE SAFETY						
Disease Screening	Organization	Date	Population	Recommendations	Comments	Source
Motor Vehicle Safety	ICSI	2010	Children and adolescents	Recommend that all health-care providers ask about: 1. Car seats 2. Booster seats 3. Seat belt use 4. Helmet use while riding motorcycles	One study demonstrated a 21% reduction in mortality with the use of child restraint systems versus seat belts in children aged 2–6 years involved in motor vehicle collisions (*Arch Ped Adolesc Med.* 2006;160:617–621).	http://www.icsi.org/preventive_services_for_children_guideline_/preventive_services_for_children_and_adolescents_2531.html

Disease Screening	Organization	Date	Population	Recommendations	Comments	Source
OBESITY						
Obesity	AAFP USPSTF	2010 2010	Children aged ≥ 6 years	The AAFP recommends that clinicians screen children aged 6 years and older for obesity.	Obese children should be offered intensive counseling and behavioral interventions to promote improvement in weight status.	http://www.guidelines.gov/content.aspx?id=34005 http://www.uspreventiveservicestaskforce.org/uspstf/uspschobes.htm
	ICSI	2010	Children aged ≥ 2 years	Height, weight, and body mass index (BMI) should be recorded annually starting at age 2 years.	1. Children with a BMI ≥ 25 are five times more likely to be overweight as adults compared with their normal-weight counterparts. 2. Overweight children should be counseled about wholesome eating, 30–60 minutes of daily physical activity, and avoiding soft drinks.	http://www.icsi.org/preventive_services_for_children_guideline_/preventive_services_for_children_and_adolescents_2531.html
	AAFP	2010	Adults aged > 18 years	Recommends screening all adults and offering intensive counseling and behavioral interventions to promote sustained weight loss in obese adults.	Intensive counseling involves more than 1 session per month for at least 3 months.	http://www.guidelines.gov/content.aspx?id=34005

	OBESITY					
Disease Screening	**Organization**	**Date**	**Population**	**Recommendations**	**Comments**	**Source**
Obesity (continued)	ICSI	2010	Adults aged > 18 years	Height, weight, and BMI should be measured at least annually.	Intensive intervention to promote weight loss should be offered to all obese adults (BMI ≥ 30 or waist circumference ≥ 40 in [men] or ≥ 35 in [women]).	http://www.icsi.org/preventive_services_for_adults/preventive_services_for_adults_4.html
	VA/DoD	2006	Adults	1. Height, weight, and BMI should be measured at least annually. 2. Waist circumference should be measured at least annually.	1. Intensive intervention to promote weight loss should be offered to: a. Obese adults (BMI ≥ 30 or waist circumference ≥ 40 in [men] or ≥ 35 in [women]) b. overweight adults (BMI 25–29.9) with an obesity-associated condition[a]	http://www.healthquality.va.gov/obesity/obe06_final1.pdf

[a]HTN, DM type 2, dyslipidemia, obstructive sleep apnea, degenerative joint disease, or metabolic syndrome.

Disease Screening	Organization	Date	Population	Recommendations	Comments	Source
OSTEOPOROSIS						
Osteoporosis	USPSTF ACPM	2011 2009	Women aged ≥ 65 years or younger women whose fracture risk is ≥ that of a 65-year-old white woman	Routine screening for women using either dual-energy x-ray absorptiometry (DXA) of the hip and lumbar spine or quantitative ultrasonography of the calcaneus.	1. The optimal screening interval is unclear. 2. Screening should not be performed more frequently than every 2 years. 3. Ten-year risk for osteoporotic fractures can be calculated for individuals by using the FRAX tool (http://www.shef.ac.uk/FRAX/). 4. Quantitative ultrasonography of the calcaneus predicts fractures of the femoral neck, hip, and spine as effectively as does DXA. 5. The criteria for treatment of osteoporosis rely on DXA measurements.	http://www.uspreventiveservicestaskforce.org/uspstf10/osteoporosis/osteors.htm http://www.guideline.gov/content.aspx?id=15270
	AAFP	2010	Women aged ≥ 65 years or aged ≥ 60 years at an increased risk for osteoporotic fracture	Routine screening for osteoporosis.		http://www.guidelines.gov/content.aspx?id=34005
	USPSTF	2011	Older men	Insufficient evidence to recommend for or against routine osteoporosis screening.		http://www.uspreventiveservicestaskforce.org/uspstf10/osteoporosis/osteors.htm
	ICSI	2010	Women aged ≥ 65 years	Routine screening for osteoporosis.		http://www.icsi.org/preventive_services_for_adults/preventive_services_for_adults_4.html
	NOF ACPM	2008 2009	Men aged ≥ 70 years	Recommends routine screening via bone mineral density (BMD).	Repeat every 3–5 years if "normal" baseline score; if high risk, then every 1–2 years.	http://www.guideline.gov/content.aspx?id=15270

	PHENYLKETONURIA				
Disease Screening	Organization	Date	Population	Recommendations	Comments	Source
Phenylketonuria (PKU)	AAFP USPSTF	2010 2007	Newborns	Recommend screening all newborns for PKU.	Newborn screen tests for PKU, hemoglobinopathies, and hypothyroidism.	http://www.guidelines.gov/content.aspx?id=34005 http://www.uspreventiveservicestaskforce.org/uspstf07/sicklecell/sicklers.htm

RH (D) INCOMPATIBILITY

Disease Screening	Organization	Date	Population	Recommendations	Comments	Source
Rh (D) Incompatibility	AAFP USPSTF	2010 2007	Pregnant women	1. Recommend blood typing and Rh (D) antibody testing for all pregnant women at their first prenatal visit. 2. Repeat Rh (D) antibody testing for all unsensitized Rh (D)-negative women at 24–28 weeks' gestation.	Rh (D) antibody testing at 24–28 weeks can be skipped if the biological father is known to be Rh (D)-negative.	http://www.guidelines.gov/content.aspx?id=34005 http://www.uspreventiveservicestaskforce.org/3rduspstf/rh/rhrs.htm

Disease Screening	Organization	Date	Population	Recommendations	Comments	Source
Scoliosis	AAFP USPSTF	2010 2004	Adolescents	Recommend against routine screening of asymptomatic adolescents for idiopathic scoliosis.		http://www.guidelines.gov/content.aspx?id=34005 http://www.uspreventiveservicestaskforce.org/3rduspstf/scoliosis/scoliors.htm

SCOLIOSIS

SPEECH & LANGUAGE DELAY

Disease Screening	Organization	Date	Population	Recommendations	Comments	Source
Speech & Language Delay	AAFP	2008	Preschool children	Evidence is insufficient to recommend for or against routine use of brief, formal screening instruments in primary care to detect speech and language delay in children up to age 5 years.	1. Fair evidence suggests that interventions can improve the results of short-term assessments of speech and language skills; however, no studies have assessed long-term consequences.	http://www.aafp.org/online/en/home/clinical/exam.html
	USPSTF	2006			2. In a study of 9000 toddlers in the Netherlands, two-time screening for language delays reduced the number of children who required special education (2.7% vs 3.7%) and reduced deficient language performance (8.8% vs 9.7%) at age 8 years. (*Pediatrics.* 2007;120:1317).	http://www.ahrq.gov/clinic/uspstf/uspschdv.htm
					3. Studies have not fully addressed the potential harms of screening or interventions for speech and language delays, such as labeling, parental anxiety, or unnecessary evaluation and intervention.	

SYPHILIS

Disease Screening	Organization	Date	Population	Recommendations	Comments	Source
Syphilis	CDC AAFP USPSTF	2010 2010 2009	Pregnant women	Strongly recommends routine screening of all pregnant women at the first prenatal visit.	1. A nontreponemal test (Venereal Disease Research Laboratory [VDRL] or rapid plasma reagent [RPR] test) should be used for initial screening. 2. All reactive nontreponemal tests should be confirmed with a fluorescent treponemal antibody absorption (FTA-ABS) test.	http://www.cdc.gov/mmwr/pdf/rr/rr5912.pdf http://www.guidelines.gov/content.aspx?id=34005 http://www.uspreventiveservicestaskforce.org/uspstf/uspssyphpg.htm
	AAFP CDC USPSTF	2010 2010 2004	Persons at increased risk[a]	Recommends screening high-risk persons.	3. Women at high risk for syphilis or who are previously untested, should be tested again at 28 gestational weeks. Consider testing a third time at the time of delivery. 4. Syphilis is a reportable disease in every state.	http://www.guidelines.gov/content.aspx?id=34005 http://www.cdc.gov/mmwr/pdf/rr/rr5912.pdf

[a]High-risk includes commercial sex workers, persons who exchange sex for money or drugs, persons with other STDs (including HIV), sexually active homosexual men, and sexual contacts of persons with syphilis, gonorrhea, chlamydia, or HIV infection.

THYROID DISEASE

Disease Screening	Organization	Date	Population	Recommendations	Comments	Source
Thyroid Disease	AAFP ICSI	2010 2010	Adults	Insufficient evidence to recommend for or against routine screening for thyroid disease.	Individuals with symptoms and signs potentially attributable to thyroid dysfunction and those with risk factors for its development may require thyroid-stimulating hormone (TSH) testing.	http://www.guidelines.gov/content.aspx?id=34005 http://www.icsi.org/preventive_services_for_adults/preventive_services_for_adults_4.html
	ICSI	2010	Newborns	Recommends screening for congenital hypothyroidism in newborns.		http://www.icsi.org/preventive_services_for_children_guideline_/preventive_services_for_children_and_adolescents_2531.html

	TOBACCO USE				
Disease Screening	**Organization**	**Date**	**Population**	**Recommendations**	**Comments**	**Source**

Disease Screening	**Organization**	**Date**	**Population**	**Recommendations**	**Comments**	**Source**
Tobacco Use	AAFP USPSTF ICSI	2010 2009 2010	Adults	Recommends screening all adults for tobacco use and provide tobacco cessation interventions for those who use tobacco products.	The "5-A" framework is helpful for smoking cessation counseling: a. Ask about tobacco use. b. Advise to quit through clear, individualized messages. c. Assess willingness to quit. d. Assist in quitting. e. Arrange follow-up and support sessions.	http://www.guidelines.gov/content.aspx?id=34005 http://www.uspreventiveservicestaskforce.org/uspstf/uspstbac2.htm http://www.icsi.org/preventive_services_for_adults/preventive_services_for_adults_4.html
	AAFP USPSTF ICSI	2010 2009 2010	Pregnant women	Recommends screening all pregnant women for tobacco use and provide pregnancy-directed counseling and literature for those who smoke.		http://www.guidelines.gov/content.aspx?id=34005 http://www.uspreventiveservicestaskforce.org/uspstf/uspstbac2.htm http://www.icsi.org/preventive_services_for_adults/preventive_services_for_adults_4.html

TOBACCO USE						
Disease Screening	**Organization**	**Date**	**Population**	**Recommendations**	**Comments**	**Source**
Tobacco Use (continued)	AAFP	2010	Children and adolescents	Evidence is insufficient to recommend for or against routine screening.	The avoidance of tobacco products by children and adolescents is desirable. It is uncertain whether advice and counseling by health care professionals in this area is effective.	http://www.guidelines.gov/content.aspx?id=34005
	ICSI	2010	Children and adolescents aged ≥ 10 years	Screen for tobacco use and reassess at every opportunity.	Provide ongoing cessation services to all tobacco users at every opportunity.	http://www.icsi.org/preventive_services_for_children__guideline_/preventive_services_for_children_and_adolescents_2531.html

TUBERCULOSIS, LATENT

Disease Screening	Organization	Date	Population	Recommendations	Comments	Source
Tuberculosis, Latent	CDC	2010	Persons at increased risk of developing tuberculosis (Tb)	Screening by tuberculin skin test (TST) or interferon-gamma release assay (IGRA) is recommended. Frequency of testing is based on likelihood of further exposure to Tb and level of confidence in the accuracy of the results.	1. Typically, a TST is used to screen for latent Tb. 2. IGRA is preferred if: a. Testing persons who have a low likelihood of returning to have their TST read b. Testing persons who have received a Bacille Calmette-Guérin (BCG) vaccination	http://www.cdc.gov/mmwr/pdf/rr/rr5905.pdf

Disease Screening	Organization	Date	Population	Recommendations	Comments	Source
VISUAL IMPAIRMENT, GLAUCOMA, OR CATARACT						
Visual Impairment, Glaucoma, or Cataract	USPSTF AAFP	2009 2010	Older adults	Insufficient evidence to recommend for or against visual acuity screening or glaucoma screening in older adults.		http://www.uspreventiveservicestaskforce.org/uspstf09/visualscr/viseldrs.htm http://www.guidelines.gov/content.aspx?id=34005
	ICSI	2010	Older adults	Objective vision testing (Snellen chart) recommended for adults aged ≥ 65 years.		http://www.icsi.org/preventive_services_for_adults/preventive_services_for_adults_4.html
	ICSI	2010	Children	Vision screening recommended for children aged ≤ 4 years.	Screen for amblyopia, strabismus, or decreased visual acuity.	http://www.icsi.org/preventive_services_for_children_guideline_/preventive_services_for_children_and_adolescents_2531.html

2
Disease Prevention

PRIMARY PREVENTION OF CANCER (CA): NCI EVIDENCE SUMMARY 2011

CA Type[a,b]	Minimize Risk Factor Exposure	Strength of Evidence That Modifying or Avoiding Risk Factor Will Reduce CA	Therapeutic	Strength of Evidence
Breast[a,b]	Hormone replacement therapy —About 24% increased incidence of invasive breast CA with combination hormone replacement therapy (HRT) (estrogen and progesterone) —Estrogen alone with mixed evidence—unlikely to increase risk significantly	Solid	Tamoxifen (postmenopausal and high-risk premenopausal women) —Treatment with tamoxifen for 5 years reduced breast CA risk by 40%–50% —Meta-analysis shows relative risk (RR) = 2.4 (95% confidence interval [CI], 1.5–4.0) for endometrial CA and 1.9 (95% CI, 1.4–2.6) for venous thromboembolic events	Solid
	Ionizing radiation —Increased risk occurs about 10 years after exposure. Risk depends on dose and age at exposure	Solid	Raloxifene (postmenopausal women) —Similar effect as tamoxifen in reduction of invasive breast CA but does not reduce the incidence of noninvasive tumors—studied only in postmenopausal women —Similar risks as tamoxifen for venous thrombosis, but no risk of endometrial CA	Solid
	Obesity —In WHI, RR = 2.85 for breast CA for women > 82.2 kg compared to women < 58.7 kg	Solid	Aromatase inhibitors —Anastrozole reduces the incidence of new primary breast CAs by 50% compared with tamoxifen; similar results have been reported with letrozole and exemestane treatment	Fair
	Alcohol —RR for intake of four alcoholic drinks/day is 1.32 —RR increases about 7% for each drink per day	Solid	—There is a 65% reduction in the risk of breast CA occurrence in postmenopausal women treated with exemestane for 5 years (*NEJM.* 2011;364:2381). —Harmful effects of aromatase inhibitors include decreased bone mineral density, increased falls, and decreased cognitive function, fibromyalgia, and carpal tunnel syndrome	Fair

	PRIMARY PREVENTION OF CANCER (CA): NCI EVIDENCE SUMMARY 2011 (CONTINUED)		
CA Type[a,b]	Minimize Risk Factor Exposure	Strength of Evidence That Modifying or Avoiding Risk Factor Will Reduce CA	Therapeutic	Strength of Evidence
Breast[a,b] (Continued)	Factors of unproven or disproven association —Abortions —Environmental factors —Diet and vitamins —Active and passive cigarette smoking —Use of statin drugs		—Fracture rate for women being treated with anastrozole was 5.9% compared with 3.7% for those being treated with tamoxifen Prophylactic bilateral mastectomy (high-risk women) —Reduces risk as much as 90% —About 6% of women were dissatisfied with their decision; regrets about mastectomy were less among women who opted not to have reconstruction	Solid
			Prophylactic salpingo-oophorectomy among *BRCA*-positive women —Breast CA incidence decreased as much as 50% —Nearly all women experience some sleep disturbances, mood changes, hot flashes, and bone demineralization, but the severity of these symptoms varies greatly.	Fair
			Exercise —Exercising > 4 hours/week results in average risk reduction of 30%–40% The effect may be greatest for premenopausal women of normal or low body weight Breast-feeding —The RR of breast CA is decreased 4.3% for every 12 months of breast-feeding, in addition to 7% for each birth Pregnancy before age 20 years —About 50% decrease in breast CA compared to nulliparous women or those who give birth after age 35 years	Solid

PRIMARY PREVENTION OF CANCER (CA): NCI EVIDENCE SUMMARY 2011 (CONTINUED)

CA Type	Minimize Risk Factor Exposure	Strength of Evidence That Modifying or Avoiding Risk Factor Will Reduce CA	Therapeutic	Strength of Evidence
Cervical	Human papillomavirus (HPV) infection[c] —Abstinence of sexual activity; condom and/or spermicide use (RR, 0.4)	Solid	HPV-16/HPV-18 vaccination[d] —Reduces incident and persistent infections with efficacy of 91.6% (95% CI, 64.5–98.0) and 100% (95% CI, 45–100), respectively; duration of efficacy is not yet known; impact on long-term cervical CA rates also unknown but likely to be significant	Solid
	Cigarette smoke (active or passive) —Increases risk of high-grade cervical intraepithelial neoplasia (CIN) or invasive CA 2- to 3-fold among HPV-infected women	Solid	Screening with Pap smears	Solid
	High parity —HPV-infected women with seven or more full-term pregnancies have a 4-fold increased risk of squamous cell CA of the cervix compared with nulliparous women	Solid	—Estimates from population studies suggest that screening may decrease CA incidence and mortality by more than 80%. Adding screening for HPV after age 30 years increases sensitivity	Fair
	Long-term use of oral contraceptives —Increases risk by 3- to 4-fold —Longer use related to higher risk	Solid		Solid

	PRIMARY PREVENTION OF CANCER (CA): NCI EVIDENCE SUMMARY 2011 (CONTINUED)		
CA Type	Minimize Risk Factor Exposure	Strength of Evidence That Modifying or Avoiding Risk Factor Will Reduce CA	Therapeutic	Strength of Evidence
Colorectal[b,c]	Excessive alcohol use, RR is 1.44 for > 45 g/day (>4.5 drinks/day)	Solid	*Nonsteroidal anti-inflammatory drugs* —Based on solid evidence, nonsteroidal inflammatory drugs (NSAIDs) reduce the risk of adenomas, but how much this reduces the risk of CRC is uncertain. Harms include upper gastrointestinal (UGI) bleeding (4–5/1000 people/year), chronic kidney disease (CKD), and cardiovascular (CV) events	*Inadequate[1]* Solid
	Cigarette smoking—RR for current smokers versus never smokers, 1.18	Solid	—Based on solid evidence, daily aspirin use for at least 5 years reduces CRC incidence and mortality (37%). Harm of low-dose aspirin use includes about 20–30 extra cases of UGI complications per 1000 users over a 1-year period	
	Obesity—RR for woman with a body mass index (BMI) > 29 is 1.45. Similar increase seen in colorectal CA (CRC) mortality	Solid	Postmenopausal combination hormone replacement (not estrogen alone). —Based on solid evidence (WHI), 44% reduction seen in CRC incidence among HRT users	
	Regular physical activity-a meta-analysis of 52 studies showed a 24% reduction in incidence of CRC	Solid	—Based on solid evidence (WHI), combination HRT users have a 26% increased invasive breast CA risk, a 29% increase in coronary heart disease (CHD) events, and a 41% increase in stroke rates *Polyp removal* —Based on fair evidence, removal of adenomatous polyps reduces the risk of CRC (especially polyps > 1 cm) —Based on fair evidence, complications of polyp removal include perforation of the colon and bleeding estimated at 7–9 events per 1000 procedures *Low-fat, high-fiber diet does not reduce the risk of CRC* Statins do not reduce the incidence or mortality of CRC Data are inadequate to show a reduction in the risk of CRC from calcium or vitamin D supplementation	Solid

PRIMARY PREVENTION OF CANCER (CA): NCI EVIDENCE SUMMARY 2011 (CONTINUED)

CA Type	Minimize Risk Factor Exposure	Strength of Evidence That Modifying or Avoiding Risk Factor Will Reduce CA	Therapeutic	Strength of Evidence
Endometrial	Unopposed estrogen		Oral contraception (estrogen and progesterone containing)	Fair
	—Use in postmenopausal women (≥ 5 years of use = 10-fold higher risk)	Solid	—Use of oral contraceptions for 4 years reduces the risk of endometrial CA by 56%; 8 years, by 67%; and 12 years, by 72%	
	—Obesity—risk increases 1.59-fold for each 5 kg/m² change in body mass	Solid		
	—Lack of exercise—regular exercise with 38%–48% decrease in risk	Solid		Fair
	—Tamoxifen—used for > 2 years has a 2.3–7.5-fold increased risk of endometrial CA (usually stage I—95% cure rate with surgery). Nulliparous women have a 35% increased risk of endometrial CA	Solid		Inadequate
				Solid
Gastric	*Helicobacter pylori* infection	Solid	Anti-*H. pylori* therapy	*Inadequate*
	Excessive salt intake	Fair	*Dietary interventions*	*Inadequate*
	Deficient consumption of fruits/ vegetables	Fair		

	PRIMARY PREVENTION OF CANCER (CA): NCI EVIDENCE SUMMARY 2011 (CONTINUED)		
CA Type	Minimize Risk Factor Exposure	Strength of Evidence That Modifying or Avoiding Risk Factor Will Reduce CA	Therapeutic	Strength of Evidence
Liver	Avoidance of cirrhosis (hepatitis B and C, excessive alcohol use, hepatic steatosis in diabetes mellitus [DM])	Fair	Hepatitis B virus (HBV) vaccination (newborns of mothers infected with HBV) —HBV vaccination of newborns of Taiwanese mothers reduced the incidence of hepatocellular carcinoma (HCC) from 0.7 to 0.36 per 100,000 children after about 10 years	Solid
Lung	Cigarette smoking and second-hand exposure to tobacco smoke	Solid	No evidence that vitamin E/tocopherol, retinoids, vitamin C, or beta carotene in any dose reduces the risk of lung CA	
	Beta carotene, pharmacologic doses, actually increases the risk of lung CA especially in high-intensity smokers.	Solid		
	Radon gas exposure	Solid		
Oral	Tobacco	Solid	Oropharyngeal squamous cell CAs (tonsil and base of tongue) are related to HPV infection (type 16 and 18) in 60% of patients—related to sexual practices, number of partners, and may be prevented by HPV vaccine. (*NEJM.* 2010;363:24)	
	Alcohol & Dietary Factors	*Inadequate*		

PRIMARY PREVENTION OF CANCER (CA): NCI EVIDENCE SUMMARY 2011 (CONTINUED)

CA Type	Minimize Risk Factor Exposure	Strength of Evidence That Modifying or Avoiding Risk Factor Will Reduce CA	Therapeutic	Strength of Evidence
Ovarian	Postmenopausal use of HRT (estrogen replacement only) with a 3.2-fold increased risk after ≥20 years of use	Fair	Oral contraceptives —5%–10% reduction in ovarian CA per year of use, up to 80% maximum RR reduction —Increased risk of deep venous thrombosis (DVT) with oral contraceptive pill (OCP) use of about three events per 10,000 women per year; increased breast CA risk among long-term OCP users of about one extra case per 100,000 women per year	Solid
	Obesity —Elevated BMI including during adolescence associated with increased mortality from ovarian CA	Fair	Prophylactic salpingo-oophorectomy—in high-risk women (eg, BRCA1 or BRCA2) —Ninety percent reduction in ovarian CA risk —When prior to menopause, about 50% of women experience vasomotor symptoms; 4.5-fold increased RR of heart disease	Solid
Prostate	Family history of prostate CA in men aged < 60 years defines risk. One first-degree relative with prostate CA increases the risk 3-fold, two first-degree relatives increase the risk 5-fold.		Finasteride —Decreased 7-year prostate CA incidence from 25% (placebo) to 18% (finasteride), but no change in mortality —Trial participants report reduced ejaculate volume (47% → 60%); increased erectile dysfunction (62% → 67%); increased loss of libido (60% → 65%); increased gynecomastia (3% → 4.5%)	Solid

		PRIMARY PREVENTION OF CANCER (CA): NCI EVIDENCE SUMMARY 2011 (CONTINUED)		
CA Type	Minimize Risk Factor Exposure	Strength of Evidence That Modifying or Avoiding Risk Factor Will Reduce CA	Therapeutic	Strength of Evidence
	—Incidence of prostate CA in African Americans increased, occurs at a younger age, and is more virulent		Dutasteride —Absolute risk reduction of 22.8% —No difference in prostate CA-specific or overall mortality. Increase in more aggressive CA (Gleason 7–10) in dutasteride group. Vitamin E/alpha-tocopherol—inadequate data Selenium —No study shows benefit in reducing risk of prostate CA Lycopene —Inadequate data	Inadequate Inadequate Inadequate
Skin	Sunburns (melanoma)	Inadequate	Sunscreen (squamous cell carcinoma of the skin)	Inadequate

[a]National Surgical Adjuvant Breast and Bowel Project (NSABP) Study of Tamoxifen and Raloxifene (STAR) trial: raloxifene is as effective as tamoxifen in reducing the risk of invasive breast CA among postmenopausal women with at least a 5-year predicted breast CA risk of 1.66% based on the Gail model (http://bcra.nci.nih.gov/brc). Raloxifene does not reduce the risk of noninvasive CA and is not associated with endometrial CA.

[b]Women's Health Initiative (WHI): alternate-day use of low-dose aspirin (100 mg) for an average of 10 years of treatment does not lower the risk of total, breast, colorectal, or other site-specific CAs. There was a trend toward reduction in risk for lung CA (*JAMA.* 2005;294:47–55).

[c]Methods to minimize risk of HPV infection include abstinence from sexual activity and the use of barrier contraceptives and/or spermicidal gel during sexual intercourse.

[d]On June 8, 2006, the U.S. Food and Drug Administration (FDA) announced approval of Gardasil, the first vaccine developed to prevent cervical CA, precancerous genital lesions, and genital warts due to HPV types 6, 11, 16, and 18. The vaccine is approved for use in females aged 9–26 years (http://www.fda.gov). A bivalent vaccine, Cervarix, is also FDA approved with activity against HPV subtypes 16 and 18 (*NEJM.* 2006;354:1109–1112).

[e]Cereal fiber supplementation and diets low in fat and high in fiber, fruits, and vegetables do not reduce the rate of adenoma recurrence over a 3- to 4-year period.

[f]There is solid evidence that NSAIDs reduce the risk of adenomas, but the extent to which this translates into a reduction in CRC is uncertain.

Source: http://www.cancer.gov/cancertopics/pdq/prevention.

DENTAL CARIES						
Disease Prevention	Organization	Date	Population	Recommendations	Comments	Source
Dental Caries	AAFP	2010	Children and adolescents	Recommends fluoride supplementation to prevent dental caries for infants and children aged 6 months through 16 years residing in areas with inadequate fluoride in the water supply (< 0.6 ppm).		http://www.guidelines.gov/content.aspx?id=34005

Disease Prevention	Organization	Date	Population	Recommendations	Comments	Source
Diabetes Mellitus (DM), Type 2	**ADA**	2011	Persons with impaired glucose tolerance (IGT)[a]	1. Recommend initiation of an effective ongoing program targeting weight loss. Program should emphasize moderate activity most days of the week. 2. Consider initiation of metformin for patients at highest risk for developing diabetes (eg, HgbA1c ≥ 6%) despite lifestyle interventions).	1. Goal of program is weight loss of at least 7% of body weight and to encourage at least 30 minutes of moderate activity a minimum of 5 days/week. 2. Program should include follow-up counseling.	http://care.diabetesjournals.org/content/34/Supplement_1/S11.full.pdf+html

DIABETES MELLITUS (DM), TYPE 2

[a]IGT if fasting glucose 110–125 mg/dL, 2-hour glucose after 75-g anhydrous glucose load 140–199 mg/dL, or HgbA1c 5.7%–6.4%.

Disease Prevention	Organization	Date	Population	Recommendations	Comments	Source
DOMESTIC VIOLENCE						
Domestic Violence	WHO	2010	Adolescents and adult women	Recommend school-based programs that emphasize preventing dating violence.	1. Interventions of possible, but not proven, efficacy include: 　a. School-based programs that teach children to recognize and avoid sexually abusive situations. 　b. Empowerment and relationship skills training for women. 　c. Programs that change social and cultural gender norms.	http://www.who.int/violence_injury_prevention/publications/violence/9789241564007_eng.pdf

| | | **DRIVING RISK** | | | |

Disease Prevention	Organization	Date	Population	Recommendations	Comments	Source
Driving Risk	AAN	2010	Adults with dementia	Assess patients with dementia for the following characteristics that place them at increased risk for unsafe driving: 1. Caregiver's assessment that the patient's driving ability is marginal or unsafe. 2. History of traffic citations. 3. History of motor vehicle collisions. 4. Reduced driving mileage. 5. Self-reported situational avoidance. 6. Mini-Mental Status Exam score ≤ 24. 7. Aggressive or impulsive personality.		http://www.guidelines.gov/content.aspx?id=15853

ENDOCARDITIS

Disease Prevention	Organization	Date	Population	Recommendations	Comments	Source
Endocarditis	AHA ESC	2007 2009	Endocarditis is more likely a result of random exposure to bacteremia rather than associated with procedures. Certain persons at highest risk for adverse sequelae from endocarditis.[a]	1. Give antibiotic prophylaxis[b] before certain dental[c] as well as certain other procedures only to those patients at highest risk.[d] 2. Antibiotic prophylaxis is no longer indicated for native valvular heart disease unless previous endocarditis is present.	1. Emphasis is on providing prophylaxis to patients at greatest risk of endocarditis. 2. General consensus suggests few cases of infective endocarditis can be prevented by preprocedure prophylaxis with antibiotics.	*Circulation.* 2007;116:1736 *European Heart J.* 2009;30:2369–2413 *Circulation.* 2008;52:676–685

[a]Patients with prosthetic valves; previous endocarditis; selected patients with congenital heart disease (unrepaired cyanotic congenital heart disease [CHD]; completely repaired congenital heart defect with prosthetic material or device during first 6 months after procedure; repaired cyanotic CHD with residual defects at or near-repair site); and cardiac transplant recipients who develop valvulopathy.

[b]Standard prophylaxis regimen: amoxicillin (adults 2.0 g; children 50 mg/kg orally 1 hour before procedure). If unable to take oral medications, give ampicillin (adults 2.0 g IM or IV; children 50 mg/kg IM or IV within 30 minutes of procedure). If penicillin-allergic, give clindamycin (adults 600 mg; children 20 mg/kg orally 1 hour before procedure) or azithromycin or clarithromycin (adults 500 mg; children 15 mg/kg orally 1 hour before procedure). If penicillin-allergic and unable to take oral medications, give clindamycin (adults 600 mg; children 20 mg/kg IV within 30 minutes before procedure). If allergy to penicillin is not anaphylaxis, angioedema, or urticaria, options for non-oral treatment also include cefazolin (1 g IM or IV for adults, 50 mg/kg IM or IV for children); and for penicillin-allergic, oral therapy includes cephalexin 2 g PO for adults or 50 mg/kg PO for children (IM, intramuscular; IV, intravenous; PO, by mouth, orally).

[c]All dental procedures that involve manipulation of gingival tissue or the periapical region of teeth or perforation of oral mucosa only in high-risk patients.

[d]Antibiotic prophylaxis is recommended for procedures in the respiratory tract or infected skin, skin structures, or musculoskeletal tissue in high-risk patients. Antibiotic prophylaxis for genitourinary (GU) or gastrointestinal (GI) procedures is indicated with ongoing infection.

PREVENTION OF FALLS IN THE ELDERLY

Disease Prevention	Organization	Date	Population	Recommendations	Comments	Source
Prevention of Falls in the Elderly	USPSTF	2010	Older adults	1. Recommends vitamin D supplementation (800 international units [IUs] orally daily). 2. Recommends home-hazard modification (eg, adding nonslip tape to rugs and steps, provision of grab bars, etc) for all homes of persons aged ≥ 65 years. 3. Recommends exercise or physical therapy interventions targeting gait and balance training. 4. Insufficient evidence to recommend a multifactorial assessment and management approach for all elderly persons.	1. 30%–40% of all community-dwelling persons aged ≥ 65 years fall at least once a year. 2. Falls are the leading cause of fatal and nonfatal injuries among persons aged ≥ 65 years. 3. A review and modification of chronic medications, including psychotropic medications, is important although not proven to reduce falls.	http://www.uspreventiveservicestaskforce.org/uspstf11/fallsprevention/fallspreves.pdf

GONORRHEA, OPHTHALMIA NEONATORUM					
Disease Prevention	Organization	Date	Population	Recommendations	Comments	Source
Gonorrhea, Ophthalmia Neonatorum	AAFP USPSTF	2010 2005	Newborns	Recommend prophylactic ocular topical medication against gonococcal ophthalmia neonatorum for all newborns.		http://www.guidelines.gov/content. aspx?id=34005 http://www. uspreventiveservicestaskforce.org/ uspstf/uspsgono.htm

GROUP B STREPTOCOCCAL INFECTION						

Disease Prevention	Organization	Date	Population	Recommendations	Comments	Source
Group B Streptococcal (GBS) Infection	CDC	2010	Pregnant women	1. Intrapartum antibiotic prophylaxis (IAP) to prevent early-onset invasive GBS disease in newborns is indicated for high-risk pregnancies.[a] • IAP is **not** indicated for GBS colonization or GBS bacteriuria **during a previous pregnancy**, negative vaginal-rectal GBS culture, or if a cesarean delivery is performed with intact membranes and before the onset of labor (regardless of GBS screening culture status).	1. Penicillin G is the agent of choice for IAP. 2. Ampicillin is an acceptable alternative to penicillin G. 3. Cefazolin may be used if the patient has a penicillin allergy that does not cause anaphylaxis, angioedema, urticaria, or respiratory distress. 4. Clindamycin or erythromycin may be used if the patient has a penicillin allergy that causes anaphylaxis, angioedema, urticaria, or respiratory distress.	http://www.cdc.gov/mmwr/preview/mmwrhtml/rr5910a1.htm?s_cid=rr5910a1_w

[a]Indications for IAP: previous infant with invasive GBS disease; history of GBS bacteriuria during current pregnancy; positive GBS vaginal-rectal screening culture within 5 weeks of delivery; unknown GBS status with any of the following: preterm labor at < 37 gestational weeks, amniotic membrane rupture ≥ 18 hours, intrapartum fever ≥ 100.4°F (≥ 38°C); intrapartum nucleic acid amplification test positive for GBS.

HUMAN IMMUNODEFICIENCY VIRUS (HIV), OPPORTUNISTIC INFECTIONS

Disease Prevention	Organization	Date	Population	Recommendations	Comments	Source
Human Immunodeficiency Virus (HIV), Opportunistic Infections	CDC	2009	HIV-infected adults and adolescents	See table below (from the clinical practice guidelines at http://www.cdc.gov/mmwr/preview/mmwrhtml/rr5804a1.htm)		http://www.cdc.gov/mmwr/preview/mmwrhtml/rr5804a1.htm
	CDC	2009	HIV-infected children	See table below (from the clinical practice guidelines at http://www.cdc.gov/mmwr/preview/mmwrhtml/rr5811a1.htm)		http://www.cdc.gov/mmwr/preview/mmwrhtml/rr5811a1.htm

PROPHYLAXIS TO PREVENT FIRST EPISODE OF OPPORTUNISTIC DISEASE AMONG HIV-INFECTED ADULTS			
Pathogen	**Indication**	**First Choice**	**Alternative**
Pneumocystis carinii pneumonia (PCP)	CD4+ count < 200 cells/μL (AII) or oropharyngeal candidiasis (AII) CD4+ < 14% or history of AIDS-defining illness (BII) CD4+ count > 200 but < 250 cells/μL if monitoring CD4+ count every 1–3 months is not possible (BIII)	Trimethoprim-sulfamethoxazole (TIMP-SMX), 1 DS PO daily (AII); or 1 SS daily (AII)	• TMP-SMX 1 DS PO tiw (BI); or • Dapsone 100 mg PO daily or 50 mg PO bid (BI); or • Dapsone 50 mg PO daily + pyrimethamine 50 mg PO weekly + leucovorin 25 mg PO weekly (BI); or • Aerosolized pentamidine 300 mg via Respigard III nebulized every month (BI); or • Atovaquone 1500 mg PO daily (BI); or • Atovaquone 1500 mg + pyrimethamine 25 mg + leucovorin 10 mg PO daily (CIII)
Toxoplasma gondii encephalitis	Toxoplasma IgG positive patients with CD4+ count < 100 cells/μL (AII) Seronegative patients receiving PCP prophylaxis not active against toxoplasmosis should have toxoplasma serology retested if CD4+ count decline to < 100 cells/μL (CIII) Prophylaxis should be initiated if seroconversion occurred (AII)	TMP-SMX 1 DS PO daily (AII)	• TMP-SMX 1 DS OI tiw (BIII); or • TMP-SMX 1 SS PO daily (BIII); or • Dapsone 50 mg PO daily + pyrimethamine 50 mg PO weekly + leucovorin 25 mg PO weekly (BI); or • (Dapsone 200 mg + pyrimethamine 75 mg + leucovorin 25 mg) PO weekly (BIII); • (Atovaquone 1500 mg +/– pyrimethamine 25 mg + leucovorin 10 mg) PO daily (CIII)
Mycobacterium tuberculosis infection (TB) (Treatment of latent TB infection or LTBI)	(+) diagnostic test for LTBI, no evidence of active TB, and no prior history of treatment for active or latent TB (AII); (–) diagnostic test for LTBI and no evidence of active TB, but close contact with a person with infectious pulmonary TB (AII); A history of untreated or inadequately treated healed TB (ie, old fibrotic lesions) regardless of diagnostic tests for LTBI and no evidence of active TB (AII)	Isoniazid (INH) 300 mg PO daily (AII) or 900 mg PO biw (BII) for 9 months–both plus pyridoxine 50 mg PO daily (BIII); or For persons exposed to drug-resistant TB, selection of drugs after consultation with public health authorities (AII)	• Rifampin (RIF) 600 mg PO daily × 4 months (BIII); or • Rifabutin (RFB) (dose adjusted based on concomitant ART) × 4 months (BIII)

PROPHYLAXIS TO PREVENT FIRST EPISODE OF OPPORTUNISTIC DISEASE AMONG HIV-INFECTED ADULTS (CONTINUED)

Pathogen	Indication	First Choice	Alternative
Disseminated *Mycobacterium axium* complex (MAC) disease	CD4+ count < 50 cells/μL—after ruling out active MAC infection (AI)	Azithromycin 1200 mg PO once weekly (AI); or Clarithromycin 500 mg PO bid (AI); or azithromycin 600 mg PO twice weekly (BIII)	• RFB 300 mg PO daily (BI) (dosage adjustment based on drug-drug interactions with ART); rule out active TB before starting RFB
Streptococcus pneumonia infection	CD4+ count > 200 cells/μL and no receipt of pneumococcal vaccine in the past 5 years (AII) CD4+ count < 200 cells/μL—vaccination can be offered (CIII) In patients who received polysaccharide pneumococcal vaccination (PPV) when CD4+ count < 200 cells/μL but has increased to > 200 cells/μL in response to ART (CIII)	23-valent PPV 0.5 mL IM × 1 (BII) Revaccination every 5 years may be considered (CIII)	
Influenza A and B virus infection	All HIV-infected patients (AII)	Inactivated influenza vaccine 0.5 mL IM annually (AIII)	
Histoplasma capsulatum infection	CD4+ count ≥ 150 cells/μL and at high risk because of occupational exposure or live in a community with a hyperendemic rate of histo plasmosis (> 10 cases/100 patient-years) (CI)	Itraconazole 200 mg PO daily (CI)	
Coccidioidomycosis	Positive IgM or IgG serologic test in a patient from a disease-endemic area; and CD4+ count < 250 cells/μL (CIII)	Fluconazole 400 mg PO daily (CIII) Itraconazole 200 mg PO bid (CIII)	

PROPHYLAXIS TO PREVENT FIRST EPISODE OF OPPORTUNISTIC DISEASE AMONG HIV-INFECTED ADULTS (CONTINUED)

Pathogen	Indication	First Choice	Alternative
Varicella-zoster virus (VZV) infection	*Pre-exposure prevention:* Patient with CD4+ count ≥ 200 cells/μL who have not been vaccinated, have no history of varicella or herpes zoster, or who are seronegative for VZV (CIII) Note: routine VZV serologic testing in HIV-infected adults is not recommended *Post-exposure–close contact with a person who has active varicella or herpes zoster:* For susceptible patients (those who have no history of vaccination or infection with either condition, or are known to be VZV seronegative (AIII)	*Pre-exposure prevention:* Primary varicella vaccination (Varivax), two doses (0.5 mL SQ) administered 3 months apart (CIII) If vaccination results in disease because of vaccine virus, treatment with acyclovir is recommended (AIII) *Postexposure therapy:* Varicella-zoster immune globulin (VariZIG) 125 IU per 10 kg (maximum of 625 IU) IM, administered within 96 hours after exposure to a person with active varicella or herpes zoster (AIII) Note: As of June 2007, VariZIG can be obtained only under a treatment IND (1-800-843-7477, FFF Enterprises)	• VZV-susceptible household contacts of susceptible HIV-infected persons should be vaccinated to prevent potential transmission of VZV to their HIV-infected contacts (BIII) *Alternative postexposure therapy:* • Postexposure varicella vaccine (Varivax) 0.5 mL SO × 2 doses, 3 months apart if CD4+ count >200 cells/μL (CIII); or • Preemptive acyclovir 800 mg PO 5×/day for 5 days (CIII) • These two alternatives have not been studied in the HIV population
Human papillomavirus (HPV) infection	Women aged 15–26 years (CIII)	HPV quadrivalent vaccine 0.5 mL IM months 0, 2, and 6 (CIII)	
Hepatitis A virus (HAV) infection	HAV-susceptible patients with chronic liver disease, or who are injection-drug users, or men who have sex with men (AII). Certain specialists might delay vaccination until CD4+ count > 200 cells/μL (CIII)	Hepatitis A vaccine 1 mL IM × 2 doses—at 0 & 6–12 months (AII) IgG antibody response should be assessed 1 month after vaccination: nonresponders should be revaccinated (BIII)	

PROPHYLAXIS TO PREVENT FIRST EPISODE OF OPPORTUNISTIC DISEASE AMONG HIV-INFECTED ADULTS (CONTINUED)

Pathogen	Indication	First Choice	Alternative
Hepatitis B virus (HBV) infection	All HIV patients without evidence of prior exposure to HBV should be vaccinated with HBV vaccine, including patients with CD4+ count < 200 cells/μL (AII) *Patients with isolated anti-HBc:* (BIII) (consider screening for HBV DNA before vaccination to rule out occult chronic HBV infection)	Hepatitis B vaccine IM (Engerix-B[a] 20 μg/mL or Recombivax HB[b] 10 μg/mL) at 0,1, and 6 months (AII) Anti-HBs should be obtained 1 month after receipt of the vaccine series (BIII)	Some experts recommend vaccinating with 40 μg doses of either vaccine (CIII)
	Vaccine non responders: Defined as anti-HBs < 10 IU/mL 1 month after a vaccination series. For patients with low CD4+ count at the time of first vaccination series, certain specialists might delay revaccination until after a sustained increase in CD4+ count with ART.	Revaccinate with a second vaccine series (BIII)	Some experts recommend revaccinating with 40 μg doses of either vaccine (CIII)
Malaria	Travel disease-endemic area	Recommendations are the some for HIV-infected and noninfected patients. One of the following three drugs is usually recommended depending on location: atovaquone/proguanil, doxycycline, or mefloquine. Refer to the following website for the most recent recommendations based on region and drug susceptibility. http://www.cdc.gov/malaria/(AII)	

DS, double strength; PO, by mouth; SS, single strength; bid, twice daily; tiw, three times weekly; SQ, subcutaneous; IM, intramuscular

PROPHYLAXIS TO PREVENT FIRST EPISODE OF OPPORTUNISTIC INFECTIONS AMONG HIV-EXPOSED AND HIV-INFECTED INFANTS AND CHILDREN, UNITED STATES[a,b]

Pathogen	Indication	Preventive Regimen	
		First Choice	Alternative
		STRONGLY RECOMMENDED AS STANDARD OF CARE	
Pneumocystis pneumonia[c]	HIV-infected or HIV- indeterminate infants aged 1–12 months; HIV-infected children aged 1–5 years with CD4 count of < 500 cells/mm³ or CD4 percentage of < 15%; HIV-infected children aged 6–12 years with CD4 count of < 200 cells/mm³ or CD4 percentage of < 15%	• TMP-SMX, 150/750 mg/m² body surface area per day (max: 320/1600 mg) orally divided into two doses daily and administered three times weekly on consecutive days (AI) • Acceptable alternative dosage schedules for same dose (AI): single dose orally three times weekly on consecutive days; two divided doses orally daily; or two divided doses orally three times weekly on alternate days	• Dapsone: children aged ≥ 1 month, 2 mg/kg body weight (max 100 mg) orally daily; or 4 mg/kg body weight (max 200 mg) orally weekly (BI) • Atovaquone: children aged 1–3 months and > 24 months, 30 mg/kg body weight orally daily; children aged 4–24 months, 45 mg/kg body weight orally daily (BI) • Aerosolized pentamidine: children aged ≥ 5 years, 300 mg every month by Respirgard I™ (Marquest, Englewood, CO) nebulizer (BI)
Malaria	Travel to area in which malaria is endemic	Recommendations are the same for HIV-infected and HIV-uninfected children. Refer to http://www.cdc.gov/malaria/ for the most recent recommendations based on region and drug susceptibility. • Mefloquine, 5 mg/kg body weight orally 1 time weekly (max 250 mg) • Atovaquone/proguanil (Malarone) 1 time daily 11–20 kg = 1 pediatric tablet (62.5 mg/25 mg) 21–30 kg = 2 pediatric tablets (125 mg/50 mg) 31–40 kg = 3 pediatric tablets (187.5 mg/75 mg) > 40 kg = 1 adult tablet (250 mg/100 mg)	• Doxycycline, 100 mg orally daily for children > 8 years (2.2 mg/kg/day). • Chloroquine base, 5 mg/kg base orally up to 300 mg weekly for sensitive regions only (7.5 mg/kg chloroquine phosphate)

PROPHYLAXIS TO PREVENT FIRST EPISODE OF OPPORTUNISTIC INFECTIONS AMONG HIV-EXPOSED AND HIV-INFECTED INFANTS AND CHILDREN, UNITED STATES[a,b] (CONTINUED)

Pathogen	Indication	Preventive Regimen		
		First Choice	Alternative	
		STRONGLY RECOMMENDED AS STANDARD OF CARE		
Mycobacterium tuberculosis	TST reaction ≥ 5 mm or prior positive TST result without treatment; or regardless of current	• Isoniazid, 10–15 mg/kg body weight (max 300 mg) orally daily for 9 months (AII); or 20–30 mg/kg body weight (max 900 mg) orally 2 times weekly for 9 months (BII)	• Rifampin, 10–20 mg/kg body weight (max 600 mg) orally daily for 4–6 months (BIII)	
Isoniazid-sensitive	TST result and previous treatment, close contact with any person who has contagious TB. TB disease must be excluded before start of treatment.			
Isoniazid-resistant	Same as previous pathogen; increased probability of exposure to isoniazid-resistant TB	• Rifampin, 10–20 mg/kg body weight (max 600 mg) orally daily for 4–6 months (BIII)	• Uncertain	
Multidrug-resistant (isoniazid and rifampin)	Same as previous pathogen; increased probability of exposure to multidrug-resistant TB	• Choice of drugs requires consultation with public health authorities and depends on susceptibility of isolate from source patient		
Mycobacterium avium complex[d]	For children aged ≥ 6 years with CD4 count of < 50 cells/mm³; aged 2–5 years with CD4 count of < 75 cells/mm³; aged 1–2 years with CD4 count of < 500 cells/mm³; aged < 1 year with CD4 count of < 750 cells/mm³	• Clarithromycin, 7.5 mg/kg body weight (max 500 mg) orally 2 times daily (AII), or azithromycin, 20 mg/kg body weight (max 1200 mg) orally weekly (AII)	• Azithromycin, 5 mg/kg body weight (max 250 mg) orally daily (AII); children aged ≥ 6 years, rifabutin, 300 mg orally daily (BI)	

PROPHYLAXIS TO PREVENT FIRST EPISODE OF OPPORTUNISTIC INFECTIONS AMONG HIV-EXPOSED AND HIV-INFECTED INFANTS AND CHILDREN, UNITED STATES[a,b] (CONTINUED)

Pathogen	Indication	Preventive Regimen	
		First Choice	Alternative
		STRONGLY RECOMMENDED AS STANDARD OF CARE	
Varicella-zoster virus[c]	Substantial exposure to varicella or shingles with no history of varicella or zoster or seronegative status for VZV by a sensitive, specific antibody assay or lack of evidence for age-appropriate vaccination	• Varicella-zoster immune globulin (VariZIG), 125 IU per 10 kg (max 625 IU) IM, administered within 96 hours after exposure[d] (AIII)	• If VariZIG is not available or > 96 hours have passed since exposure, some experts recommend prophylaxis with acyclovir 20 mg/kg body weight (max 800 mg) per dose orally 4 times a day for 5–7 days. Another alternative to VariZIG is intravenous immune globulin (IVIG), 400 mg/kg, administered once. IVIG should be administered within 96 hours after exposure (CIII)
Vaccine-preventable pathogens	Standard recommendations for HIV-exposed and HIV-infected children	Routine vaccinations	
Toxoplasma gondii[g]	Immunoglobulin G (IgG) antibody to *Toxoplasma* and severe immunosuppression: HIV-infected children aged < 6 years with CD4 <15%; HIV-infected children aged ≥ 6 years with CD4 <100 cells/mm³ (BIII)	• TMP-SMX, 150/750 mg/m² body surface area daily orally in 2 divided doses (BIII) • Acceptable alternative dosage schedules for same dosage (AI): single dose orally 3 times weekly on consecutive days; 2 divided doses orally daily; or 2 divided doses orally 3 times weekly on alternate days	• Dapsone (children aged ≥ 1 month), 2 mg/kg body weight or 15 mg/m² body surface area (max 25 mg) daily; PLUS pyrimethamine, 1 mg/kg body weight (max 25 mg) orally daily; PLUS leucovorin, 5 mg orally every 3 days (BI) • Atovaquone (children aged 1–3 months and > 24 months, 30 mg/kg body weight orally daily; children aged 4–24 months, 45 mg/kg body weight orally daily) with or without pyrimethamine, 1 mg/kg body weight or 15 mg/m² body surface area (max 25 mg) orally daily; PLUS leucovorin, 5 mg orally every 3 days (CIII)

PROPHYLAXIS TO PREVENT FIRST EPISODE OF OPPORTUNISTIC INFECTIONS AMONG HIV-EXPOSED AND HIV-INFECTED INFANTS AND CHILDREN, UNITED STATES[a,b] (CONTINUED)

Pathogen	Indication	Preventive Regimen	
		First Choice	Alternative
		STRONGLY RECOMMENDED AS STANDARD OF CARE	
		NOT RECOMMENDED FOR MOST CHILDREN; INDICATED FOR USE ONLY IN UNUSUAL CIRCUMSTANCES	
Invasive bacterial infections	Hypogammaglobulinemia (ie, IgG < 400 mg/dL)	• IVIG (400 mg/kg body weight every 2–4 weeks) (AI)	
Cytomegalovirus (CMV)	CMV antibody positivity and severe immunosuppression (CD4 < 50 cells/mm[3])	• Valganciclovir, 900 mg orally 1 time daily with food for older children who can receive adult dosing (CIII)	

[a]Abbreviations: HIV, human immunodeficiency virus; PCP, *Pneumocystis* pneumonia; TMP-SMX, trimethoprim-sulfamethoxazole; TST, tuberculin skin test; TB, tuberculosis; IM, intramuscularly; IVIG, intravenous immune globulin; IgG, immunoglobulin G; CMV, cytomegalovirus; VZV, varicella-zoster virus; FDA, Food and Drug Administration.
[b]Information in these guidelines might not represent FDA approval or FDA-approved labeling for products or indications. Specifically, the terms "safe" and "effective" might not be synonymous with the FDA-defined legal standards for product approval. Letters and roman numerals in parentheses after regimens indicate the strength of the recommendation and the quality of the evidence supporting it.
[c]Daily trimethoprim-sulfamethoxazole (TMP-SMX) reduces the frequency of certain bacterial infections. TMP-SMX, dapsone-pyrimethamine, and possibly atovaquone (with or without pyrimethamine) protect against toxoplasmosis; however, data have not been prospectively collected. Compared with weekly dapsone, daily dapsone is associated with lower incidence of PCP but higher hematologic toxicity and mortality. Patients receiving therapy for toxoplasmosis with sulfadiazine-pyrimethamine are protected against PCP and do not need TMP-SMX.
[d]Substantial drug interactions can occur between rifamycins (ie, rifampin and rifabutin) and protease inhibitors and nonnucleoside reverse transcriptase inhibitors. A specialist should be consulted.
[e]Children routinely being administered intravenous immune globulin (IVIG) should receive VariZIG if the last dose of IVIG was administered > 21 days before exposure.
[f]As of 2007, VariZIG can be obtained only under a treatment Investigational New Drug protocol.
[g]Protection against toxoplasmosis is provided by the preferred anti-*Pneumocystis* regimens and possibly by atovaquone.

HYPERTENSION (HTN)						
Disease Prevention	Organization	Date	Population	Recommendations	Comments	Source
Hypertension (HTN)	Canadian HTN Program JNC VII ICSI 13th Edition	2007 2003 2010	Persons at risk for developing HTN[a]	Recommend weight loss, reduced sodium intake, moderate alcohol consumption, increased physical activity, potassium supplementation, and modification of eating patterns.[b]	1. A 5-mm Hg reduction in systolic blood pressure in the population would result in a 14% overall reduction in mortality due to stroke, a 9% reduction in mortality due to CHD, and a 7% decrease in all-cause mortality.	http://www.hypertension.ca *JAMA.* 2003;289:2560–2572
	ACCF/AHA	2011	Patients aged >65 years	Lifestyle management is effective in all ages.	2. Weight loss of as little as 10 lb (4.5 kg) reduces blood pressure and/or prevents HTN in a large proportion of overweight patients.	*J Am Coll Cardiol.* 2011;57(20):2037–2114

[a]Family history of HTN; African American (black race) ancestry; overweight or obesity; sedentary lifestyle; excess intake of dietary sodium; insufficient intake of fruits, vegetables, and potassium; excess consumption of alcohol.
[b]See Lifestyle Modifications for Primary Prevention of Hypertension on page 122.

LIFESTYLE MODIFICATIONS FOR PRIMARY PREVENTION OF HYPERTENSION

- Maintain healthy body weight for adults (BMI, 18.5–24.9 kg/m^2; waist circumference < 102 cm for men and < 88 cm for women).
- Reduce dietary sodium intake to no more than 100 mmol/day (approximately 6 g of sodium chloride or 2.4 g of sodium/day).
- Engage in regular aerobic physical activity, such as brisk walking, jogging, cycling, or swimming (30–60 minutes/day, 4–7 days/week), in addition to the routine activities of daily living. Higher intensities of exercise are not more effective.
- Limit alcohol consumption to no more than 2 drinks (eg, 24 oz [720 mL] of beer, 10 oz [300 mL] of wine, or 3 oz [90 mL] of 100-proof whiskey) per day in most men and to no more than one drink per day in women and lighter-weight persons.
- Maintain adequate intake of dietary potassium (> 90 mmol [3500 mg]/day).
- Consume a diet that is rich in fruits and vegetables and in low-fat dairy products with a reduced content of saturated and total fat (Dietary Approaches to Stop Hypertension [DASH] eating plan).
- Maintain a smoke-free environment.

Sources: http://www.hypertension.ca and *Hypertension.* 2003;42:1206–1252.
Trials of Hypertension Prevention (TDHP) long-term follow-up: risk of CV event 25% lower in sodium-reduction group. (RR, 0.75; 95% CI, 0.57–0.99) (*BMJ.* 2007;334:885–892)

IMMUNIZATIONS, ADULTS

Disease Prevention	Organization	Date	Population	Recommendations	Comments	Source
Immunizations, Adults	CDC ICSI	2011 2010	Adults	Recommend immunizing adults according to the Centers for Disease Control and Prevention (CDC) recommendations unless contraindicated (see Appendix IX).		http://www.cdc.gov/vaccines/recs/ schedules/downloads/adult/ mmwr-adult-schedule.pdf http://www.icsi.org/preventive_ services_for_adults/preventive_ services_for_adults_4.html

IMMUNIZATIONS, INFANTS AND CHILDREN

Disease Prevention	Organization	Date	Population	Recommendations	Comments	Source
Immunizations, Infants and Children	CDC ICSI	2011 2010	Infants and children aged 0–6 years	Recommend immunizing infants and children according to the CDC recommendations unless contraindicated. (See Appendix IX)		http://www.cdc.gov/vaccines/recs/ schedules/downloads/ child/0-6yrs-schedule-pr.pdf http://www.cdc.gov/vaccines/recs/ schedules/downloads/child/ catchup-schedule-pr.pdf http://www.icsi.org/preventive_ services_for_children_guideline_/ preventive_services_for_children_ and_adolescents_2531.html

IMMUNIZATIONS, CHILDREN AND ADOLESCENTS

Disease Prevention	Organization	Date	Population	Recommendations	Comments	Source
Immunizations, Children and Adolescents	CDC ICSI	2011 2010	Children and adolescents aged 7–18 years	Recommend immunizing children and adolescents according to the CDC recommendations unless contraindicated (see Appendix IX).		http://www.cdc.gov/vaccines/recs/ schedules/downloads/child/7-18yrs-schedule-pr.pdf http://www.cdc.gov/vaccines/recs/ schedules/downloads/child/ catchup-schedule-pr.pdf http://www.icsi.org/preventive_ services_for_children_guideline_/ preventive_services_for_children_ and_adolescents_2531.html

INFLUENZA, CHEMOPROPHYLAXIS

Disease Prevention	Organization	Date	Population	Recommendations	Comments	Source
Influenza, Chemoprophylaxis	IDSA CDC	2009 2011	Children and adults	1. Consider antiviral chemoprophylaxis for adults and children aged ≥ 1 year at high risk of influenza complications (see Influenza, Vaccination section) when any of the following conditions are present: a. Influenza vaccination is contraindicated.[a] b. Unvaccinated adults or children when influenza activity has been detected in the community. Vaccinate simultaneously. c. Unvaccinated adults and children in close contact with people diagnosed with influenza. d. Residents of extended-care facilities with an influenza outbreak.	1. Influenza vaccination is the best way to prevent influenza. 2. Antiviral chemoprophylaxis is not a substitute for influenza vaccination. 3. Duration of chemoprophylaxis is 2 weeks postvaccination in most persons but is indicated for 6 weeks in children who were not previously vaccinated or who require two vaccine doses. 4. Chemoprophylaxis for 10 days in a household in which a family member has influenza. 5. Agents for chemoprophylaxis of influenza A (H1N1) and B: zanamivir or oseltamivir.	http://www.guidelines.gov/content.aspx?id=14173 http://www.cdc.gov/mmwr/preview/mmwrhtml/rr6001a1.htm?s_cid=rr6001a1_w

[a]Contraindications for influenza vaccination: anaphylactic hypersensitivity to eggs, acute febrile illness, history of Guillain-Barré syndrome within 6 weeks of a previous influenza vaccination.

INFLUENZA, VACCINATION

Disease Prevention	Organization	Date	Population	Recommendations	Comments	Source

Influenza, Vaccination	CDC	2010	All persons aged ≥ 6 months	1. All persons aged ≥ 6 months should receive the seasonal influenza vaccine annually.
				 2. All children aged 6 months–8 years should receive two doses of the 2011–2012 seasonal influenza vaccine (≥ 4 weeks apart) if:
				   a. Vaccination status is unknown.
				   b. Persons have never received the influenza vaccine before.
				   c. Those who did not receive the 2009 H1N1 vaccine.
					1. Highest-risk groups for influenza complications are:
					   a. Pregnant women
					   b. Children aged 6 months–4 years
					   c. Children aged 6 months–18 years who are on chronic aspirin therapy
					   d. Adults aged ≥ 50 years
					   e. Persons with chronic medical conditions[a]
					   f. Residents of extended-care facilities
					   g. American Indians/Alaska natives
					   h. Morbidly obese (BMI ≥ 40) persons
					   i. Healthcare personnel
					   j. Household contacts or caregivers of children aged < 5 years or adults aged ≥ 50 years
						http://www.cdc.gov/mmwr/preview/mmwrhtml/rr59e0729a1.htm?s_cid=rr59e0729a1_w

[a]Chronic heart, lung, renal, liver, hematologic, cancer, neuromuscular, or seizure disorders, severe cognitive dysfunction, diabetes, HIV infection, or immunosuppression.

MOTOR VEHICLE INJURY, PREVENTION

Disease Prevention	Organization	Date	Population	Recommendations	Comments	Source
Motor Vehicle Injury, Prevention	ICSI	2010	Infants, children, and adolescents	1. Providers should ask the family about the use of car seats, booster seats, and seat belts. 2. Ask children and adolescents about helmet use in recreational activities.	1. Head injury rates are reduced by about 75% in motorcyclists who wear helmets compared with those who do not. 2. Properly used child restraint systems can reduce mortality up to 21% compared with seat belt usage in children aged 2–6 years.	http://www.icsi.org/preventive_services_for_children_guideline_/preventive_services_for_children_and_adolescents_2531.html

	MYOCARDIAL INFARCTION (MI)				
Disease Prevention	Organization	Date	Population	Recommendations	Comments	Source
Myocardial Infarction (MI)	*In a report showing a 50% reduction in the population's CHD mortality rate, 81% was attributable to primary prevention of CHD through tobacco cessation and lipid- and blood pressure-lowering activities. Only 19% of CHD mortality reduction occurred in patients with existing CHD (secondary prevention).*					*BMJ.* 2005;331(7517):614
	USPSTF	2009	Adults at increased risk of CHD events	1. Recommends aspirin (ASA) usage for MI prevention in men aged 45–79 years when the potential benefit outweighs the risk. 2. Recommends against ASA usage for MI prevention in men aged <45 years. 3. No recommendations for ASA usage for MI prevention in women. 4. Insufficient evidence to recommend ASA usage for CV disease prevention in men and women aged ≥80 years.	1. Meta-analysis concludes ASA prophylaxis reduces ischemic stroke risk in women (−17%) and MI events in men (−32%). No mortality benefit is seen in either group. Risk of bleeding is increased in both groups to a similar degree as the event rate reduction (*JAMA.* 2006; 295:306–313).	http://www.uspreventiveservicestaskforce.org/uspstf/uspsasmi.htmh
	ADA	2011	Diabetics type 1 or 2	Consider ASA (75–162 mg/day) if at increased CV risk (10-year > 10% based on Framingham risk score (see Appendix VI and VII), and in men aged > 50 years or women aged > 60 years with one additional risk factor.		*Diabetes Care.* 2011;34(S1): S11–S61

MYOCARDIAL INFARCTION (MI)						
Disease Prevention	**Organization**	**Date**	**Population**	**Recommendations**	**Comments**	**Source**
Myocardial Infarction (MI) (continued)	AHA	2006	All children and adults	*Dietary guidelines:* (1) Balance calorie intake and physical activity to achieve or maintain a healthy body weight. (2) Consume a diet rich in vegetables and fruit. (3) Choose whole grain, high-fiber foods. (4) Consume fish, especially oily fish, at least twice a week. (5) Limit intake of saturated fats to < 7% energy, trans fats to < 1% energy, and cholesterol to < 300 mg per day by: • Choosing lean meats and vegetable alternatives • Selecting fat-free (skim), 1% fat, and low-fat dairy products • Minimizing intake of partially hydrogenated fats. (6) Minimize intake of beverages and foods with added sugars. (7) Choose and prepare foods with little or no salt. (8) If you consume alcohol, do so in moderation. (9) Follow these recommendations for food consumed/prepared inside *and* outside of the home. *Avoid use of and exposure to tobacco products.*		*Circulation.* 2006;114:82–96

MYOCARDIAL INFARCTION (MI)

Disease Prevention	Organization	Date	Population	Recommendations	Comments	Source
Myocardial Infarction (MI) (continued)	AHA NCEP III	2002 2002	Hyperlipidemia[a]	For screening recommendations, see page 40; also see NCEP III screening and management (page 133) recommendations.	1. Short-term reduction in low-density lipoprotein (LDL) using dietary counseling by dietitians is superior to that achieved by physicians (*Am J Med.* 2000;109:549). 2. Lowest rate of recurrent events related to absolute LDL reduction (*Lancet.* 2005;366(9493): 1267–1278).	*Circulation.* 2002;106:338 *Circulation.* 2004;110: 227–239
	JNC VII	2003	HTN	See page 148 for JNC VII treatment algorithms.		*Hypertension.* 2003;42:1206–1252
	AHA	2007	HTN	Goal: Blood pressure (BP) < 140/90 mm Hg for general population; < 130/80 mm Hg if high CHD risk (DM, CKD, CHD or CHD equivalent [carotid artery disease, peripheral arterial disease, abdominal aortic aneurysm], or 10-year Framingham risk score ≥ 10%) (see Appendix VI and VII).		*Circulation.* 2007;115:2761–2788

MYOCARDIAL INFARCTION (MI)						
Disease Prevention	Organization	Date	Population	Recommendations	Comments	Source
Myocardial Infarction (MI) (continued)	ACP	2004	Diabetes mellitus	Statins should be used for primary prevention of macrovascular complications if patient has type 2 DM and other CV risk factors (aged > 55 years, left ventricular hypertrophy, previous cerebrovascular disease, peripheral arterial disease, smoking, or HTN).		*Ann Intern Med.* 2004;140:644–649 http://www.acponline.org/clinical/guidelines/?hp - acg
	ADA	2011	Diabetes mellitus	Goals: Normal fasting glucose (≤ 100 mg/dL) and near-normal HbA1c (< 7%), BP < 130/80 mm Hg; low-density-lipoprotein cholesterol (LDL-C) < 100 mg/dL (or < 70 for high risk), high-density-lipoprotein cholesterol (HDL-C) > 50 mg/dL and triglycerides < 150 mg/dL.	1. Intensive glucose lowering HbA1c < 7 should be avoided in patients with a history of hypoglycemic spells, advanced microvascular or macrovascular complications, long-standing DM, or if extensive comorbid conditions are present.	*Diabetes Care.* 2011;34 (S11–S61) *Diabetes Care.* 2009;32(1):187–192 *Circulation.* 2006;114:82–96

MYOCARDIAL INFARCTION (MI)

Disease Prevention	Organization	Date	Population	Recommendations	Comments	Source
Myocardial Infarction (MI) (continued)	AHA	2006		ASA therapy (75–162 mg/day) for those at increased risk (10-year risk > 10%). Advise all patients not to smoke.	2. DM with BP readings of 130–139/80–89 mm Hg that persist after 3 months of lifestyle and behavioral therapy should be treated with agents that block the renin-angiotensin system. If BP > 140/90 mm Hg, treat with drug class demonstrated to reduce CHD events in diabetics (angiotensin-converting enzyme [ACE] inhibitors, angiotensin receptor blockers [ARBs], beta-blockers, diuretics, and calcium channel blockers). No advantage of combining ACE inhibitor and ARB in HTN Rx (ONTARGET Trial). 3. Stroke and nonfatal stroke are reduced by lower BP targets (< 130/80 mm Hg). In the absence of harm, this benefit appears to justify the lower BP goal.	*Circulation.* 2006;114:82–96 *N Engl J Med.* 2008;358:1547–1559 *N Engl J Med.* 2008;358:2545–2559 *N Engl Med.* 2008;358:2560–2572

	MYOCARDIAL INFARCTION (MI)					
Disease Prevention	Organization	Date	Population	Recommendations	Comments	Source
Myocardial Infarction (MI) (continued)	AHA	2011	Women	Standard CVD lifestyle recommendations, PLUS: Waist circumference ≤ 35 in Omega-3 fatty acids if high risk (EPA 1800 mg/d)[a] BP < 120/80 mm Hg Lipids: LDL-C < 100 mg/dL, HDL-C > 50 mg/dL, triglycerides < 150 mg/dL ASA (75–325 mg/day) indicated only in high-risk women.[a] In women aged ≥ 65 years, *consider* ASA (81 mg daily or 100 mg every other day) if BP is controlled and the benefit of ischemic stroke and MI prevention is likely to outweigh the risk of a GI bleed and hemorrhagic stroke.	Estrogen plus progestin hormone therapy should not be used or continued. Antioxidants (vitamin E, C, and beta carotene), folic acid, and B_{12} supplementation are not recommended to prevent CHD. ASA is not indicated to prevent MI in low-risk women aged < 65 years.	*J Am Coll Cardiol.* 2011;57(12):1404–1423

| | | | | MYOCARDIAL INFARCTION (MI) | | |

Disease Prevention	Organization	Date	Population	Recommendations	Comments	Source
Myocardial Infarction (MI) (continued)	ESC	2007	Adults at risk of CV disease	Smoking cessation	European Society of Cardiology recommends using the SCORE Risk System to estimate risk of atherosclerotic CV disease.	*European Heart J.* 2007;28:2375
				Weight reduction if BMI ≥ 25 kg/m² or waist circumference ≥ 88 cm in women and ≥ 102 cm in men.		
				No further weight gain if waist circumference 80–88 cm in women and 94–102 cm in men.		
				Thirty minutes of moderately vigorous exercise on most days of the week		
				Healthy diet		
				Antihypertensives when BP ≥ 140/90 mm Hg		
				Statins when total cholesterol ≥ 190 mg/dL or LDL ≥ 115 mg/dL		
				In patients with known CV disease: ASA and statins		
				In patients with DM: glucose-lowering drugs		

ᵃHigh risk: CHD or risk equivalent or 10-year absolute CHD risk > 20% based on Framingham risk score (see Appendix VI and VII).

NEURAL TUBE DEFECTS					
Disease Prevention	Organization	Date	Population	Recommendations	Comments	Source
Neural Tube Defects	AAFP USPSTF ICSI	2010 2009 2010	Women planning or capable of pregnancy	Recommend that all women of childbearing age take a daily supplement containing 400–800 mcg of folic acid.	1. Women planning a pregnancy should start folic acid supplementation at least 1 month before conception and continue through the first 2–3 months of pregnancy. 2. The ACOG and AAFP recommend 4 mg/day folic acid for women with a history of a child affected by a neural tube defect.	http://www.guidelines.gov/content.aspx?id=34005 http://www.uspreventiveservicestaskforce.org/uspstf09/folicacid/folicacidrs.htm http://www.icsi.org/preventive_services_for_adults/preventive_services_for_adults_4.html

Disease Prevention	Organization	Date	Population	Recommendations	Comments	Source
OBESITY						
Obesity	ICSI	2009	Adolescents and adults	1. Recommends a team approach for weight management in all persons of normal weight (BMI 18.5–24.9) or overweight (BMI 25–29.9) including: a. Nutrition b. Physical activity c. Lifestyle changes d. Screen for depression e. Screen for eating disorders f. Review medication list and assess if any medications can interfere with weight loss 2. Recommend regular follow-up to reinforce principles of weight management.	1. Recommend 30–60 minutes of moderate physical activity on most days of the week. 2. Nutrition education focused on decreased caloric intake, encouraging healthy food choices, and managing restaurant and social eating situations. 3. Weekly weight checks 4. Encourage non-food rewards for positive reinforcement. 5. Stress management techniques.	http://www. guidelines.gov/ content. aspx?id=14178
	Endocrine Society	2008	Children	1. Recommends exclusive breast-feeding for at least 6 months. 2. Educate children and parents about healthy diets and the importance of regular physical activity. 3. Encourage school systems to promote healthy eating habits and provide health education courses. 4. Clinicians should help to educate communities about healthy dietary and activity habits.	1. Avoid the consumption of calorie-dense, nutrient-poor foods (eg, juices, soft drinks, "fast food" items, and calorie-dense snacks). 2. Control calorie intake by portion control. 3. Reduce saturated dietary fat intake for children aged > 2 years. 4. Increase dietary fiber, fruits, and vegetables. 5. Eat regular, scheduled meals and avoid snacking. 6. Limit television, video games, and computer time to 2 hours daily.	http://www. guidelines.gov/ content. aspx?id=13572

OSTEOPOROTIC HIP FRACTURES						
Disease Prevention	Organization	Date	Population	Recommendations	Comments	Source
Osteoporotic Hip Fractures	AAFP USPSTF	2010 2005	Postmenopausal women	Recommend against the routine use of combined estrogen and progestin for the prevention of osteoporotic fractures.	The results of studies including the WHI and the Heart and Estrogen/Progestin Replacement Study reveal that HRT probably reduces	http://www.guidelines.gov/content.aspx?id=34005 http://www.uspreventiveservicestaskforce.org/uspstf/uspspmho.htm
	AAFP USPSTF	2010 2005	Postmenopausal women who have had a hysterectomy	Recommend against the routine use of estrogen for the prevention of osteoporotic fractures in postmenopausal women who have had a hysterectomy.	osteoporotic hip and vertebral fractures and may decrease the risk of colon CA; however, HRT may lead to an increased risk of breast CA, stroke, cholecystitis, dementia, and venous thromboembolism. HRT does not decrease the risk of coronary artery disease.	http://www.guidelines.gov/content.aspx?id=34005 http://www.uspreventiveservicestaskforce.org/uspstf/uspspmho.htm

PRESSURE ULCERS

Disease Prevention	Organization	Date	Population	Recommendations	Comments	Source
Pressure Ulcers	ICSI WONCA	2010 2010	Adults or children with impaired mobility	1. Recommend a risk assessment of all persons in both outpatient and inpatient settings (eg, the Braden Scale in adults and Braden Q Scale in children). 2. Recommend education of patient, family, and caregivers regarding the causes and risk factors of pressure ulcers. 3. Recommend caution when using compression stockings with lower extremity arterial disease. 4. Avoid thigh-high stockings when compression stockings are used. 5. Recommend minimizing friction and shear on skin during transfers. a. Avoid dragging patient when moving. b. Pad skin-to-skin contact. c. Lubricate or powder bed pans prior to placing under patient. d. Keep skin moisturized.	4. Outpatient risk assessment for pressure ulcers: a. Is the patient bed- or wheelchair-bound? b. Does the patient require assistance for transfers? c. Is the patient incontinent of urine or stool? d. Any history of pressure ulcers? e. Does the patient have a clinical condition placing him/her at risk for pressure ulcers? i. DM ii. Peripheral vascular disease iii. Stroke iv. Polytrauma v. Musculoskeletal disorders (fractures or contractures)	http://www.guidelines.gov/content.aspx?id=16004 http://www.guidelines.gov/content.aspx?id=23868

PRESSURE ULCERS					
Disease Prevention	Organization	Date	Population	Recommendations	Comments	Source
Pressure Ulcers (continued)				6. Recommend minimizing pressure on skin, especially areas with bony prominences. 　a. Turn patient side-to-side every 2 hours. 　b. Pad areas over bony prominences. 　c. Use heel protectors or place pillows under calves. 　d. Consider a bariatric bed for patients weighing over 300 lb. 7. Recommend managing moisture. 　a. Moisture barrier protectant on skin 　b. Frequent diaper changes 　c. Scheduled toileting 　d. Treat candidiasis if present 　e. Consider a rectal tube for stool incontinence with diarrhea 8. Recommend maintaining adequate nutrition and hydration. 9. Recommend keeping the head of the bed at or less than 30° elevation.	vi.　Spinal cord injury vii.　Guillain-Barré syndrome viii.　Multiple sclerosis ix.　CA x.　Chronic obstructive pulmonary disease xi.　Coronary heart failure xii.　Dementia xiii.　Preterm neonate xiv.　Cerebral palsy 　f. Does the patient appear malnourished? 　g. Is equipment in use that could contribute to ulcer development (eg, oxygen tubing, prosthetic devices, urinary catheter)?	

Disease Prevention	Organization	Date	Population	Recommendations	Comments	Source
Sexually Transmitted Infections (STIs)	AAFP USPSTF	2010 2008	Sexually active adolescents and high-risk adults	Recommend high-intensity behavioral counseling to prevent sexually transmitted infections for all sexually active adolescents and for adults at increased risk for STIs.		http://www.guidelines.gov/content.aspx?id=34005 http://www.uspreventiveservicestaskforce.org/uspstf/uspsstds.htm

SEXUALLY TRANSMITTED INFECTIONS

STROKE						

Disease Prevention	Organization	Date	Population	Recommendations	Comments	Source
Stroke[a]	AHA/ASA AHA/ASA	2011 2006	Treat all known CV risk factors HTN	Screen and treat BP to < 140/90 mm Hg. If HTN with diabetes or renal disease, treat to < 130/80 mm Hg.	1. Strokes and nonfatal strokes are reduced in diabetic patients by lower BP targets (< 130/80 mm Hg). In the absence of harm, this benefit appears to justify the lower BP goal.	*Stroke.* 2011;42:517–584 *Stroke.* 2006;37:1583–1633 *Chest.* 2004;126: 429S–456S
			Atrial fibrillation	1. Prioritize rate control; consider rhythm control if this is the first event, if it occurs in a young patient with minimal heart disease, or if symptomatic. 2. Rate control goal is < 110 beats per minute (bpm) in patient with stable ventricular function (ejection fraction [EF] > 40%).	2. Average stroke rate in patients with risk factors is about 5% per year. 3. Adjusted-dose warfarin and antiplatelet agents reduce absolute risk of stroke.	*J Am Coll Cardiol.* 2011;57(2):223–242

Disease Prevention[a]	Organization	Date	Population	Recommendations	Comments	Source
STROKE						
Stroke[a] (continued)				3. Antithrombotic therapy is required. Anticoagulation or antiplatelet therapy is determined by ACC/AHA or CHASD2 (nonvalvular atrial fibrillation) Guidelines. 4. Patients with prior CV accident, mitral stenosis, a mechanical valve, or two risk factors require warfarin.[b] 5. Patients with one risk factor may receive either ASA or warfarin.[c] 6. Therapeutic warfarin international normalized ratio (INR) goal is 2.5 (+/− 0.5). In high-risk patient unsuitable for anticoagulation, dual antiplatelet therapy (ASA plus clopidogrel) is reasonable. See Management algorithm, page 122–125, for pharmacologic and antithrombotic recommendations.	Absolute cerebrovascular accident (CVA) risk reduction with dual antiplatelet Rx is 0.8%/year balanced by increased bleeding risk 0.7% ACTIVE A/W Trials.	*J Am Coll Cardiol.* 2006;48:e149–e246 *Circulation.* 2006;114:e257–e354 *Lancet.* 2006;367: 1903–212 *European Heart J.* 2010;31:2369–2429

Disease Prevention[a]	Organization	Date	Population	Recommendations	Comments	Source
STROKE						
Stroke[a] (continued)			DM	1. Six-fold increase of stroke. 2. Short-term glycemic control does not lower macrovascular events. 3. HgA1c goal is < 7%. 4. BP goal is < 130/80 mm Hg. 5. Statin therapy. 6. Consider ACE inhibitor or ARB therapy for further stroke risk reduction.		*Stroke.* 2011;42:517–584
			Asymptomatic carotid artery stenosis (CAS)	1. No indication for general screening for CAS with ultrasonography. 2. Screen for other stroke risk factors and treat aggressively. 2. ASA unless contraindicated. 3. Prophylactic carotid endarterectomy (CEA) for patients with high-grade (> 70%) CAS by ultrasonography when performed by surgeons with low (< 3%) morbidity/mortality rates may be useful in selected cases depending on life expectancy, age, sex, and comorbidities. 4. However, recent studies have demonstrated that "best" medical therapy results in a stroke rate ≤ 1%.	Consensus statement on treatment of asymptomatic CAS is controversial.[d] Atherosclerotic intracranial stenosis: ASA should be used in preference to warfarin. Warfarin—significantly higher rates of adverse events with no benefit over ASA (*NEJM.* 2005 Mar 31;352(13): 1305–1316).	*Neurology.* 2005;65(6):794–801

				STROKE		
Disease Prevention[a]	Organization	Date	Population	Recommendations	Comments	Source
Stroke (continued)				5. The number needed to treat (NNT) in published trials to prevent one stroke in 1 year in this asymptomatic group varies from 84 up to 2000 (*JACC.* 2011;57;e16–e94).		*J Am Coll Cardiol.* 2011;57(20)
	ASA/ACCF/ AHA/AANN AANS/ACR CNS		Symptomatic CAS	Optimal timing for CEA is within 2 weeks post-transient ischemic attack. CEA plus medical therapy is effective within 6 months of symptom onset with > 70% CAS. Intense medical therapy alone is indicated if the occlusion is < 50%. Intensive medical therapy plus CEA may be considered with obstruction 50%–69%. Surgery should be *limited* to male patients with a low perioperative stroke/death rate (< 6%) and should have a life expectancy of at least 5 years. Carotid artery stenting is associated with increased nonfatal stroke frequency but this is offset by decreased risk of MI post CEA.		
			Cryptogenic CVA	Cryptogenic CVA with patent foramen ovale should receive ASA 81 mg/day	Consider referral to tertiary center for enrollment in randomized trial to determine optimal Rx	*J Am Coll Cardiol.* 2009;53(21): 2014–2018

Disease Prevention[a]	Organization	Date	Population	Recommendations	Comments	Source
Stroke[a] (continued)			Hyperlipidemia	See screening recommendations on page 40. See Cholesterol and Lipid Management (pages 133–135). Statin therapy post-CVA with intensive lipid-lowering goal after an ischemic stroke or transient ischemic attack with or without CHD reduced the risk of stroke and CV events (SPARCL Trial)		*Stroke.* 2011;42:517–584 *Stroke.* 2008;39: 1647–1652
			Sickle cell disease	Begin screening with transcranial Doppler (TCD) at age 2 years. Transfusion therapy is recommended for patients at high-stroke risk per TCD (high cerebral blood flow velocity > 200 cm/s). Frequency of screening not determined.	Transfusion therapy decreased stroke rates from 10% to < 1% per year (*NEJM.* 1998;339:5).	*Stroke.* 2006;37: 1583–1633
			Smoking	Strongly encourage patient and family to stop smoking. Provide counseling, nicotine replacement, and formal programs as available. Avoid environmental smoke.		

[a]Assess risk of stroke in all patients. See Appendix VIII and IX for risk assessment tool.

[b]High-risk factors for stroke in patients with atrial fibrillation include previous transient ischemic attack or stroke or embolus, HTN, poor left ventricular function, age > 75 years, DM, rheumatic mitral valve disease, and prosthetic heart valves.

[c]Moderate risk factors for stroke are ages 65–75 years, DM, and coronary artery disease with preserved left ventricular function.

[d]Net benefit of CEA requires treatment by surgical team with low perioperative risk of stroke/death (< 3%) and is enhanced for patients with symptomatic CAS when performed early (within 2 weeks of last ischemic event) (*Lancet.* 2004;363:915). CEA remains the standard of care, even in high-risk surgical patients (*Ann Surg.* 2005;241(2):356–363).

[e]*Chest.* 2008;133(suppl 6):546S–592S

SUDDEN INFANT DEATH SYNDROME

Disease Prevention	Organization	Date	Population	Recommendations	Comments	Source
Sudden Infant Death Syndrome (SIDS)	ICSI	2010	Newborns and infants	Counsel all parents to place their infants on their backs to sleep.	Stomach and side sleeping have been identified as major risk factors for SIDS.	http://www.icsi.org/ preventive_services_ for_children_ guideline_/ preventive_services_ for_children_and_ adolescents_2531.html

Disease Prevention	Organization	Date	Population	Recommendations	Comments	Source
TOBACCO USE						
Tobacco Use	AAFP	2010	Children and adolescents	Recommends counseling that avoidance of tobacco products is desirable.	The efficacy of counseling to prevent tobacco use in children and adolescents is uncertain.	http://www.guidelines.gov/content.aspx?id=34005

3
Disease Management

ADRENAL INCIDENTALOMAS						
Disease Management	Organization	Date	Population	Recommendations	Comments	Source
Adrenal Incidentalomas	AACE	2009	Adults	1. Recommends clinical, biochemical, and radiographic evaluation for evidence of hypercortisolism, aldosteronism, the presence of pheochromocytoma, or a malignant tumor. 2. Patients who will be managed expectantly should have reevaluation at 3–6 months and then annually for 1–2 years.	1. A 1-mg overnight dexamethasone suppression test can be used to screen for hypercortisolism. 2. Measure plasma fractionated metanephrines and normetanephrines to screen for pheochromocytoma. 3. Measure plasma renin activity and aldosterone concentration to assess for primary or secondary aldosteronism.	https://www.aace.com/sites/default/files/AdrenalGuidelines.pdf

ALCOHOL USE DISORDERS

Disease Management	Organization	Date	Population	Recommendations	Comments	Source

Alcohol Use Disorders	ICSI
	NICE
	VA/DoD
		2010
		2010
		2009
			Adults	1. For patients identified with alcohol dependence, schedule a referral to a substance use disorders specialist before the patient has left the office.
				2. Refer all patients with alcohol abstinence syndrome to a hospital for admission.
				3. Recommend prophylactic thiamine for all harmful alcohol use or alcohol dependence.
				4. Refer suitable patients with decompensated cirrhosis for consideration of liver transplantation once they have been sober from alcohol for ≥ 3 months.
				5. Recommend pancreatic enzyme supplementation for chronic alcoholic pancreatitis with steatorrhea and malnutrition.
					1. Assess all patients for a coexisting psychiatric disorder (dual diagnosis).
					2. Addiction-focused psychosocial intervention is helpful for patients with alcohol dependence.
					3. Consider adjunctive pharmacotherapy under close supervision for alcohol dependence:
					  a. Naltrexone
					  b. Acamprosate
						http://www.icsi.org/chronic_disease_risk_factors__primary_prevention_of__guideline_23506/chronic_disease_risk_factors__primary_prevention_of__guideline_23508.html
						http://www.guidelines.gov/content.aspx?id=23784
						http://www.guidelines.gov/content.aspx?id=15676

ANDROGEN DEFICIENCY SYNDROME

Disease Management	Organization	Date	Population	Recommendations	Comments	Source
Androgen Deficiency Syndrome	Endocrine Society	2010	Adult men	1. Recommends an AM total testosterone level for men with symptoms and signs of androgen deficiency.[a] 2. Measure a serum luteinizing hormone (LH) and follicular stimulating hormone (FSH) in all men with testosterone deficiency. 3. Recommends a dual-energy x-ray absorptiometry scan for all men with testosterone deficiency. 4. Testosterone therapy indicated for androgen deficiency syndromes unless contraindications exist.[b]	1. Testosterone therapy options: a. Testosterone enanthate or cypionate 150–200 mg IM every 2 weeks b. Testosterone patch 5–10 mg qhs c. 1% testosterone gel 5–10 gm daily d. Testosterone 30 mg to buccal mucosa q12h	http://www.guidelines.gov/content.aspx?id=16326

[a]Lethargy, easy fatigue, lack of stamina or endurance, reduced libido, mood changes, irritability, and loss of libido and motivation
[b]Breast CA, prostate CA, hematocrit > 50%, untreated severe obstructive sleep apnea, severe obstructive urinary symptoms, or uncontrolled heart failure

	ANXIETY				
Disease Management	**Organization**	**Date**	**Population**	**Recommendations**	**Comments**	**Source**

Disease Management	**Organization**	**Date**	**Population**	**Recommendations**	**Comments**	**Source**
Anxiety	NICE	2011	Adults	1. Recommends cognitive behavioral therapy for generalized anxiety disorder (GAD). 2. Recommends sertraline if drug treatment is needed. 3. If sertraline is ineffective, recommend a different selective serotonin reuptake inhibitor (SSRI) or (SNRI). 4. Avoid long-term benzodiazepine use or antipsychotic therapy for GAD.		http://www.nice.org.uk/nicemedia/live/13314/52599/52599.pdf

ASTHMA

Disease Management	Organization	Date	Population	Recommendations	Comments	Source

Asthma	VA/DoD
	GINA
		2009
		2009
			Children aged > 5 years, adolescents, and adults	1. Recommend classification of asthma by level of control.
				2. Recommend a chest radiograph at the initial visit to exclude alternative diagnoses.
				3. Recommend assessing for tobacco use and strongly advise smokers to quit.
				4. Recommend spirometry with bronchodilators to determine the severity of airflow limitation and its reversibility.
				  a. Repeat spirometry at least every 1–2 years for asthma monitoring.
				5. Consider allergy testing for history of atopy, rhinitis, rhinorrhea, and seasonal variation or specific extrinsic triggers.
				6. Recommend an asthma action plan based on peak expiratory flow (PEF) monitoring for all patients.
					1. Controlled asthma defined by:
					  a. Daytime symptoms $\leq 2\times$/week
					  b. No limitations of daily activities
					  c. No nocturnal symptoms
					  d. Need for reliever medicines $\leq 2\times$/week
					  e. Normal or near-normal lung function
					  f. No exacerbations
					2. Partially controlled asthma if:
					  a. Daytime symptoms $> 2\times$/week
					  b. Any limitations of daily activities or any nocturnal symptoms
					  c. Need for reliever medicines $> 2\times$/week
					  d. $< 80\%$ predicted PEF or forced expiratory volume at 1 second (FEV_1)
					  e. Any exacerbations
					3. Uncontrolled asthma if there are ≥ 3 features of partially controlled asthma in any week.
						http://www.guidelines.gov/content.aspx?id=15706
						
						http://www.guidelines.gov/content.aspx?id=15556

					ASTHMA	
Disease Management	Organization	Date	Population	Recommendations	Comments	Source
Asthma (continued)				7. Recommend allergen and environmental trigger avoidance. 8. Physicians should help educate patients, assist them in self-management, create an asthma action plan, and regularly monitor asthma control. 9. Recommend systemic glucocorticoids for asthma exacerbations. 10. Develop a chronic medication regimen for patients adjusted based on their asthma action plan.	4. Recommend an inhaled corticosteroid for partially controlled or uncontrolled asthma. 5. Add a long-acting beta-agonist or leukotriene inhibitor for incomplete control with inhaled corticosteroid alone. 6. Short-acting beta-agonists should be used as needed for relief of acute asthma symptoms or 20 minutes prior to planned exertion in exercise-induced asthma.	

ATRIAL FIBRILLATION: MANAGEMENT OVERVIEW
HEART RATE CONTROL
Source: **AMERICAN COLLEGE OF CARDIOLOGY/AMERICAN HEART**
ASSOCIATION/EUROPEAN SOCIETY OF CARDIOLOGY

Classification of Atrial Fibrillation (AF)
Paroxysmal = Self-terminating
Recurrent = Two or more episodes
Persistent = Lasts > 7 days
Silent = Detected by monitor
Lone = Unassociated with/heart disease

Initiate Treatment
Slow the ventricular rate
Establish anticoagulation
Consider rhythm conversion

Determine Etiology
Hypertension/coronary artery disease
Cardiomyopathy/heart valve disease
Pulmonary disease/hyperthyroidism
Sinus node disease

- Expected ventricular heart rate (HR) in untreated AF is between 110–210 beats per minute (bpm).
  If HR < 110 bpm, atrioventricular (AV) node disease present; If HR > 220 bpm, preexcitation syndrome (WPW) present
- Initial choice of AV nodal slowing agent to be determined by:
  Ventricular rate/Blood pressure (BP)
  Presence of heart failure (HF) or asthma
  Associated cardiovascular (CV) symptoms (chest pain/shortness of breath [SOB])

Usual Rx
Beta-blocker
Diltiazem
Verapamil
Digoxin

HF or Low BP
Digoxin
Amiodarone

Preexcitation Syndrome
Amiodarone
Propafenone

- **Urgent electrical cardioversion** should be considered if hemodynamic instability or persistent symptoms of ischemia, HF, or if inadequate HR control with optimal medications.
- **Resting HR goal and exercise HR goal** should be determined. Holter monitor best measures the adequacy of the chronic HR control. In acute medical conditions when the patient has noncardiac illness (ie, pneumonia), the resting HR may be allowed to increase to simulate physiologic demands (mimic HR if sinus rhythm was present).

Lenient Target
Resting HR < 110 bpm
May be considered in
younger or patients
without CV symptoms.

Aggressive Target
Resting HR < 80 bpm/exercise
HR < 110 bpm treatment choice if
decreased ejection fraction (EF) < 40%
if symptoms at higher rates.

ATRIAL FIBRILLATION: MANAGEMENT OVERVIEW
HEART RATE CONTROL (CONTINUED)
Source: AMERICAN COLLEGE OF CARDIOLOGY/AMERICAN HEART ASSOCIATION/EUROPEAN SOCIETY OF CARDIOLOGY

(ESC recommends HR target < 110 bpm; CCS recommends < 100 bpm; ACCF/AHA/HRS recommends HR target < 110 bpm only if EF > 40%)

- **Consider AV nodal ablation** when chronic HR target cannot be achieved with maximal medical therapy with placement of ventricular pacemaker.

ESC, European Society of Cardiology; CCS, Canadian CV Society; ACCF, American College of Cardiology Foundation; AHA, American Heart Association; HRS, Heart Rhythm Society

Sources: ACC/AHA/ESC 2006 Guidelines. *J Am Coll Cardiol.* 2006;48:858–906. ACCF/AHA/HRS. *J Am Coll Cardiol.* 2011;57:223–242. ACC/AHA. *Circulation.* 2008;117:1101–1120. ESC 2010 Guidelines. *Euro Heart J.* 2010;31:2369–2429. Comparing the 2010 NA and European AF Guidelines. *Canadian J Cardiol.* 2011;27:7–13.

ATRIAL FIBRILLATION: MANAGEMENT, ANTITHROMBOTIC THERAPY
Source: AMERICAN COLLEGE OF CARDIOLOGY/AMERICAN HEART ASSOCIATION/EUROPEAN SOCIETY OF CARDIOLOGY

Antithrombotic selection is based on stroke risk versus bleeding risk.

- Antithrombotic therapy is recommended in all atrial fibrillation (AF) or atrial flutter patients except those with LONE AF or contraindications.
- **Moderate risk factors (RF)** for embolization: Aged > 75 years, hypertension (HTN), heart failure (HF), ejection fraction (EF) ≤ 35%, diabetes mellitus (DM).
- **High risk factors (RF)** for embolization: Mechanical heart valve, mitral stenosis, prior embolization (cardiovascular accident [CVA], transient ischemic attack [TIA], systemic embolism).

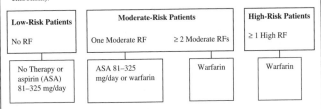

Low-Risk Patients	Moderate-Risk Patients		High-Risk Patients
No RF	One Moderate RF	≥ 2 Moderate RFs	≥ 1 High RF
No Therapy or aspirin (ASA) 81–325 mg/day	ASA 81–325 mg/day or warfarin	Warfarin	Warfarin

- Warfarin international normalized ratio (INR) goal 2.5 (+/– 0.5) in all patients unless mechanical valve present, in which case INR goal 3 (+/– 0.5).
- INR should be determined weekly during initiation of therapy and then monthly when stable.
- Warfarin reduces the relative risk (RR) of thromboembolism versus placebo by 67%. ASA reduces RR of thromboembolism versus placebo by 19%. Warfarin reduces the RR of thromboembolism versus ASA by 39%. Warfarin reduced the RR over ASA plus clopidogrel by 42%.
- The daily recommended dose of dietary vitamin K is 65–80 mcg/day. If unexplained variations noted in the INR, increase vitamin K dosage to 100–200 mcg daily. www.nal. usda.gov/fnic/foodcomp/Data/Other/IFT2002_VitK.pdf)
- Warfarin resistance should be considered if INR < 2 with a warfarin dose > 15 mg daily. Should exclude dietary and medication interference or patient nonadherence. Check Factor II and Factor X activity. If these factors are < 40% of normal, the INR is inaccurate and the patient is therapeutically anticoagulated. If these factors are > 40%, check warfarin level.
- The ESC recommends the **CHA₂DS₂-VASc score**, a new risk factor-based approach to be used in nonvalvular AF (high-risk score > 3). It goes beyond the **CHADS₂ score** by adjusting the importance of age and adding factors of female gender and vascular disease (coronary artery disease [CAD] or peripheral arterial disease [PAD]). The ACC/AHA and the Canadian Cardiovascular Society recommend the CHADS₂ score (high-risk score ≥ 2). Comparative efficacy to the present system awaits further evaluation.
- **HAS-BLED bleeding risk score** is utilized to determine the risk of bleeding while taking warfarin. Risk factors include: **H**ypertension (≥ 160 mm Hg); **A**bnormal kidney function (creatinine ≥ 2, chronic dialysis, transplant); **A**bnormal liver function (cirrhosis, bilirubin > 2×, aspartate transaminase [AST] > 3×); **S**troke; **B**leeding history or anemia; **L**abile INR (< 60% within range); **E**lderly (aged ≥ 65 years); **D**rugs/alcohol (use of ASA or clopidogrel) or alcohol (8 or more alcoholic drinks/week). Each risk factor is assigned 1 point for a total of 9 points. A high risk of bleeding is considered ≥ 3 points.

ATRIAL FIBRILLATION: MANAGEMENT, ANTITHROMBOTIC THERAPY (CONTINUED)
Source: AMERICAN COLLEGE OF CARDIOLOGY/AMERICAN HEART ASSOCIATION/EUROPEAN SOCIETY OF CARDIOLOGY

- In high-risk patients unable to take warfarin, may consider dual antiplatelet therapy (ASA + clopidogrel). (*Lancet.* 2006;367:1903–1912) The absolute CVA risk reduction was 0.8%, which was offset by a 0.7% increased risk of bleeding.
- Dabigatran (Pradaxa @ 150 mg bid) maybe a useful alternative to warfarin in high-risk patients who **do not have** a mechanical heart valve, significant valve disease, renal failure (creatinine clearance < 15 mL/min), or advanced liver disease (impaired baseline clotting). Dabigatran required twice-daily dosing, has a higher risk of nonhemorrhagic complications than does warfarin, a higher rate of drug discontinuation, and no difference in mortality. Consider use in patients with labile INR measurements on warfarin or in patients with a high risk of bleeding. (*J Am Coll Cardiol.* 2011;57:1330–1337)

ESC, European Society of Cardiology; ACC, American College of Cardiology; AHA, American Heart Association; CCS, Canadian Cardiovascular Society

Sources: ACC/AHA/ESC 2006 Guidelines. *J Am Coll Cardiol.* 2006;48:858–906. ACCF/AHA/HRS. *J Am Coll Cardiol.* 2011;57:223–242. ACC/AHA. *Circulation.* 2008;117:1101–1120. ESC Guidelines. 2010;31:2369–2429. ACCF/AHA/HRS Focus Update. *J Am Coll Cardiol.* 2011;57(2):223–242. Comparing the 2010 NA and European AF Guidelines. *Can J Cardiol.* 2011;27:7–13.

ANTITHROMBOTIC STRATEGIES FOLLOWING CORONARY ARTERY STENTING IN PATIENTS WITH AF AT MODERATE TO HIGH THROMBO-EMBOLIC RISK (IN WHOM ORAL ANTICOAGULATION THERAPY IS REQUIRED)

Haemorrhagic Risk	Clinical Setting	Stent Implanted	Anticoagulation Regimen
Low or intermediate (e.g. HAS-BLED score 0–2)	Elective	Bare-metal	1 month: triple therapy of VKA (INR 2.0–2.5) + aspirin ≤100 mg/day + clopidogrel 75 mg/day Up to 12th month: combination of VKA (INR 2.0–2.5) + clopidogrel 75 mg/day[b] (or aspirin 100 mg/day) Lifelong: VKA (INR 2.0–3.0) alone
	Elective	Drug-eluting	3 (-olimus[a] group) to 6 (paclitaxel) months: triple therapy of VKA (INR 2.0–2.5) + aspirin ≤100 mg/day + clopidogrel 75 mg/day Up to 12th month: combination of VKA (INR 2.0–2.5) + clopidogrel 75 mg/day[b] (or aspirin 100 mg/day) Lifelong: VKA (INR 2.0–3.0) alone
	ACS	Bare-metal/drug-eluting	6 months: triple therapy of VKA (INR 2.0–2.5) + aspirin ≤100 mg/day + clopidogrel 75 mg/day Up to 12th month: combination of VKA (INR 2.0–2.5) + clopidogrel 75 mg/day[b] (or aspirin 100 mg/day) Lifelong: VKA (INR 2.0–3.0) alone
High (e.g. HAS-BLED score ≥3)	Elective	Bare-metal[c]	2–4 weeks: triple therapy of VKA (INR 2.0–2.5) + aspirin ≤100 mg/day + clopidogrel 75 mg/day Lifelong: VKA (INR 2.0–3.0) alone
	ACS	Bare-metal[c]	4 weeks: triple therapy of VKA (INR 2.0–2.5) + aspirin ≤100 mg/day + clopidogrel 75 mg/day Up to 12th month: combination of VKA (INR 2.0–2.5) + clopidogrel 75 mg/day[b] (or aspirin 100 mg/day) Lifelong: VKA (INR 2.0–3.0) alone

ACS, acute coronary syndrome; AF, atrial fibrillation; INR, international normalized ratio; VKA, vitamin K antagonist.

Gastric protection with a proton pump inhibitor (PPI) should be considered where necessary.

[a]Sirolimus, everolimus, and tacrolimus.

[b]Combination of VKA (INR 2.0–3.0)+aspirin ≤100 mg/day (with PPI, if indicated) may be considered as an alternative.

[c]Drug-eluting stents should be avoided as far as possible, but, if used, consideration of more prolonged (3–6 months) triple antithrombotic therapy is necessary.

Adapted from Lip et al.

ATRIAL FIBRILLATION: MANAGEMENT, RHYTHM CONTROL DRUG NONPHARMACOLOGIC THERAPY
Source: AMERICAN COLLEGE OF CARDIOLOGY/AMERICAN HEART ASSOCIATION/EUROPEAN SOCIETY OF CARDIOLOGY

- **AFFIRM, RACE, PIAF, and STAF Trials** found **no difference** in quality of life between rate and rhythm control in atrial fibrillation (AF). The AFFIRM and RACE Trials demonstrated no difference in stroke rate or mortality between rate and rhythm control in AF.

Favors Rate Control	versus	**Favors Rhythm Control**
Asymptomatic in AF		Continued symptoms in AF
Older patients		Younger patients
Advanced heart disease		LONE or minimal heart disease
Comorbid conditions		Few comorbid conditions
Persistent AF		Recent onset/paroxysmal AF

- **Rhythm Control**
  Fifty percent of patients with new-onset AF spontaneously convert to sinus in 48 hours.
- **2, 3, 4 Cardioversion Rule**
  - New-onset AF < **2 days** in duration—may be considered for acute electrical or drug conversion to sinus rhythm while on heparin.
  - Onset of AF > **2 days** or of unknown duration—require either **3 weeks** of therapeutic oral anticoagulation (international normalized ratio [INR] 2–3) or a negative transesophageal echocardiogram (TEE) to exclude clot before conversion while on heparin should be considered.
  - In either approach to conversion, oral anticoagulation (OAC) must be continued at least **4 weeks** postconversion due to the possibility of delayed return of atrial contraction and clot release. In high-risk patients, lifelong OAC should be considered.

- **Pharmacologic Approach:** Choice based on etiology of heart disease
  - LONE: flecainide, propafenone, sotalol, amiodarone
  - HTN: flecainide, propafenone, sotalol, amiodarone (LVH)
  - CAD: sotalol, dofetilide, amiodarone
  - HF: amiodarone, dofetilide

(LONE; HTN, hypertension; CAD, coronary artery disease; HF, heart failure; LVH, left ventricular hypertrophy)
- **Nonpharmacologic Approach:**
- AF catheter ablation/MAZE procedure (open surgical approach)
  Consider if antiarrhythmic drug therapy fails or if AF coexists with preexcitation pathway. AF ablation is more effective in younger patients with paroxysmal AF; catheter ablation maintains sinus rhythm ~ 80% as opposed to ~ 40% with drugs @ 5 years.
  May require repeat procedures (average 1.8 procedures).
  Long-term anticoagulation should be continued even after successful ablation in patients at high risk for thromboembolism. In low-embolic-risk patients, warfarin may be converted to aspirin (ASA) therapy after 3 months. (*J Am Coll Cardiol.* 2010;55:735–743)
- Consider MAZE procedure if performing open heart surgery for other reasons or if vascular or cardiac anatomy prevents the less-invasive catheter approach.
- Consider implantable atrial defibrillators: least commonly used treatment.

ATRIAL FIBRILLATION: MANAGEMENT, RHYTHM CONTROL DRUG/NONPHARMACOLOGIC THERAPY (CONTINUED)
Source: AMERICAN COLLEGE OF CARDIOLOGY/AMERICAN HEART ASSOCIATION/EUROPEAN SOCIETY OF CARDIOLOGY

- **Prevention of Atrial Remodeling**
  - Calcium channel blockers
  - Angiotensin-converting enzyme (ACE) inhibitors
  - Angiotensin receptor blocker (ARB) agents
  - Statins

Sources: ACC/AHA/ESC 2006 Guidelines. *J Am Coll Cardiol.* 2006;48:858–906. ACCF/AHA/HRS. *J Am Coll Cardiol.* 2011;57:223–242. ACC/AHA. *Circulation.* 2008;117:1101–1120. ESC 2010 Guidelines. *Euro Heart J.* 2010;31:2369–2429. *Circulation.* 2009;119:606–618.

BENIGN PROSTATIC HYPERPLASIA (BPH)						
Disease Management	Organization	Date	Population	Recommendations	Comments	Source

Benign Prostatic Hyperplasia (BPH)	AUA	2010	Adult men	1. Routine measurement of serum creatinine is not indicated in men with BPH.
				2. Do not recommend dietary supplements or phytotherapeutic agents for lower urinary tract symptoms (LUTS) management.
				3. Patients with LUTS with no signs of bladder outlet obstruction by flow study should be treated for detrusor overactivity.
				  a. Alter fluid intake
				  b. Behavioral modification
				  c. Anticholinergic medications
				4. Options for moderate-severe LUTS from BPH
				(AUA symptom index score ≥ 8)
				  a. Watchful waiting
				  b. Medical therapies
				    i. Alpha-blockers[a]
				    ii. 5-alpha reductase inhibitors[b]
				    iii. Anticholinergic agents
				    iv. Combination therapy
				  c. Transurethral needle ablation
				  d. Transurethral microwave thermotherapy
					1. Combination therapy with alpha-blocker and 5-alpha reductase inhibitor is effective for moderate-severe LUTS with significant prostate enlargement.
					2. Men with planned cataract surgery should have cataract surgery before initiating alpha-blockers.
					3. 5-alpha reductase inhibitors should not be used for men with LUTS from BPH without prostate enlargement.
					4. Anticholinergic agents are appropriate for LUTS that are primarily irritative symptoms and patient does not have an elevated post-void residual (> 250 mL).
					5. The choice of surgical method should be based on the patient's presentation, anatomy, surgeon's experience, and patient's preference.
						http://www.guidelines.gov/content.aspx?id=25635&search=aua+2010+bph

	BENIGN PROSTATIC HYPERPLASIA (BPH)					
Disease Management	Organization	Date	Population	Recommendations	Comments	Source
Benign Prostatic Hyperplasia (BPH) (continued)				e. Transurethral laser ablation or enucleation of the prostate f. Transurethral incision of the prostate g. Transurethral vaporization of the prostate h. Transurethral resection of the prostate i. Laser resection of the prostate j. Photoselective vaporization of the prostate k. Prostatectomy 5. Surgery is recommended for BPH causing renal insufficiency, recurrent urinary tract infections (UTIs), bladder stones, gross hematuria, or refractory LUTS.		

[a]Alpha-blockers: alfuzosin, doxazosin, tamsulosin, and terazosin. All have equal clinical effectiveness.
[b]5-alpha reductase inhibitors: dutasteride and finasteride.

BRONCHITIS, ACUTE

Disease Management	Organization	Date	Population	Recommendations	Comments	Source
Bronchitis, Acute	Michigan Quality Improvement Consortium	2010	Adults aged ≥ 18 years	1. Recommends against a chest x-ray if all the following are present: a. Heart rate < 100 bpm b. Respiratory rate < 24 breaths/min c. Temperature < 38°C 2. Recommends against antibiotics	1. Consider antitussive agents for short-term relief of coughing. 2. Beta$_2$-agonists or mucolytic agents should not be used routinely to alleviate cough.	http://www.guidelines.gov/content.aspx?id=16317

CA SURVIVORSHIP

CA SURVIVORSHIP: LATE EFFECTS OF CA TREATMENTS

CA or CA Treatment History	Late Effect Type	Periodic Evaluation
Any CA experience	Psychosocial disorders[b]	
Any chemotherapy	Oral and dental abnormalities	Dental exam and cleaning (every 6 months)
Chemotherapy (alkylating agents)[a]	Gonadal dysfunction	Pubertal assessment (yearly) in adults if symptoms of hypogonadism present
	Hematologic disorders[c]	History, exam for bleeding disorder; CBC/differential (yearly)
	Ocular toxicity[d]	Visual acuity, funduscopic exam, evaluation by ophthalmologist (if radiation) (yearly if ocular tumors, total body irradiation (TBI), or ≥30 Gy; otherwise, every 3 years)
	Pulmonary toxicity[e]	CXR, PFTs (at entry into long-term follow-up, then as clinically indicated)
	Renal toxicity[f]	Blood pressure (yearly); electrolytes, BUN, creatinine, Ca^{++}, Mg^{++}, PO_4^-, urinalysis (at entry into long-term follow-up, then clinically as indicated)
	Urinary tract toxicity[g]	
Chemotherapy (anthracycline antibiotics)[a]	Cardiac toxicity[h]	ECHO or MUGA; EKG at entry into long-term follow-up, periodic thereafter (↑ frequency if chest radiation); fasting glucose, lipid panel (every 3–5 years)
	Hematologic disorders[c]	See "Chemotherapy (alkylating agents)"
Chemotherapy anti-tumor antibiotics (mitomycin C)[f]	Pulmonary toxicity[e]	CXR and PFTs end of exposure then reevaluation as clinically indicated
Chemotherapy-antimetabolites (cytarabine, high-dose IV; MTX, high-dose intravenous IV; intrathecal IT)	Clinical leukoencephalopathy[i]	Full neurologic examination (yearly)
	Neurocognitive deficits	Neuropsychological evaluation (at entry into long-term follow-up, then as clinically indicated)
Chemotherapy (epipodophyllotoxins)[a]	Hematologic disorders (causes acute myelocytic leukemia [AML] with specific 11q 23 translocation)[c]	See "Chemotherapy (alkylating agents)"

CA SURVIVORSHIP		
CA SURVIVORSHIP: LATE EFFECTS OF CA TREATMENTS (CONTINUED)		
CA or CA Treatment History	**Late Effect Type**	**Periodic Evaluation**
Chemotherapy (heavy metals)[a]	Dyslipidemia/hypertension and increased risk of cardiovascular disease	Fasting lipid panel at entry
	Gonadal dysfunction	See "Chemotherapy (alkylating agents)"
	Hematologic disorders[c]	See "Chemotherapy (alkylating agents)"
	Ototoxicity[j]	Complete pure tone audiogram or brainstem auditory-evoked response (yearly × 5 years, then every 5 years)
	Peripheral sensory neuropathy	Examination yearly for 2–3 years
	Renal toxicity[f]	See "Chemotherapy (alkylating agents)"
Chemotherapy—microtubular inhibitors (taxanes, ixabepilone, eribulin)	Peripheral neuropathy	Examination yearly for 2–3 years
Chemotherapy (nonclassical alkylators)[a]	Gonadal dysfunction	See "Chemotherapy (alkylating agents)"
	Hematologic disorders[c]	
Chemotherapy (plant alkaloids)[a]	Peripheral sensory neuropathy	See "Chemotherapy (heavy metals)"
	Raynaud's phenomenon	Yearly history/examination
Chemotherapy (purine agonists)[a]	Hematologic disorders[c]	See "Chemotherapy (alkylating agents)"
	Reduction in CD4 count	Monitor for infection
Corticosteroids (dexamethasone, prednisone)	Ocular toxicity[d]	Musculoskeletal examination (yearly)
	Avascular osteonecrosis	
	Osteopenia/osteoporosis	

	CA SURVIVORSHIP	
CA SURVIVORSHIP: LATE EFFECTS OF CA TREATMENTS (CONTINUED)		
CA or CA Treatment History	**Late Effect Type**	**Periodic Evaluation**
Targeted biological therapy —Trastuzumab (anti-Her-2) —Rituximab (antilymphocyte CD20)	Cardiac dysfunction is usually reversible Reduction in immunoglobulins and increased risk of infection	Monitor 2D echo for ejection fraction every 3 months during therapy and as needed for symptoms Monitor quantitative immunoglobulins if increased frequency of infection
Hematopoietic cell (bone marrow) transplant	Hematologic disorders[c] Oncologic disorders[k] Avascular osteonecrosis Osteopenia/osteoporosis	See "Chemotherapy (alkylating agents)"[a] Inspection/exam targeted to irradiation fields (yearly) See "Corticosteroids (dexamethasone, prednisone)"[a] See "Chemotherapy (antimetabolites)"[a]
Chemotherapy drugs with minimal long-term toxicity effects Topoisomerase I inhibitors (Camptosar, topotecan) Antibiotics (actinomycin) Antimetabolites (L-asparaginase, 5 FU, capecitabine, gemcitabine, 6 mercaptopurine)	Mild reduction in bone marrow reserve	Routine monitoring for end-organ dysfunction is not indicated
Radiation therapy (field- and dose-dependent)	Cardiac toxicity[b] Central adrenal insufficiency (pediatric brain tumors) Cerebrovascular complications[l] Chronic sinusitis Functional asplenia	See "Chemotherapy (alkylating agents)"[a] 8 AM serum cortisol (yearly × 15 years, and as clinically indicated) Neurologic exam (yearly) Head/neck exam (yearly) Blood culture when temperature ≥ 101°F, rapid institution of empiric antibiotics

CA SURVIVORSHIP

CA SURVIVORSHIP: LATE EFFECTS OF CA TREATMENTS (CONTINUED)

CA or CA Treatment History	Late Effect Type	Periodic Evaluation
	Gonadal dysfunction	See "Chemotherapy (alkylating agents)"
	Growth hormone deficiency (children and adolescents)	Height, weight, BMI (every 6 months until growth completed, then yearly); Tanner staging (every 6 months until sexually mature)
	Hyperthyroidism	TSH, free T_4 (yearly)
	Hyperprolactinemia	Prolactin level (as clinically indicated)
	Hypothyroidism	TSH, free T_4
	Neurocognitive deficits	See "Chemotherapy (cytarabine)"
	Ocular toxicity[d]	See "Chemotherapy (alkylating agents)"
	Oncologic disorders[g]	See "Hematopoietic cell (bone marrow) transplant"
	Oral and dental abnormalities	See "Any chemotherapy"
	Ototoxicity[j]	See "Chemotherapy (heavy metals)"
	Overweight/obesity/metabolic syndrome	Fasting glucose, fasting serum insulin, fasting lipid profile (every 2 years if overweight or obese; every 5 years if normal weight)
	Pulmonary toxicity[e]	See "Chemotherapy (alkylating agents)"
	Renal toxicity[f]	See "Chemotherapy (alkylating agents)"
	Urinary tract toxicity[g]	See "Chemotherapy (alkylating agents)"

CBC, complete blood count; TBI, total body irradiation; MTX, methotrexate; CXR, chest x-ray; PFTs, pulmonary function tests; BUN, blood urea nitrogen; ECHO, echocardiogram; MUGA, multiple-gated acquisition scan; EKG, electrocardiogram; IV, intravenous; IT, intrathecal; AML, acute myelocytic leukemia; BMI, body mass index; TSH, thyroid stimulating hormone

[a]Chemotherapeutic agents, by mechanism of action:
- Alkylating agents: busulfan, carmustine (BCNU), chlorambucil, cyclophosphamide, ifosfamide, lomustine (CCNU), mechlorethamine, melphalan, procarbazine, thiotepa
- Antimetabolites: MTX, cytosine arabinoside, gemcitabine
- Heavy metals: carboplatin, cisplatin, oxaliplatin
- Nonclassical alkylators: dacarbazine (DTIC), temozolomide
- Anthracycline antibiotics: daunorubicin, doxorubicin, epirubicin, idarubicin, mitoxantrone
- Antitumor antibiotics: bleomycin, mitomycin C
- Plant alkaloids: vinblastine, vincristine, vinorelbine
- Purine agonists: fludarabine, pentostatin, cladribine
- Microtubular inhibitors: docetaxel, paclitaxel, cabazitaxel, ixabepilone
- Epipodophyllotoxins: etoposide (VP16), teniposide (VM26)

CA SURVIVORSHIP

CA SURVIVORSHIP: LATE EFFECTS OF CA TREATMENTS (CONTINUED)

[b]Psychosocial disorders: mental health disorders, risky behaviors, psychosocial disability due to pain, fatigue, limitations in healthcare/insurance access, "chemo brain" syndrome.

[c]Hematologic disorders: acute myeloid leukemia, myelodysplasia

[d]Ocular toxicity: cataracts, orbital hypoplasia, lacrimal duct atrophy, xerophthalmia, keratitis, telangiectasias, retinopathy, optic chiasm neuropathy, endophthalmos, chronic painful eye, maculopathy, glaucoma

[e]Pulmonary toxicity: pulmonary fibrosis, interstitial pneumonitis, restrictive lung disease, obstructive lung disease. Increased sensitivity to oxygen toxicity—keep $FiO_2 \leq 28\%$ in patients with bleomycin exposure

[f]Renal toxicity: glomerular and tubular renal insufficiency, hypertension, hemolytic uremic syndrome

[g]Urinary tract toxicity: hemorrhagic cystitis, bladder fibrosis, dysfunctional voiding, vesicoureteral reflux, hydronephrosis, bladder malignancy

[h]Cardiac toxicity: cardiomyopathy, arrhythmias, left ventricular dysfunction, congestive heart failure, pericardial fibrosis, pericarditis, valvular disease, myocardial infarction, atherosclerotic heart disease

[i]Clinical leukoencephalopathy: spasticity, ataxia, dysarthria, dysphagia, hemiparesis, seizures

[j]Ototoxicity: sensorineural hearing loss, tinnitus, vertigo, tympanosclerosis, otosclerosis, eustachian tube dysfunction, conductive hearing loss

[k]Oncologic disorders: secondary benign or malignant neoplasm, especially breast CA after mantle radiation, gastrointestinal malignancy after para-aortic radiation for seminoma of the testis

[l]Cerebrovascular complications: stroke, and occlusive cerebral vasculopathy

Note: Guidelines for surveillance and monitoring for late effects after treatment for adult CAs available via the National Comprehensive Cancer Network, Inc. (NCCN). (http://www.nccn.org/professionals/physician_gls)

Source: Long-Term Follow-Up Guidelines for Survivors of Childhood, Adolescent, and Young Adult Cancers. Children's Oncology Group, Version 2.0, March 2006. (For full guidelines and references, see http://www.survivorshipguidelines.org)

See also: *NEJM.* 2006;355:1722–1782, *J Clin Onc.* 2007;25:3991–4008.

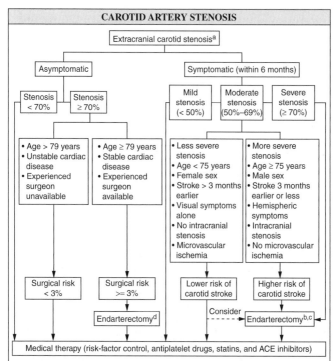

CAROTID ARTERY STENOSIS

Extracranial carotid stenosis[a]

Asymptomatic
- Stenosis < 70%
- Stenosis ≥ 70%

Symptomatic (within 6 months)
- Mild stenosis (< 50%)
- Moderate stenosis (50%–69%)
- Severe stenosis (≥ 70%)

Stenosis < 70%:
- Age > 79 years
- Unstable cardiac disease
- Experienced surgeon unavailable

→ Surgical risk < 3%

Stenosis ≥ 70%:
- Age ≥ 79 years
- Stable cardiac disease
- Experienced surgeon available

→ Surgical risk >= 3% → Endarterectomy[d]

Mild / Moderate (Less severe):
- Less severe stenosis
- Age < 75 years
- Female sex
- Stroke > 3 months earlier
- Visual symptoms alone
- No intracranial stenosis
- Microvascular ischemia

→ Lower risk of carotid stroke → Consider - - - →

Severe (More severe):
- More severe stenosis
- Age ≥ 75 years
- Male sex
- Stroke 3 months earlier or less
- Hemispheric symptoms
- Intracranial stenosis
- No microvascular ischemia

→ Higher risk of carotid stroke → Endarterectomy[b,c]

Medical therapy (risk-factor control, antiplatelet drugs, statins, and ACE inhibitors)

[a]Critical stenosis defined as > 70% by noninvasive imaging or > 50% by catheter angiography.

[b]Carotid endarterectomy (CEA) in symptomatic patients with average or low surgical risk should generally be reserved for patients with > 5 years' expectancy, and perioperative stroke/death rate < 6%. When CEA is indicated, it should be performed within 2 weeks after an ischemic central nervous system (CNS) event.

[c]Carotid artery stenting (CAS) with an embolic protection device is an alternative to CEA in symptomatic patients with average or low surgical risk when > 70% obstruction is present, and the periprocedural stroke and mortality rate is < 6%. CAS may be chosen over CEA if the neck anatomy is surgically unfavorable or if comorbid conditions make CEA a very high risk.

[d]The annual rate of stroke in asymptomatic patients treated with optimal medical therapy for carotid artery stenosis has decreased to < 1%. Therefore the benefit of CEA or CAS remains controversial in asymptomatic patients. (*Stroke*. 2010;41:975–979)

Source: AHA/ASA 2005 Guidelines. *Circulation*. 2006;113:e872. *Stroke*. 2006;37:577. ASA/ACCF/AHA/AANN/AANS/ACR/ASNR/CNS/SAIP/SCAI/SIR/SNIS/SVM/SVS 2011 Guidelines. *J Am Coll Cardiol*. 2011;57:e16–e94. ACCF/SCAI/SVMB/SIR/ASITN 2007 Consensus. *J Am Coll Cardiol*. 2007;49(1):126–168.

CATARACT IN ADULTS: EVALUATION & MANAGEMENT ALGORITHM
Source: AAO & AOA

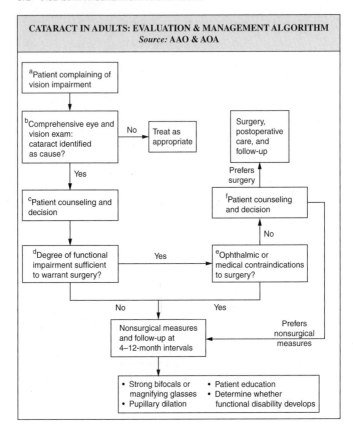

Notes:

[a]Begin evaluation only when patients complain of a vision problem or impairment. Identifying impairment in visual function during routine history and physical exam constitutes sound medical practice.

[b]Essential elements of the comprehensive eye and vision exam:

- *Patient history:* Consider cataract if: acute or gradual onset of vision loss; vision problems under special conditions (eg, low contrast, glare); difficulties performing various visual tasks.

  Ask about: refractive history, previous ocular disease, amblyopia, eye surgery, trauma, general health history, medications, and allergies. It is critical to describe the actual impact of the cataract on the person's function and quality of life. There are several instruments available for assessing functional impairment related to cataract, including VF-14, Activities of Daily Vision Scale, and Visual Activities Questionnaire.

- *Ocular exam:* Including: Snellen acuity and refraction; measurement of intraocular pressure; assessment of pupillary function; external exam; slit-lamp exam; and dilated exam of fundus.

- *Supplemental testing:* May be necessary to assess and document the extent of the functional disability and to determine whether other diseases may limit preoperative or postoperative vision.

  Most elderly patients presenting with visual problems do not have a cataract that causes functional impairment. Refractive error, macular degeneration, and glaucoma are common alternative etiologies for visual impairment.

[c]Once cataract has been identified as the cause of visual disability, patients should be counseled concerning the nature of the problem, its natural history, and the existence of both surgical and nonsurgical approaches to management. The principal factor that should guide decision making with regard to surgery is *the extent to which the cataract impairs the ability to function in daily life.* The findings of the physical exam should corroborate that the cataract is the major contributing cause of the functional impairment, and that there is a reasonable expectation that managing the cataract will positively impact the patient's functional activity. Preoperative visual acuity is a poor predictor of postoperative functional improvement: The decision to recommend cataract surgery should not be made solely on the basis of visual acuity.

[d]Patients who complain of mild to moderate limitation in activities due to a visual problem, those whose corrected acuities are near 20/40, and those who do not yet wish to undergo surgery may be offered nonsurgical measures for improving visual function. Treatment with nutritional supplements is not recommended. Smoking cessation retards cataract progression. Indications for surgery: cataract-impaired vision no longer meets the patient's needs; evidence of lens-induced disease (eg, phacomorphic glaucoma, phacolytic glaucoma); necessary to visualize the fundus in an eye that has the potential for sight (eg, diabetic patient at risk of diabetic retinopathy).

[e]*Contraindications to surgery:* the patient does not desire surgery; glasses or vision aids provide satisfactory functional vision; surgery will not improve visual function; the patient's quality of life is not compromised; the patient is unable to undergo surgery because of coexisting medical or ocular conditions; a legal consent cannot be obtained; or the patient is unable to obtain adequate postoperative care. Routine preoperative medical testing (12-lead EKG, CBC, measurement of serum electrolytes, BUN, creatinine, and glucose), while commonly performed in patients scheduled to undergo cataract surgery, does not appear to measurably increase the safety of the surgery.

[f]Patients with significant functional and visual impairment due to cataract who have no contraindications to surgery should be counseled regarding the expected risks and benefits of and alternatives to surgery.

Source: American Academy of Ophthalmology Preferred Practice Pattern: Cataract in the Adult Eye. (2006) (http://www.aao.org/PPP)

American Optometric Association Consensus Panel on Care of the Adult Patient with Cataract. Optometric Clinical practice guideline: Care of the Adult Patient with Cataract. (2004) (http://www.aoa.org)

	CERUMEN IMPACTION				
Disease Management	Organization	Date	Population	Recommendations	Comments	Source
Cerumen Impaction	AAO-HNS	2008	Children and adults	1. Strongly recommended treating cerumen impaction when it is symptomatic or prevents a needed clinical exam. 2. Clinicians should treat the patient with cerumen impaction with an appropriate intervention: a. Ceruminolytic agents b. Irrigation c. Manual removal	Ceruminolytic agents include Cerumenex, Addax, Debrox, or dilute solutions of acetic acid, hydrogen peroxide, or sodium bicarbonate.	http://www.entnet.org/Practice/upload/FINAL-CerumenImpaction-Journal-2008.pdf

CHOLESTEROL & LIPID MANAGEMENT IN ADULTS

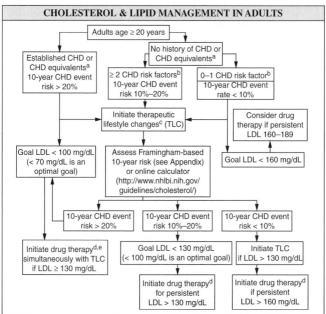

[a]CHD risk equivalents carry a risk for major coronary events equal to that of established CHD (ie, > 20% per 10 years) and include: diabetes, other clinical forms of atherosclerotic disease (peripheral arterial disease, abdominal aortic aneurysm, and symptomatic carotid artery disease).

[b]Age (men aged ≥ 45 years, women ≥ 55 years or postmenopausal), hypertension (BP ≥ 140/90 mm Hg or on antihypertensive medication), cigarette smoking, HDL < 40 mg/dL, family history of premature CHD in first-degree relative (males < 55 years, females < 65 years). For HDL ≥ 60 mg/dL, subtract 1 risk factor from above.

[c]Reduce saturated fat (< 7% total calories) and cholesterol (< 200 mg/day intake); increase physical activity; and achieve appropriate weight control. Assess effects of TLC on lipid levels after 3 months.

[d]Drug therapy response should be monitored and modified at 6-week intervals to achieve goal LDL levels; after goal LDL met, monitor response and adherence every 4–6 months.

[e]Addition of fibrate or nicotinic acid is also an option if ↑ TGs or ↓ HDL.

Source: Executive summary of the third report of the National Cholesterol Education Project (NCEP) expert panel on detection, evaluation and treatment of high blood cholesterol in adults (Adult Treatment Panel III). Implications of Recent Clinical Trials for the National Cholesterol Education Program Adult Treatment Panel III Guidelines. *Circulation*. 2004; 110:227–239.

Note: West of Scotland Coronary Prevention Study: 5 years of pravastatin treatment associated with significant reduction in coronary events for subsquent 10 years in men with hypercholesterolemia and no history of myocardial infarction. *NEJM*. 2007; 357(15):1477–1486.

2004 MODIFICATIONS TO THE
ATP III TREATMENT ALGORITHM FOR LDL-C

In high-risk persons (10-year CHD risk > 20%), the recommended LDL-C goal is < 100 mg/dL.

An LDL-C goal of < 70 mg/dL is a therapeutic option, especially for patients at very high risk.

If LDL-C is ≥ 100 mg/dL, an LDL-lowering drug is indicated as initial therapy simultaneously with lifestyle changes.

If baseline LDL-C is < 100 mg/dL, institution of an LDL-lowering drug to achieve an LDL-C level < 70 mg/dL is a therapeutic option.

If a high-risk person has high triglycerides or low HDL-C, consideration can be given to combining a fibrate or nicotinic acid with an LDL-lowering drug. When triglycerides are ≥ 200 mg/dL, non-HDL-C is a secondary target of therapy, with a goal 30 mg/dL higher than the identified LDL-C goal.

For **moderately high-risk persons** (2+ risk factors and 10-year risk 10%–20%), the recommended LDL-C goal is < 130 mg/dL; an LDL-C goal < 100 mg/dL is a therapeutic option. When LDL-C level is 100–129 mg/dL, at baseline or on lifestyle therapy, initiation of an LDL-lowering drug to achieve an LDL-C level < 100 mg/dL is a therapeutic option.

Any person at high risk or moderately high risk who has lifestyle-related risk factors (eg, obesity, physical inactivity, elevated triglycerides, low HDL-C, or metabolic syndrome) is a candidate for TLC to modify these risk factors regardless of LDL-C level.

When LDL-lowering drug therapy is employed in high-risk or moderately high-risk persons, intensity of therapy should be sufficient to achieve at least a 30%–40% reduction in LDL-C levels.

Source: Implications of Recent Clinical Trials for the National Cholesterol Education Program Adult Treatment Panel III Guidelines. *Circulation*. 2004;110:227–239.

CHOLESTEROL AND LIPID MANAGEMENT IN CHILDREN
Source: AHA, 2007

Children:
- Consider drug therapy if, after 6–12 month trial of fat- and cholesterol-restricted dietary management
- LDL ≥ 190 mg/dL or
- LDL > 160 mg/dL and positive family history of premature CHD; ≥ 2 other risk factors are present
- Treatment goal < 110 mg/dL (ideal) or < 130 mg/dL (minimal)
- Do not start before age 10 years in boys and until after menarche in girls
- Statins (HMG-CoA reductase inhibitors) as first-line drug therapy

Source: Circulation. 2007;115:1948–1967.

CONSTIPATION

Disease Management	Organization	Date	Population	Recommendations	Comments	Source
Constipation, Idiopathic	NICE	2010	Children aged ≤ 18 years	1. Assess all children for fecal impaction. 2. Recommends polyethylene glycol (PEG) as first-line agent for oral disimpaction. 3. Add a stimulant laxative if PEG therapy is ineffective after 2 weeks. 4. Recommends sodium citrate enemas for disimpaction only if all oral medications have failed. 5. Recommends a maintenance regimen with PEG for several months after a regular bowel pattern has been established. 6. Recommends gradually tapering maintenance dose over several months as bowel pattern allows. 7. Recommends adequate fluid intake.	Minimal fluid intake for age: *Age Volume* 1–3 years 1300 mL 4–8 years 1700 mL 9–13 years 2200 mL 14–18 years 2500 mL	http://www.nice.org.uk/nicemedia/live/12993/48741/48741.pdf

PERCENTAGE OF WOMEN EXPERIENCING AN UNINTENDED PREGNANCY DURING THE FIRST YEAR OF TYPICAL USE AND THE FIRST YEAR OF PERFECT USE OF CONTRACEPTION AND THE PERCENTAGE CONTINUING USE AT THE END OF THE FIRST YEAR—UNITED STATES

| Method | Women Experiencing an Unintended Pregnancy Within the First Year of Use | | |
	Typical Use*	Perfect Use[†]	Women Continuing Use at 1 Year[§]
No method[¶]	85%	85%	
Spermicides**	29%	18%	42%
Withdrawal	27%	4%	43%
Fertility awareness–based methods	25%		51%
Standard Days method[††]		5%	
TwoDay method™[††]		4%	
Ovulation method[††]		3%	
Sponge			
Parous women	32%	20%	46%
Nulliparous women	16%	9%	57%
Diaphragm[‡§]	16%	6%	57%
Condom[¶]			
Female (Reality®)	21%	5%	49%
Male	15%	2%	53%
Combined pill and progestin-only pill	8%	0.3%	68%
Evra patch®	8%	0.3%	68%
NuvaRing®	8%	0.3%	68%
Depo-Provera®	3%	0.3%	56%
Intrauterine device			
ParaGard® (copper T)	0.8%	0.6%	78%
Mirena® (LNG-IUS)	0.2%	0.2%	80%

PERCENTAGE OF WOMEN EXPERIENCING AN UNINTENDED PREGNANCY DURING THE FIRST YEAR OF TYPICAL USE AND THE FIRST YEAR OF PERFECT USE OF CONTRACEPTION AND THE PERCENTAGE CONTINUING USE AT THE END OF THE FIRST YEAR—UNITED STATES (CONTINUED)

| Method | Women Experiencing an Unintended Pregnancy Within the First Year of Use | | | Women Continuing Use at 1 Year[§] |
	Typical Use[*]	Perfect Use[†]		
Implanon[®]	0.05%	0.05%		84%
Female sterilization	0.5%	0.5%		100%
Male sterilization	0.15%	0.10%		100%
Emergency contraceptive pills[***]	Not applicable	Not applicable		Not applicable
Lactational amenorrhea methods[†††]	Not applicable	Not applicable		Not applicable

Adapted from Trussell J. Contraceptive efficacy. In Hatcher RA, Trussell J, Nelson AL, Cates W, Stewart FH, Kowal D. Contraceptive technology. 19th revised ed. New York, NY: Ardent Media; 2007.

[*] Among typical couples who initiate use of a method (not necessarily for the first time), the percentage who experience an unintended pregnancy during the first year if they do not stop use for any other reason. Estimates of the probability of pregnancy during the first year of typical use for spermicides, withdrawal, fertility awareness-based methods, the diaphragm, the male condom, the pill, and Depo-Provera are taken from the 1995 National Survey of Family Growth corrected for underreporting of abortion; see the text for the derivation of estimates for the other methods.

[†] Among couples who initiate use of a method (not necessarily for the first time) and who use it *perfectly* (both consistently and correctly), the percentage who experience an unintended pregnancy during the first year if they do not stop use for any other reason. See the text for the derivation of the estimate for each method.

[§] Among couples attempting to avoid pregnancy, the percentage who continue to use a method for 1 year.

[¶] The percentages becoming pregnant in the typical use and perfect use columns are based on data from populations where contraception is not used and from women who cease using contraception to become pregnant. Of these, approximately 89% become pregnant within 1 year. This estimate was lowered slightly (to 85%) to represent the percentage who would become pregnant within 1 year among women now relying on reversible methods of contraception if they abandoned contraception altogether.

[***] Foams, creams, gels, vaginal suppositories, and vaginal film.

[†††] The TwoDay and Ovulation methods are based on evaluation of cervical mucus. The Standard Days method avoids intercourse on cycle days 8–19.

[‡‡] With spermicidal cream or jelly.

[¶¶] Without spermicides.

PERCENTAGE OF WOMEN EXPERIENCING AN UNINTENDED PREGNANCY DURING THE FIRST YEAR OF TYPICAL USE AND THE FIRST YEAR OF PERFECT USE OF CONTRACEPTION AND THE PERCENTAGE CONTINUING USE AT THE END OF THE FIRST YEAR—UNITED STATES (CONTINUED)

Method	Women Experiencing an Unintended Pregnancy Within the First Year of Use		Women Continuing Use at 1 Year[§]
	Typical Use*	Perfect Use[†]	

***Treatment initiated within 72 hours after unprotected intercourse reduces the risk for pregnancy by at least 75%. The treatment schedule is 1 dose within 120 hours after unprotected intercourse and a second dose 12 hours after the first dose. Both doses of Plan B can be taken at the same time. Plan B (1 dose is 1 white pill) is the only dedicated product specifically marketed for emergency contraception. The Food and Drug Administration has in addition declared the following 22 brands of oral contraceptives to be safe and effective for emergency contraception: Ogestrel or Ovral (1 dose is 2 white pills); Levlen or Nordette (1 dose is 4 light-orange pills); Cryselle, Levora, Low-Ogestrel, Lo/Ovral, or Quasense (1 dose is 4 white pills); Tri-Levlen or Triphasil (1 dose is 4 yellow pills); Jolessa, Portia, Seasonale, or Trivora (1 dose is 4 pink pills); Seasonique (1 dose is 4 light blue-green pills); Empresse (1 dose is 4 orange pills); Alesse, Lessina, or Levlite (1 dose is 5 pink pills); Aviane (1 dose is 5 orange pills); and Lutera (1 dose is 5 white pills).

[††]Lactational amenorrhea method is a highly effective temporary method of contraception. However, to maintain effective protection against pregnancy, another method of contraception must be used as soon as menstruation resumes, the frequency or duration of breastfeeding is reduced, bottle feeds are introduced, or the baby reaches 6 months of age.

CHRONIC OBSTRUCTIVE PULMONARY DISEASE (COPD), EXACERBATIONS

Disease Management	Organization	Date	Population	Recommendations	Comments	Source
Chronic Obstructive Pulmonary Disease (COPD), Exacerbations	NICE	2010	Adults	1. Recommends noninvasive positive pressure ventilation for moderate-severe hypercapnic respiratory failure. 2. Prednisolone 30 mg orally, or its equivalent IV, should be prescribed for 7–14 days. 3. Recommends antibiotics for COPD exacerbations associated with more purulent sputum. 4. Bronchodilators can be delivered by either nebulizers or meter-dosed inhalers depending on the patient's ability to use the device during a COPD exacerbation.	Initial empiric antibiotics should be an aminopenicillin, macrolide, or a tetracycline.	http://www.nice.org.uk/nicemedia/live/13029/49397/49397.pdf

CHRONIC OBSTRUCTIVE PULMONARY DISEASE (COPD), STABLE

Disease Management	Organization	Date	Population	Recommendations	Comments	Source

Chronic Obstructive Pulmonary Disease (COPD), Stable	NICE	2010	Adults	1. Recommends confirming all suspected COPD with postbronchodilator spirometry.
				2. Recommends spirometry in all persons aged > 35 years who are current or ex-smokers and have a chronic cough to evaluate for early-stage COPD.
				3. Recommends smoking cessation counseling.
				4. Stepwise medication approach[a]:
				  a. Short-acting beta-agonist (SABA) as needed (prn)
				  b. If persistent symptoms, add:
				    i. $FEV_1 \geq 50\%$, add either a long-acting beta-agonist (LABA) or long-acting muscarinic agonist (LAMA)
				    ii. $FEV_1 < 50\%$, add either LABA + inhaled corticosteroid (ICS), or LAMA
				  c. If persistent symptoms, add:
				    i. LAMA to LABA + ICS
				5. Recommends pulmonary rehabilitation for symptomatic patients with moderate-severe COPD ($FEV_1 < 50\%$).
				6. Recommends calculating the BODE index (BMI, airflow obstruction, dyspnea, and exercise capacity on a 6-minute walk test) to calculate the risk of death in severe COPD.[b]
						http://www.nice.org.uk/nicemedia/live/13029/49397/49397.pdf

[a]SABA, short-acting beta-agonist: albuterol, fenoterol, levalbuterol, metaproterenol, pirbuterol, and terbutaline.
LABA, long-acting beta-agonists: arformoterol, formoterol, or salmeterol.
LAMA, long-acting muscarinic agonists: tiotropium.
ICS, inhaled corticosteroids: beclomethasone, budesonide, ciclesonide, flunisolide, fluticasone, mometasone, and triamcinolone.
[b]See http://www.nejm.org/doi/full/10.1056/NEJMoa021322#=article

SUMMARY OF CHANGES IN CLASSIFICATIONS FROM WHO MEDICAL ELIGIBILITY CRITERIA FOR CONTRACEPTIVE USE, 4TH EDITION*†

Condition	COC/P/R	POP	DMPA	Implants	LNG-IUD	Cu-IUD	Clarification
Breastfeeding a. <1 mo postpartum {WHO: <6 wks postpartum} b. 1 mo to <6 mos {WHO: ≥6 wks to <6 mos postpartum}	3§ {4} 2§ {3}	2§ {3}	2§ {3}	2§ {3}			The US Department of Health and Human Services recommends that infants be exclusively breastfed during the first 4–6 months of life, preferably for a full 6 months. Ideally, breastfeeding should continue through the first year of life (1). {Not included in WHO MEC}
Postpartum (in breastfeeding or nonbreastfeeding women), including post caesarean section a. <10 min after delivery of the placenta {WHO: <48 hrs, including insertion immediately after delivery of the placenta} b. 10 min after delivery of the placenta to <4 wks {WHO: ≥48 hrs to <4 wks}					2 {1 if not breastfeeding and 3 if breastfeeding} 2 {3}	 2 {3}	

SUMMARY OF CHANGES IN CLASSIFICATIONS FROM WHO MEDICAL ELIGIBILITY CRITERIA FOR CONTRACEPTIVE USE, 4TH EDITION[*] (CONTINUED)

Condition	COC/P/R	POP	DMPA	Implants	LNG-IUD	Cu-IUD	Clarification
Deep venous thrombosis (DVT)/ pulmonary embolism (PE)							
a. History of DVT/PE, not on anticoagulant therapy							
ii. Lower risk for recurrent DVT/PE (no risk factors)	3 {4}						
b. Acute DVT/PE		2 {3}	2 {3}	2 {3}	2 {3}	2 {1}	
c. DVT/PE and established on anticoagulant therapy for at least 3 mos						2 {1}	
i. Higher risk for recurrent DVT/PE (≥1 risk factors)							
• Known thrombophilia, including antiphospholipid syndrome							
• Active cancer (metastatic, on therapy, or within 6 mos after clinical remission), excluding non-melanoma skin cancer							
• History of recurrent DVT/PE							

SUMMARY OF CHANGES IN CLASSIFICATIONS FROM WHO MEDICAL ELIGIBILITY CRITERIA FOR CONTRACEPTIVE USE, 4TH EDITION*†

Condition	COC/P/R	POP	DMPA	Implants	LNG-IUD	Cu-IUD	Clarification
ii. Lower risk for recurrent DVT/ PE (no risk factors)	3§ [4]					2 [1]	Women on anticoagulant therapy are at risk for gynecologic complications of therapy such as hemorrhagic ovarian cysts and severe menorrhagia. Hormonal contraceptive methods can be of benefit in preventing or treating these complications. When a contraceptive method is used as a therapy, rather than solely to prevent pregnancy, the risk/benefit ratio may be different and should be considered on a case-by-case basis. [Not included in WHO MEC]
Valvular heart disease b. Complicated¶ (pulmonary hypertension, risk for atrial fibrillation, history of subacute bacterial endocarditis)						1 [2]	1 [2]
Ovarian cancer¶						1 [Initiation = 3, Continuation = 2]	1 [Initiation = 3, Continuation = 2]

SUMMARY OF CHANGES IN CLASSIFICATIONS FROM WHO MEDICAL ELIGIBILITY CRITERIA FOR CONTRACEPTIVE USE, 4TH EDITION*† (CONTINUED)							
Condition	COC/P/R	POP	DMPA	Implants	LNG-IUD	Cu-IUD	Clarification
Uterine fibroids						2 {1 if no uterine distortion and 4 if uterine distortion is present}	2 {1 if no uterine distortion and 4 if uterine distortion is present}

*For conditions for which classification changed for ≥1 methods or the condition description underwent a major modification, WHO conditions and recommendations appear in curly brackets.

†Abbreviations: WHO, World Health Organization; COC, combined oral contraceptive; P, combined hormonal contraceptive patch; R, combinedhormonal vaginal ring; POP, progestin-only pill; DMPA, depot medroxyprogesterone acetate; LNG-IUD, levonorgestrel-releasing intrauterine device; Cu-IUD, copper intrauterine device; DVT, deep venous thrombosis; PE, pulmonary embolism; VTE, venous thromboembolism.

‡Consult the clarification column for this classification.

¶Condition that exposes a women to increased risk as a result of unintended pregnancy.

SUMMARY OF RECOMMENDATIONS FOR MEDICAL CONDITIONS ADDED TO THE U.S. MEDICAL ELIGIBILITY CRITERIA FOR CONTRACEPTIVE USE*

Condition	COC/P/R	POP	DMPA	Implants	LNG-IUD	Cu-IUD	Clarification
History of bariatric surgery†							
a. Restrictive procedures: decrease storage capacity of the stomach (vertical banded gastroplasty, laparoscopic adjustable gastric band, laparoscopic sleeve gastrectomy)	1	1	1	1	1	1	
b. Malabsorptive procedures: decrease absorption of nutrients and calories by shortening the functional length of the small intestine (Roux-en-Y gastric bypass, biliopancreatic diversion)	COCs: 3 P/R: 1	3	1	1	1	1	
Peripartum cardiomyopathy†							
a. Normal or mildly impaired cardiac function (New York Heart Association Functional Class I or II: patients with no limitation of activities or patients with slight, mild limitation of activity) (2)							
i <6 mos	4	1	1	1	2	2	
ii ≥6 mos	3	1	1	1	2	2	
b. Moderately or severely impaired cardiac function (New York Heart Association Functional Class III or IV: patients with marked limitation of activity or patients who should be at complete rest) (2)	4	2	2	2	2	2	

SUMMARY OF RECOMMENDATIONS FOR MEDICAL CONDITIONS ADDED TO THE U.S. MEDICAL ELIGIBILITY CRITERIA FOR CONTRACEPTIVE USE*

Condition	COC/P/R	POP	DMPA	Implants	LNG-IUD		Cu-IUD		Clarification
					Initiation	Continua-tion	Initiation	Continua-tion	
Rheumatoid arthritis									
a. On immunosuppressive therapy	2	1	2/3§	1	2	1	2	1	DMPA use among women on long-term corticosteroid therapy with a history of, or risk factorsfor, nontraumatic fractures is classified as Category 3. Otherwise, DMPA use for women with rheumatoid arthritis is classified as Category 2.
b. Not on immunosuppressive therapy	2	1	2	1	1		1		
Endometrial hyperplasia	1	1	1	1	1		1		

SUMMARY OF RECOMMENDATIONS FOR MEDICAL CONDITIONS ADDED TO THE U.S. MEDICAL ELIGIBILITY CRITERIA FOR CONTRACEPTIVE USE*

Condition	COC/P/R	POP	DMPA	Implants	LNG-IUD	Cu-IUD	Clarification
Inflammatory bowel disease (IBD) (ulcerative colitis, Crohn disease)	2/3§	2	2	1	1	1	For women with mild IBD, with no other risk factors for VTE, the benefits of COC/P/R use generally outweigh the risks (Category 2). However, for women with IBD with increased risk for VTE (e.g., those with active or extensive disease, surgery, immobilization, corticosteroid use, vitamin deficiencies, fluid depletion), the risks for COC/P/R use generally outweigh the benefits (Category 3).
Solid organ transplantation†					Initiation / Continuation	Initiation / Continuation	
a. Complicated: graft failure (acute or chronic), rejection, cardiac allograft vasculopathy	4	2	2	2	2 / 3	2 / 3	

SUMMARY OF RECOMMENDATIONS FOR MEDICAL CONDITIONS ADDED TO THE U.S. MEDICAL ELIGIBILITY CRITERIA FOR CONTRACEPTIVE USE*

Condition	COC/P/R	POP	DMPA	Implants	LNG-IUD	Cu-IUD	Clarification
b. Uncomplicated	2§	2	2	2	2	2	Women with Budd-Chiari syndrome should not use COC/P/R because of the increased risk for thrombosis.

* Abbreviations: COC, combined oral contraceptive; P, combined hormonal contraceptive patch; R, combined hormonal vaginal ring; POP, progestin-only pill; DMPA, depotmedroxyprogesterone acetate; LNG-IUD, levonorgestrel-releasing intrauterine device; Cu-IUD, copper intrauterine device; IBD, inflammatory bowel disease; VTE, venousthromboembolism.

† Condition that exposes a women to increased risk as a result of unintended pregnancy.

§ Consult the clarification column for this classification.

SUMMARY OF ADDITIONAL CHANGES TO THE U.S. MEDICAL ELIGIBILITY CRITERIA FOR CONTRACEPTIVE USE	
Condition/Contraceptive Method	**Change**
Emergency contraceptive pills	History of bariatric surgery, rheumatoid arthritis, inflammatory bowel disease, and solid organ transplantation were added to Appendix D and given a Category 1.
Barrier methods	For 6 conditions—history of bariatric surgery, peripartum cardiomyopathy, rheumatoid arthritis, endometrial hyperplasia, inflammatory bowel disease, and solid organ transplantation—the barrier methods are classified as Category 1.
Sterilization	In general, no medical conditions would absolutely restrict a person's eligibility for sterilization. Recommendations from the World Health Organization (WHO) Medical Eligibility Criteria for Contraceptive Use about specific settings and surgical procedures for sterilization are not included here. The guidance has been replaced with general text on sterilization.
Other deleted items	Guidance for combined injectables, levonorgestrel implants, and norethisterone enanthate has been removed because these methods are not currently available in the United States. Guidance for "blood pressure measurement unavailable" and "history of hypertension, where blood pressure CANNOT be evaluated (including hypertension in pregnancy)" has been removed.
Unintended pregnancy and increased health risk	The following conditions have been added to the WHO list of conditions that expose a woman to increased risk as a result of unintended pregnancy: history of bariatric surgery within the past 2 years, peripartum cardiomyopathy, and receiving a solid organ transplant within 2 years.

CORONARY ARTERY STENT THERAPY
USE OF TRIPLE ANTICOAGULATION TREATMENT
Source: AMERICAN COLLEGE OF CARDIOLOGY/AMERICAN HEART ASSOCIATION/EUROPEAN SOCIETY OF CARDIOLOGY

The prudent use of triple anticoagulation therapy with aspirin, clopidogrel, and warfarin in AF patients at high risk of thromboembolism and recent coronary stent placement remains a *matter of clinical judgment*, balancing the risk of thrombotic versus bleeding events.

Facts:

- Bare metal stents are the stent of choice if TAT is required.
- Drug eluting stents should be reserved for high-risk clinical or anatomic situations (diabetic patients or if the coronary lesions are unusually long, totally occlusive, or in small blood vessels) if TAT is required.
- Dual antiplatelet therapy with clopidogrel (75 mg/day) and ASA (81 mg/day) is the most effective therapy to *prevent coronary stent thrombosis*.
- Warfarin anticoagulation is the most effective therapy to *prevent thromboembolism* in high-risk AF patients as defined by the $CHADS_2$ risk score (≥ 2) or the CHA_2DS_2-VAS_C risk score (≥ 3).
- TAT is the most effective therapy to *prevent* both *coronary stent thrombosis* and the *occurrence* of embolic strokes in high-risk patients.
- However, the addition of DAPT to warfarin increases the bleeding risk by 3.7-fold.
- Therefore, awaiting a definitive clinical trial (WOEST Trial), risk stratification of patients to evaluate the *thromboembolic potential of AF* versus the *bleeding potential* should be performed.
- The HAS-BLED (see box below) bleeding risk score is the best measure of bleeding risk. A high risk of bleeding is defined by a score ≥ 3.

Hypertension (≥ 160 mm Hg), **A**bnormal kidney function (creatinine ≥ 2, chronic dialysis, transplant), **A**bnormal liver function (cirrhosis, bilirubin > 2×, AST > 3×), **S**troke, **B**leeding history or anemia, **L**abile INR (< 60% within range), **E**lderly (aged ≥ 65 years), **D**rugs/alcohol (use of ASA or clopidogrel) or alcohol (≥ 8 alcoholic drinks/week). *Each risk factor is assigned 1 point for a total of 9 points.*

- If DAPT or TAT is required, *prophylactic GI therapy* with an H_2 blocker (except cimetidine) or PPI agent should be maintained. If omeprazole (Prilosec) is considered, the risk-to-benefit ratio needs to be considered due to its possible interference with clopidogrel function.
- In patients with a high risk of bleeding, TAT should be reserved for AF patients with a high thromboembolic risk. If the bleeding risk is high but the AF thromboembolic risk is low, DAPT therapy is suggested.

TAT, triple anticoagulation therapy; AF, atrial fibrillation; ASA, aspirin; BMS, bare metal stents; DES, drug eluting stents; DAPT, dual antiplatelet therapy; AST, aspartate transaminase; INR, international normalized ratio; GI, gastrointestinal; H_2, histamine; PPI, proton pump inhibitor

Sources: Adopted from European Society of Cardiology Guidelines for the Management of Atrial Fibrillation. *Euro Heart J.* 2010;31:2369–2429. Managing the anticoagulated patient with atrial fibrillation at high risk of stroke who needs coronary intervention. *BMJ.* 2008;337a840. Coronary Stent Implantation in Patients Committed to Long-term Oral Anticoagulation. *CHEST.* 2011;139(5):981–987. ACC/AHA/SCAI 2007 Focused Update of the 2005 Guidelines for PCI. *J Am Coll Cardiol.* 2008;51(2):172–208. ACC/AHA 2011 Guidelines for the Management of Patients With Unstable Angina/Non-ST-Elevation Myocardial Infarction. *J Am Coll Cardiol.* 2011; 57:1920–1959. ACCF/ACG/AHA 2010 Expert Consensus Document on the Concomitant Use of Protein Pump Inhibitors and Thienopyridines. *J Am Coll Cardiol.* 2010;56(24):2051–2066. Combined Antiplatelet and Anticoagulation Therapies. *J Am Coll Cardiol.* 2009;54(2):95–109.

CORONARY ARTERY STENT THERAPY
USE OF TRIPLE ANTICOAGULATION TREATMENT

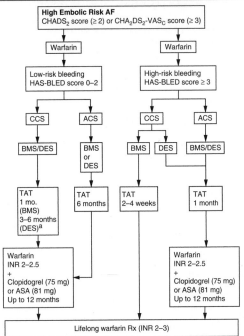

AF, atrial fibrillation; CCS, patient with chronic coronary syndrome (stable coronary artery disease); ACS, acute coronary syndrome; BMS, bare metal stent; DES, drug eluting stent; TAT, triple anticoagulation therapy; DES, drug eluting stent; ASA, aspirin; INR, international normalized ratio; Rx, therapy [warfarin (INR 2–2.5) + aspirin (81 mg daily) + clopidogrel (75 mg daily)].

[a] DES stents if sirolimus, everolimus or tacrolimus require 3-month dual platelet therapy (aspirin plus clopidogrel). If DES stent is paclitaxel, 6-month dual therapy is required.

Sources: Adopted from European Society of Cardiology Guidelines for the Management of Atrial Fibrillation. *Euro Heart J.* 2010;31:2369–2429. Managing the anticoagulated patient with atrial fibrillation at high risk of stroke who needs coronary intervention. *BMJ.* 2008;337a840. Coronary Stent Implantation in Patients Committed to Long-term Oral Anticoagulation. *CHEST.* 2011;139(5):981–987. ACC/AHA/SCAI 2007 Focused Update of the 2005 Guidelines for PCI. *J Am Coll Cardiol.* 2008;51(2):172–208. ACC/AHA 2011 Guidelines for the Management of Patients With Unstable Angina/Non-ST-Elevation Myocardial Infarction. *J Am Coll Cardiol.* 2011; 57:1920–1959. ACCF/ACG/AHA 2010 Expert Consensus Document on the Concomitant Use of Protein Pump Inhibitors and Thienopyridines. *J Am Coll Cardiol.* 2010;56(24):2051–2066. Combined Antiplatelet and Anticoagulation Therapies. *J Am Coll Cardiol.* 2009;54(2):95–109.

Disease Management	Organization	Date	Population	Recommendations	Comments	Source
				DELIRIUM		
Delirium	NICE	2010	Adults aged ≥ 18 years in the hospital or in long-term care facilities	1. Perform a short Confusion Assessment Method (CAM) screen to confirm the diagnosis of delirium. 2. Recommended approach to the management of delirium: 　a. Treat the underlying cause 　b. Provide frequent reorientation and reassurance to patients and their families 　c. Provide cognitively stimulating activities 　d. Ensure adequate hydration 　e. Prevent constipation 　f. Early mobilization 　g. Treat pain if present 　h. Provide hearing aids or corrective lenses if sensory impairment is present 　i. Promote good sleep hygiene 　j. Consider short-term antipsychotic use (< 1 week) for patients who are distressed or considered at risk to themselves or others	Recommended antipsychotics are haloperidol or olanzapine given at the lowest effective dose.	http://www.nice.org.uk/nicemedia/live/13060/49909/49909.pdf

					DEMENTIA	
Disease Management	Organization	Date	Population	Recommendations	Comments	Source
Dementia	ACP AAFP	2008 2008	Adults with dementia	1. Recommend a trial of therapy with a cholinesterase inhibitor or memantine based on individual assessment of relative risks versus benefits. 2. The choice of medication is based on tolerability, side effect profile, ease of use, and medication cost. 3. The evidence is insufficient to compare the relative efficacy of different medications for dementia. 4. Evidence is insufficient to determine the optimal duration of therapy.	1. A beneficial effect of cholinesterase inhibitors or memantine is generally observed within 3 months. 2. Good quality data in mild-moderate Alzheimer's and vascular dementia showed that cholinesterase inhibitors provide a modest improvement in global assessment, but no clinically important cognitive improvement. Subsets of patients may have significant cognitive improvement. 3. Five high-quality studies evaluated memantine use in moderate-severe Alzheimer's and vascular dementia and showed statistically significant improvement in global assessment, but no clinically important cognitive improvement.	http://www.annals.org/content/148/5/370.full.pdf

	DEPRESSION					
Disease Management	**Organization**	**Date**	**Population**	**Recommendations**	**Comments**	**Source**
Depression	USPSTF	2009	Children and adolescents	1. Adequate evidence showed that SSRIs, psychotherapy, and combined therapy will decrease symptoms of major depressive disorder in adolescents aged 12–18 years. 2. Insufficient evidence to support screening and treatment of depression in children aged 7–11 years.	1. Good evidence showed that SSRIs may increase absolute risk of suicidality in adolescents by 1%–2%. Therefore, SSRIs should be used only if close clinical monitoring is possible. 2. Fluoxetine and citalopram yielded statistically significant higher response rates than did other SSRIs.	http://www.uspreventiveservicestaskforce.org/uspstf09/depression/chdeprrs.pdf

	DIABETES MELLITUS (DM), TYPE 1				
Disease Management	Organization	Date	Population	Recommendations	Comments	Source

Diabetes Mellitus (DM), Type 1	ADA	2011	Adults and children	1. Recommends intensive insulin therapy with ≥ 3 injections daily using both basal and prandial insulin or an insulin pump.
				2. Self-monitoring blood glucose ≥ 3 times daily in all patients using multiple insulin injections or an insulin pump.
				3. Recommends assessment of psychological and social situation as part of diabetic evaluation.
				4. Recommends glucose (15–20 g) for all conscious patients with hypoglycemia.
				5. Advise all patients not to smoke.
				6. Recommends beginning these screening tests after 5 years with type 1 DM
				  a. Urine albumin/creatinine ratio and serum creatinine annually
				  b. Dilated funduscopic exam annually
				  c. Monofilament screening for diabetic neuropathy annually
				  d. Comprehensive foot exam at least annually
				7. Recommends screening at diagnosis for other autoimmune conditions:
				  a. Tissue transglutaminase IgA antibodies
				  b. Thyroperoxidase and thyroglobulin antibodies
					1. Glycemic control recommendations for **toddlers (aged 0–6 years):**
					  a. Before meals, CPG 100–180 mg/dL
					  b. Bedtime CPG, 110–200 mg/dL
					  c. HgbA1c < 8.5%
					2. Glycemic control recommendations for **school-aged (aged 6–12 years):**
					  a. Before meals, CPG 90–180 mg/dL
					  b. Bedtime CPG, 100–180 mg/dL
					  c. HgbA1c < 8%
						http://care.diabetesjournals.org/content/34/Supplement_1/S11.full

DIABETES MELLITUS (DM), TYPE 1					
Disease Management	**Organization**	**Date**	**Population**	**Recommendations**	**Comments**	**Source**

Diabetes Mellitus (DM), Type 1 (continued)				7. Fasting lipid panel at age 10 years or at puberty (consider as early as age 2 years for a strong family history of hyperlipidemia).
				  a. Repeat annually if results abnormal or every 5 years if results acceptable
				8. Consider statin therapy if aged ≥ 10 years and LDL > 160 mg/dL despite good glycemic control and lifestyle modification.
					3. Glycemic control recommendations for **adolescents (aged 13–19 years):**
					  a. Before meals, CPG 90–130 mg/dL
					  b. Bedtime CPG, 90–150 mg/dL
					  c. HgbA1c < 7.5%	

				DIABETES MELLITUS (DM), TYPE 2		
Disease Management	Organization	Date	Population	Recommendations	Comments	Source
Diabetes Mellitus (DM), Type 2	AACE	2010	Nonpregnant adults	1. Endorsed the use of HgbA1c ≥6.5% as a means of diagnosing type 2 DM. 2. HgbA1c is not recommended for diagnosing type 1 DM or gestational diabetes.		http://www.aace.com/pub/pdf/guidelines/AACEpositionA1cfeb2010.pdf
	NICE	2009	Adults	1. Consider adding a (dipeptidyl peptidase-4) DPP-4 inhibitor[a] or pioglitazone to metformin as a second-line agent if glycemic control is inadequate and a significant risk of hypoglycemia or sulfonylurea contraindications exist 2. Consider adding a DPP-4 inhibitor[b] or pioglitazone to a sulfonylurea as a second-line agent if glycemic control is inadequate and a metformin contraindication exists 3. Consider a glucagon-like peptide-1 (GLP-1) mimetic (eg, exenatide) as a third-line agent when glycemic control is inadequate (HgbA1c ≥7.5%) with metformin and a sulfonylurea 4. Consider adding insulin when glycemic control is inadequate (HgbA1c ≥7.5%) with oral agents alone	1. Avoid pioglitazone in people with heart failure or who have a higher risk of fracture. 2. Avoid metformin if the glomerular filtration rate (GFR) is <45 mL/min/1.73 m².	http://www.nice.org.uk/nicemedia/live/12165/44318/44318.pdf

	DIABETES MELLITUS (DM), TYPE 2					
Disease Management	Organization	Date	Population	Recommendations	Comments	Source
Diabetes Mellitus (DM), Type 2 (continued)	ADA	2011	Adults and children	1. Self-monitoring blood glucose ≥ 3 times daily in all patients using multiple insulin injections or an insulin pump 2. Recommends HgbA1c every 3 months if therapy has changed or if blood glucose control is inadequate 3. Provide diabetes self-management education, including education about hypoglycemia management and adjustments during illness 4. Provide family planning for women of reproductive age 5. Provide medical nutrition therapy 6. Weight loss is recommended for all overweight or obese diabetic patients 7. Keep saturated fat intake < 7% of total calories 8. Recommends at least 150 min/week of moderate physical activity 9. Recommends the following: a. Immunizations: annual influenza vaccination if aged ≥ 6 months, pneumococcal polysaccharide vaccine if aged ≥ 2 years, and 1 × revaccination if aged ≥ 65 years b. Target blood pressure (BP) < 130/80 mm Hg	1. Glycemic control recommendations: a. Preprandial capillary blood gas (CPG) 70–130 mg/dL b. Postprandial CPG < 180 mg/dL (1–2 hour post-meals) c. HgbA1c < 7% 2. Consider bariatric surgery if BMI > 35 kg/m² and if diabetes is difficult to control with lifestyle modification and medications. 3. Angiotensin-converting enzyme inhibitors (ACEIs) or angiotensin receptor blockers (ARBs) are first-line antihypertensives. 4. Second-line antihypertensives are a thiazide diuretic if GFR ≥ 30 mL/min/1.73m² or a loop diuretic if GFR < 30 mL/min/1.73m².	http://care.diabetesjournals.org/content/34/Supplement_1/S11.full

DIABETES MELLITUS (DM), TYPE 2						
Disease Management	Organization	Date	Population	Recommendations	Comments	Source

Diabetes Mellitus (DM), Type 2 (continued)				c. Statin therapy if:
				  i. Overt cardiovascular disease (CVD) present
				  ii. Aged > 40 years and ≥ 1 cardiovascular (CV) risk factor[c]
				  iii. Low-density lipoprotein (LDL) > 100 mg/dL despite lifestyle modification
				d. Aspirin 75–162 mg/day if:
				  i. Primary prevention of CVD if 10-year risk of coronary artery disease (CAD) > 10%
				  ii. Secondary prevention of CVD
				e. Annual check of urine albumin/creatinine ratio and serum creatinine
				f. Annual dilated funduscopic exam
				g. Annual monofilament screening for diabetic neuropathy
				h. At minimum, annual comprehensive foot exam
					5. Clopidogrel 75 mg/day is an alternative for persons ASA intolerant.
					6. Nephrology referral indicated if GFR < 60 mL/min/1.73m², or if heavy proteinuria or structural kidney disease present
					7. Consider a serum TSH in women aged > 50 years.	

[a]Sitagliptin or vildagliptin.
[b]Sitagliptin or vildagliptin.
[c]Cardiovascular risk factors: hypertension, smoking, positive family history, men aged ≥ 45 years and women aged ≥ 55 years, or hyperlipidemia.

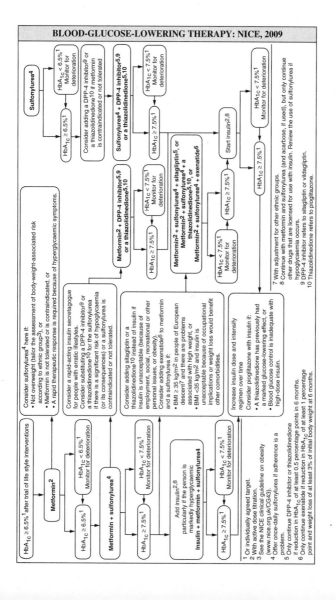

BLOOD-GLUCOSE-LOWERING THERAPY: NICE, 2009

ERECTILE DYSFUNCTION (ED)

Disease Management	Organization	Date	Population	Recommendations	Comments	Source

Erectile Dysfunction (ED)	EAU	2009	Adult men	1. Recommends a medical and psychosexual history on all patients
				2. Recommends a focused physical exam to assess CV status, neurologic status, prostate disease, penile abnormalities, and signs of hypogonadism
				3. Recommends checking a fasting glucose, lipid profile, and total testosterone levels
				4. Recommends psychosexual therapy for psychogenic ED
				5. Recommends testosterone therapy for androgen deficiency if no contraindications present[a]
				6. Selective phosphodiesterase 5 (PDE5) inhibitors are first-line therapy for idiopathic ED
					1. Selective PDE5 inhibitors:
					  a. Sildenafil
					  b. Tadalafil
					  c. Vardenafil
					2. Avoid nitrates and use alpha-blockers with caution when prescribing a selective PDE5 inhibitor
						http://www.uroweb.org/gls/EU/2010%20Male%20Sex%20Dysfunction.pdf

[a]Prostate CA, breast CA, or signs of prostatism.

Disease Management	Organization	Date	Population	Recommendations	Comments	Source
				GLAUCOMA, CHRONIC OPEN ANGLE		
Glaucoma, Chronic Open Angle	NICE	2009	Adults	1. All persons with known or suspected chronic open angle glaucoma (COAG) or ocular hypertension (OHT) should undergo the following: a. Intraocular pressure monitoring using tonometry b. Central corneal thickness measurement c. Peripheral anterior chamber depth assessments using gonioscopy d. Visual field testing e. Optic nerve assessment using slit-lamp exam 2. Recommends monitoring patients with OHT at least annually for COAG (every 6 months for high-risk patients). 3. Recommends monitoring patients with COAG every 6–12 months based on disease progression. 4. Recommends prostaglandin analogue therapy for early-moderate COAG patients at risk of visual loss. 5. Consider surgery with pharmacologic augmentation for advanced COAG. 6. Recommends beta-blocker drops for mild OHT until age 60 years. 7. Recommends prostaglandin analogue drops for any degree of OHT. 8. Recommends additional medication therapy for uncontrolled OHT despite single-agent therapy.	1. Alternative pharmacologic treatments for OHT or suspected COAG in patients whose intraocular pressures remain elevated on monotherapy include: a. Prostaglandin analogues b. Beta-blockers c. Carbonic anhydrase inhibitors d. Sympathomimetics	http://www.guidelines.gov/content.aspx?id=14444

HEADACHE DIAGNOSIS ALGORITHM: ICSI, 2011

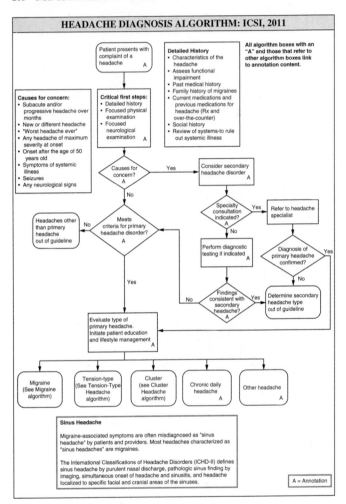

Patient presents with complaint of a headache
A

Detailed History
- Characteristics of the headache
- Assess functional impairment
- Past medical history
- Family history of migraines
- Current medications and previous medications for headache (Rx and over-the-counter)
- Social history
- Review of systems-to rule out systemic illness

All algorithm boxes with an "A" and those that refer to other algorithm boxes link to annotation content.

Causes for concern:
- Subacute and/or progressive headache over months
- New or different headache
- "Worst headache ever"
- Any headache of maximum severity at onset
- Onset after the age of 50 years old
- Symptoms of systemic illness
- Seizures
- Any neurological signs

Critical first steps:
- Detailed history
- Focused physical examination
- Focused neurological examination
A

Causes for concern?
A

Yes → Consider secondary headache disorder
A

Specialty consultation indicated?
A

Yes → Refer to headache specialist

No → Perform diagnostic testing if indicated
A

Headaches other than primary headache out of guideline

No ← Meets criteria for primary headache disorder?
A

Diagnosis of primary headache confirmed?

Yes

No → Determine secondary headache type out of guideline

Findings consistent with secondary headache?
A

No   Yes →

Yes

Evaluate type of primary headache. Initiate patient education and lifestyle management
A

Migraine (See Migraine algorithm)

Tension-type (See Tension-Type Headache algorithm)

Cluster (see Cluster Headache algorithm)

Chronic daily headache
A

Other headache
A

Sinus Headache

Migraine-associated symptoms are often misdiagnosed as "sinus headache" by patients and providers. Most headaches characterized as "sinus headaches" are migraines.

The International Classifications of Headache Disorders (ICHD-II) defines sinus headache by purulent nasal discharge, pathologic sinus finding by imaging, simultaneous onset of headache and sinusitis, and headache localized to specific facial and cranial areas of the sinuses.

A = Annotation

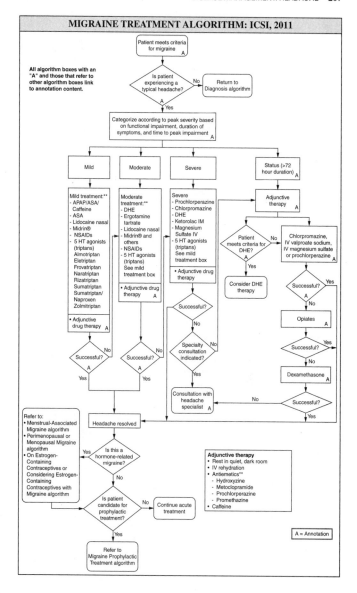

MIGRAINE TREATMENT ALGORITHM: ICSI, 2011

All algorithm boxes with an "A" and those that refer to other algorithm boxes link to annotation content.

Patient meets criteria for migraine A

Is patient experiencing a typical headache? → No → Return to Diagnosis algorithm

Yes

Categorize according to peak severity based on functional impairment, duration of symptoms, and time to peak impairment A

Mild

Mild treatment:**
- APAP/ASA/Caffeine
- ASA
- Lidocaine nasal
- Midrin®
- NSAIDs
- 5 HT agonists (triptans)
  Almotriptan
  Eletriptan
  Frovatriptan
  Naratriptan
  Rizatriptan
  Sumatriptan
  Sumatriptan/Naproxen
  Zolmitriptan
- Adjunctive drug therapy A

Successful? No / Yes

Moderate

Moderate treatment:**
- DHE
- Ergotamine tartrate
- Lidocaine nasal
- Midrin® and others
- NSAIDs
- 5 HT agonists (triptans) See mild treatment box
- Adjunctive drug therapy A

Successful? No / Yes

Severe

Severe
- Prochlorperazine
- Chlorpromazine
- DHE
- Ketorolac IM
- Magnesium Sulfate IV
- 5 HT agonists (triptans) See mild treatment box
- Adjunctive drug therapy A

Successful? No

Specialty consultation indicated? No / Yes

Consultation with headache specialist A

Status (>72 hour duration) A

Adjunctive therapy A

Patient meets criteria for DHE? A → No → Chlorpromazine, IV valproate sodium, IV magnesium sulfate or prochlorperazine A

Yes

Consider DHE therapy

Successful? A → Yes

No

Opiates A

Successful? A → Yes

No

Dexamethasone A

Successful? A → No → Consultation with headache specialist A

Yes

Headache resolved

Refer to:
- Menstrual-Associated Migraine algorithm
- Perimenopausal or Menopausal Migraine algorithm
- On Estrogen-Containing Contraceptives or Considering Estrogen-Containing Contraceptives with Migraine algorithm

Is this a hormone-related migraine? → Yes

No

Is patient candidate for prophylactic treatment? → No → Continue acute treatment

Yes

Refer to Migraine Prophylactic Treatment algorithm

Adjunctive therapy
- Rest in quiet, dark room
- IV rehydration
- Antiemetics**
  - Hydroxyzine
  - Metoclopramide
  - Prochlorperazine
  - Promethazine
- Caffeine

A = Annotation

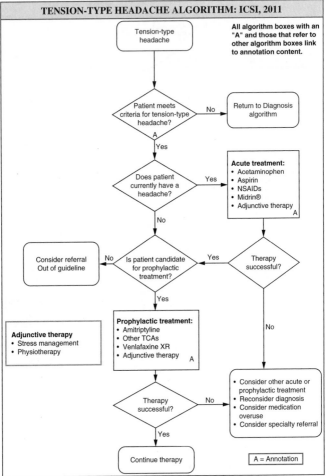

TENSION-TYPE HEADACHE ALGORITHM: ICSI, 2011

Tension-type headache

All algorithm boxes with an "A" and those that refer to other algorithm boxes link to annotation content.

Patient meets criteria for tension-type headache? — No → Return to Diagnosis algorithm

A ↓ Yes

Does patient currently have a headache? — Yes → **Acute treatment:**
• Acetaminophen
• Aspirin
• NSAIDs
• Midrin®
• Adjunctive therapy
A

↓ No

Consider referral Out of guideline ← No — Is patient candidate for prophylactic treatment? ← Yes — Therapy successful?

↓ Yes ↓ No

Prophylactic treatment:
• Amitriptyline
• Other TCAs
• Venlafaxine XR
• Adjunctive therapy A

Adjunctive therapy
• Stress management
• Physiotherapy

• Consider other acute or prophylactic treatment
• Reconsider diagnosis
• Consider medication overuse
• Consider specialty referral

Therapy successful? — No →

↓ Yes

Continue therapy

A = Annotation

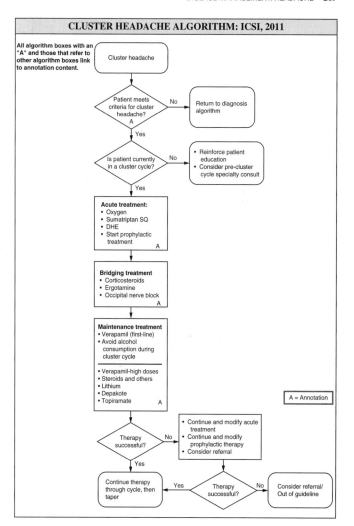

CLUSTER HEADACHE ALGORITHM: ICSI, 2011

All algorithm boxes with an "A" and those that refer to other algorithm boxes link to annotation content.

Cluster headache

Patient meets criteria for cluster headache? A — No → Return to diagnosis algorithm

Yes

Is patient currently in a cluster cycle? — No → • Reinforce patient education
• Consider pre-cluster cycle specialty consult

Yes

Acute treatment:
• Oxygen
• Sumatriptan SQ
• DHE
• Start prophylactic treatment   A

Bridging treatment
• Corticosteroids
• Ergotamine
• Occipital nerve block   A

Maintenance treatment
• Verapamil (first-line)
• Avoid alcohol consumption during cluster cycle

• Verapamil-high doses
• Steroids and others
• Lithium
• Depakote
• Topiramate   A

A = Annotation

Therapy successful? — No → • Continue and modify acute treatment
• Continue and modify prophylactic therapy
• Consider referral

Yes

Continue therapy through cycle, then taper ← Yes — Therapy successful? — No → Consider referral/ Out of guideline

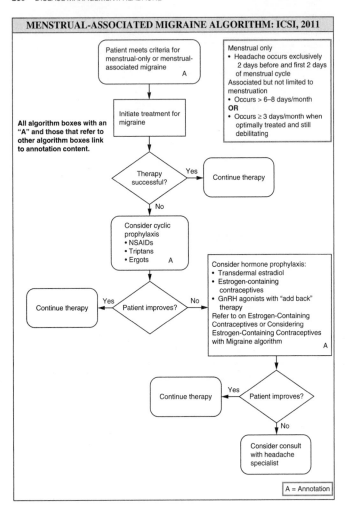

MENSTRUAL-ASSOCIATED MIGRAINE ALGORITHM: ICSI, 2011

Patient meets criteria for menstrual-only or menstrual-associated migraine — A

Menstrual only
• Headache occurs exclusively 2 days before and first 2 days of menstrual cycle
Associated but not limited to menstruation
• Occurs > 6–8 days/month
OR
• Occurs ≥ 3 days/month when optimally treated and still debilitating

Initiate treatment for migraine

All algorithm boxes with an "A" and those that refer to other algorithm boxes link to annotation content.

Therapy successful? — Yes → Continue therapy

No

Consider cyclic prophylaxis
• NSAIDs
• Triptans
• Ergots — A

Patient improves? — Yes → Continue therapy

No

Consider hormone prophylaxis:
• Transdermal estradiol
• Estrogen-containing contraceptives
• GnRH agonists with "add back" therapy
Refer to on Estrogen-Containing Contraceptives or Considering Estrogen-Containing Contraceptives with Migraine algorithm — A

Patient improves? — Yes → Continue therapy

No

Consider consult with headache specialist

A = Annotation

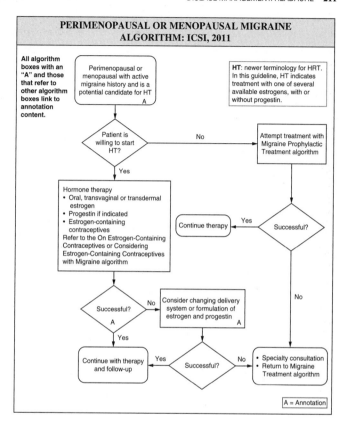

PERIMENOPAUSAL OR MENOPAUSAL MIGRAINE ALGORITHM: ICSI, 2011

All algorithm boxes with an "A" and those that refer to other algorithm boxes link to annotation content.

Perimenopausal or menopausal with active migraine history and is a potential candidate for HT   A

HT: newer terminology for HRT. In this guideline, HT indicates treatment with one of several available estrogens, with or without progestin.

Patient is willing to start HT? — No → Attempt treatment with Migraine Prophylactic Treatment algorithm

Yes

Hormone therapy
• Oral, transvaginal or transdermal estrogen
• Progestin if indicated
• Estrogen-containing contraceptives
Refer to the On Estrogen-Containing Contraceptives or Considering Estrogen-Containing Contraceptives with Migraine algorithm

Continue therapy ← Yes — Successful?

No

Successful?   A — No → Consider changing delivery system or formulation of estrogen and progestin   A

Yes

Continue with therapy and follow-up ← Yes — Successful? — No → • Specialty consultation
• Return to Migraine Treatment algorithm

A = Annotation

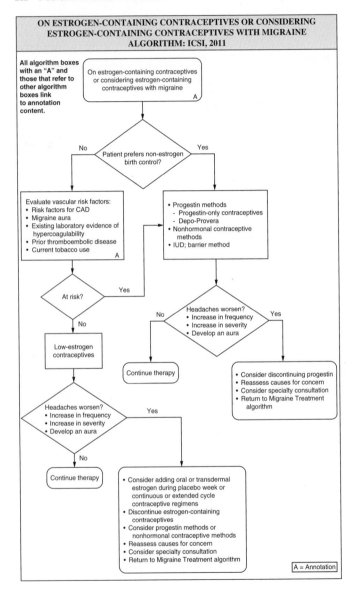

ON ESTROGEN-CONTAINING CONTRACEPTIVES OR CONSIDERING
ESTROGEN-CONTAINING CONTRACEPTIVES WITH MIGRAINE
ALGORITHM: ICSI, 2011

All algorithm boxes with an "A" and those that refer to other algorithm boxes link to annotation content.

On estrogen-containing contraceptives or considering estrogen-containing contraceptives with migraine   A

Patient prefers non-estrogen birth control?
- No
- Yes

Evaluate vascular risk factors:
- Risk factors for CAD
- Migraine aura
- Existing laboratory evidence of hypercoagulability
- Prior thromboembolic disease
- Current tobacco use   A

- Progestin methods
  - Progestin-only contraceptives
  - Depo-Provera
- Nonhormonal contraceptive methods
- IUD; barrier method

At risk?
- Yes
- No

Low-estrogen contraceptives

Headaches worsen?
- Increase in frequency
- Increase in severity
- Develop an aura
- No
- Yes

Continue therapy

- Consider discontinuing progestin
- Reassess causes for concern
- Consider specialty consultation
- Return to Migraine Treatment algorithm

Headaches worsen?
- Increase in frequency
- Increase in severity
- Develop an aura
- No
- Yes

Continue therapy

- Consider adding oral or transdermal estrogen during placebo week or continuous or extended cycle contraceptive regimens
- Discontinue estrogen-containing contraceptives
- Consider progestin methods or nonhormonal contraceptive methods
- Reassess causes for concern
- Consider specialty consultation
- Return to Migraine Treatment algorithm

A = Annotation

MIGRAINE PROPHYLACTIC TREATMENT ALGORITHM: ICSI, 2011

All algorithm boxes with an "A" and those that refer to other algorithm boxes link to annotation content.

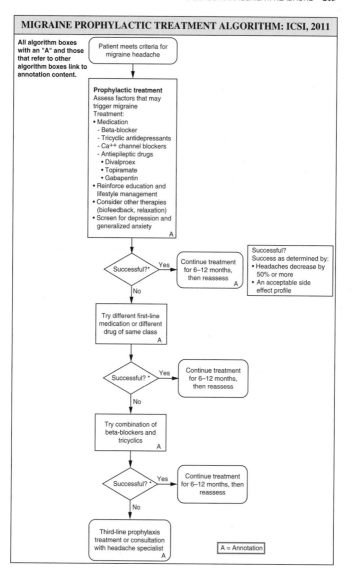

Patient meets criteria for migraine headache

Prophylactic treatment
Assess factors that may trigger migraine
Treatment:
• Medication
 - Beta-blocker
 - Tricyclic antidepressants
 - Ca++ channel blockers
 - Antiepileptic drugs
 • Divalproex
 • Topiramate
 • Gabapentin
• Reinforce education and lifestyle management
• Consider other therapies (biofeedback, relaxation)
• Screen for depression and generalized anxiety

A

Successful?* — Yes → Continue treatment for 6–12 months, then reassess A

No

Successful?
Success as determined by:
• Headaches decrease by 50% or more
• An acceptable side effect profile

Try different first-line medication or different drug of same class A

Successful? * — Yes → Continue treatment for 6–12 months, then reassess

No

Try combination of beta-blockers and tricyclics A

Successful? * — Yes → Continue treatment for 6–12 months, then reassess

No

Third-line prophylaxis treatment or consultation with headache specialist A

A = Annotation

HEART FAILURE
Source: ADAPTED FROM ACC/AHA, 2005

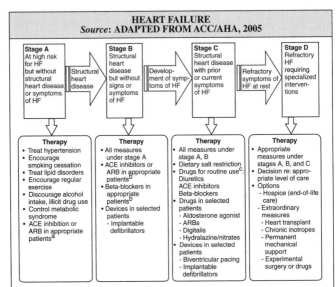

Stage A	Stage B	Stage C	Stage D
At high risk for HF but without structural heart disease or symptoms of HF	Structural heart disease but without signs or symptoms of HF	Structural heart disease with prior or current symptoms of HF	Refractory HF requiring specialized interventions

(arrows labeled: "Structural heart disease", "Development of symptoms of HF", "Refractory symptoms of HF at rest")

Therapy	**Therapy**	**Therapy**	**Therapy**

• Treat hypertension
• Encourage smoking cessation
• Treat lipid disorders
• Encourage regular exercise
• Discourage alcohol intake, illicit drug use
• Control metabolic syndrome
• ACE inhibition or ARB in appropriate patients[a]
	• All measures under stage A
	• ACE inhibitors or ARB in appropriate patients[b]
	• Beta-blockers in appropriate patients[b]
	• Devices in selected patients
	  - Implantable defibrillators
		• All measures under stage A, B
		• Dietary salt restriction
		• Drugs for routine use[c]:
		  Diuretics
		  ACE inhibitors
		  Beta-blockers
		• Drugs in selected patients
		  - Aldosterone agonist
		  - ARBs
		  - Digitalis
		  - Hydralazine/nitrates
		• Devices in selected patients
		  - Biventricular pacing
		  - Implantable defibrillators
			• Appropriate measures under stages A, B, and C
			• Decision re: appropriate level of care
			• Options
			  - Hospice (end-of-life care)
			  - Extraordinary measures
			  - Heart transplant
			  - Chronic inotropes
			  - Permanent mechanical support
			  - Experimental surgery or drugs

Stage A: Patients with hypertension, atherosclerotic disease, diabetes mellitus, metabolic syndrome, *or* those using cardiotoxins or having a family history of cardiomyopathy

Stage B: Patients with previous MI, LV remodeling including LVH and low EF, or asymptomatic valvular disease

Stage C: Patients with known structural heart disease; shortness of breath and fatigue, reduced exercise tolerance

Stage D: Patients who have marked symptoms at rest despite maximal medical therapy (eg, those who are recurrently hospitalized or cannot be safely discharged from the hospital without specialized interventions)

[a]History of atherosclerotic vascular disease, diabetes mellitus, or hypertension and associated cardiovascular risk factors.

[b]Recent or remote MI, regardless of ejection fraction; or reduced ejection fraction regardless of MI Hx. Use ARB in patients post-MI who cannot tolerate ACE inhibitors.

[c]Evidence suggests that isosorbide dinitrate plus hydralazine reduces mortality in blacks with advanced heart failure. (*NEJM.* 2004;351:2049)

Comments: Exercise training in patients with HF seems to be safe and beneficial overall in improving exercise capacity, quality of life, muscle structure, and physiologic responses to exercise. (*Circulation.* 2003;107:1210–1225)

HF, heart failure; LV, left ventricle

Source: Adapted from the American College of Cardiology, American Heart Association, Inc. *J Am Coll Cardiol.* 2005;46:1–82 and *Circulation.* 2005;112:154–235. 2009 ACCF/AHA Guidelines. *J Am Coll Cardiol.* 2009;53(150):1334–1378.

	HEPATITIS B VIRUS (HBV)				
Disease Management	Organization	Date	Population	Recommendations	Comments	Source
Hepatitis B Virus (HBV)	NIH AASLD	2009 2009	Adults and children with HBV infection	1. Recommend HBV immunoglobulin and HBV vaccine to all infants born to HBsAg-positive women. 2. Recommend antiviral therapy for adults and alanine transaminase (ALT) > 2× normal, moderate-severe hepatitis on biopsy, compensated cirrhosis or advanced fibrosis and HBV DNA > 20,000 IU/mL; or for reactivation of chronic HBV after chemotherapy or immunosuppression. 3. Recommend antiviral therapy in children for ALT > 2× normal and HBV DNA >20,000 IU/mL for at least 6 months. 4. Optimal monitoring practices have not been defined.	1. The most important predictors of cirrhosis or hepatocellular carcinoma (HCC) in chronic HBV infection are persistently elevated HBV DNA and serum ALT levels, HBV genotype C infection, male gender, older age, and coinfection with hepatitis C virus or human immunodeficiency virus (HIV). a. Persons at risk for HCC should be screened by ultrasound every 6–12 months 2. No randomized controlled trials have demonstrated a decrease in overall mortality, liver-specific mortality, or the rate of HCC with anti-HBV therapies. 3. Consider lamivudine or interferon-alpha for initial anti-HBV therapy.	http://www.guidelines.gov/content.aspx?id=14240 http://www.guidelines.gov/content.aspx?id=15475

				HEPATITIS C VIRUS (HCV)		
Disease Management	Organization	Date	Population	Recommendations	Comments	Source

Hepatitis C Virus (HCV)	AASLD	2009	Adults with HCV infection	1. Recommends education on methods to avoid transmission to others.
				2. Recommends antiviral treatment for:
				  a. Bridging fibrosis or compensated cirrhosis
				  b. Consideration of acute HCV infection
				3. Test quantitative HCV RNA before treatment and at 12 weeks of therapy.
				4. Patients who lack antibodies for hepatitis A and B viruses should receive vaccination.
				5. Recommend abstaining from alcohol consumption.
				6. Insufficient evidence to recommend herbal therapy.
					1. Optimal therapy is the combination of peginterferon-alfa and ribavirin
					  a. Duration of therapy is 48 weeks for HCV genotypes 1 and 4
					  b. Duration of therapy is 24 weeks for HCV genotypes 2 and 3
						http://www.guidelines.gov/content.aspx?id=14708

HOARSENESS					
Disease Management	Organization	Date	Population	Recommendations	Comments	Source
Hoarseness	AAO-HNS	2009	Persons with hoarseness	1. Recommends against the routine use of antibiotics to treat hoarseness. 2. Recommends voice therapy for all patients with hoarseness and a decreased voice quality of life. 3. All patients with chronic hoarseness > 3 months should undergo laryngoscopy. 4. Recommends against routine use of antireflux medications unless the patient exhibits signs or symptoms of gastroesophageal reflux disease. 5. Recommends against the routine use of corticosteroids to treat hoarseness. 6. Recommends against screening neck imaging (CT or MRI scanning) for chronic hoarseness prior to laryngoscopy. 7. Consider surgery for possible laryngeal CA, benign laryngeal soft tissue lesions, or glottis insufficiency. 8. Consider botulinum toxin injections for spasmodic dysphonia.	Nearly one-third of Americans will have hoarseness at some point in their lives.	http://www.guidelines.gov/content.aspx?id=15203

HUMAN IMMUNODEFICIENCY VIRUS (HIV)

Disease Management	Organization	Date	Population	Recommendations	Comments	Source

Human Immunodeficiency Virus (HIV)	IDSA	2009	HIV-infected adults and children	1. Recommends education to avoid high-risk behaviors to minimize risk of HIV transmission.
				2. Assess for the presence of depression, substance abuse, or domestic violence.
				3. Baseline labs: CD4 count; quantitative HIV RNA by PCR (viral load); HIV genotyping; CBCD, chemistry panel, G6PD testing; fasting lipid profile; HLA B5701 test (if abacavir is used); urinalysis; PPD; *Toxoplasma* antibodies; HBsAg, HBsAb, and HCV antibodies; VDRL; urine NAAT for gonorrhea; and urine NAAT for chlamydia (except in men aged < 25 years); Pap smear in women[a]
				4. Monitoring labs:
				  a. CD4 counts and HIV viral load every 3–4 months.
				  b. Frequency of repeat sexually transmitted disease (STD) screening is undefined.
				  c. Annual PPD test.
				  d. Persons starting antiretroviral medications should have a repeat fasting glucose and lipid panel 4–6 weeks after initiation of therapy.
					1. Homosexual men and women with abnormal cervical Pap smear results and persons with a history of genital warts should undergo anogenital human papilloma virus (HPV) screening and anal Pap testing.
					2. Serum testosterone level should be considered in men complaining of fatigue, ED, or decreased libido.
					3. Chest x-ray should be obtained in persons with pulmonary symptoms or who have a positive PPD test result.
						http://www.guidelines.gov/content.aspx?id=15440

HUMAN IMMUNODEFICIENCY VIRUS (HIV)

Disease Management	Organization	Date	Population	Recommendations	Comments	Source
Human Immunodeficiency Virus (HIV) (continued)				5. Vaccination for pneumococcal infection, influenza, varicella, hepatitis A, and hepatitis B virus according to standard immunization charts. 6. All HIV-infected women of childbearing age should be counseled regarding contraception. 7. Pap smear in women every 6 months. 8. Consider annual mammography in all women aged ≥ 40 years. 9. Hormone replacement therapy is not recommended. 10. All women aged ≥ 65 years should have a dual-energy x-ray absorptiometry (DXA) test of spine/hips.		

[a]PCR, polymerase chain reaction; CBCD, complete blood count with differential; RNA, ribonucleic acid; G6PD, glucose-6-phosphate dehydrogenase; HLA, human leukocyte antigen; PPD, purified protein derivative; HB, hepatitis B; VDRL, Venereal Disease Research Laboratory; NAAT, nucleic acid amplification test

HUMAN IMMUNODEFICIENCY VIRUS (HIV), PREGNANCY

Disease Management	Organization	Date	Population	Recommendations	Comments	Source

Human Immunodeficiency Virus (HIV), Pregnancy	CDC NIH	2010	HIV-infected pregnant women	1. Recommend combination antiretroviral (ART) regimens during the antepartum period.
				2. Women who were taking ART prior to conception should have their regimen reviewed (ie, teratogenic potential of drugs), but continue combination ART throughout the pregnancy.
				3. Initial prenatal labs should include a CD4 count, HIV viral load, and hepatitis C virus (HCV) antibody.
				  a. If HIV RNA is detectable (> 500–1000 copies/mL), perform HIV genotypic resistance testing to help guide antepartum therapy.
				4. Women who do not require ART for their own health should initiate combination ART between 14–28 gestational weeks and continue until delivery.
				  a. Zidovudine should be a component of the regimen when feasible.
				  b. Recommend against single-dose intrapartum/newborn nevirapine in addition to antepartum ART.
					1. Avoid Methergine for postpartum hemorrhage in women receiving a protease inhibitor or efavirenz.
					2. If women do not receive antepartum/ intrapartum ART prophylaxis, infants should receive zidovudine for 6 weeks.
					3. Infants born to HIV-infected women should have an HIV viral load checked at 14 days, at 1–2 months, and at 4–6 months.
						http://www.guidelines.gov/content.aspx?id=16305

Disease Management	Organization	Date	Population	Recommendations	Comments	Source
				HUMAN IMMUNODEFICIENCY VIRUS, PREGNANCY		

Human Immunodeficiency Virus (HIV), Pregnancy (continued)				5. Antepartum monitoring:
				   a. Monitor CD4 count every 3 months.
				   b. HIV viral load should be assessed 2–4 weeks after initiating or changing ART, monthly until undetectable, and then at 34–36 weeks.
				   c. Recommend a first-trimester ultrasound to confirm dating.
				   d. Screen for gestational diabetes at 24–28 weeks.
				 6. Scheduled cesarean delivery is recommended for HIV-infected women who have HIV RNA levels > 1000 copies/mL and intact membranes near term.
				 7. Intrapartum IV zidovudine is recommended for all HIV-infected pregnant women.
				 8. Avoid artificial rupture of membranes.
				 9. Avoid routine use of fetal scalp electrodes.
				 10. Breast-feeding is not recommended.		

HUMAN IMMUNODEFICIENCY VIRUS, ANTIRETROVIRAL THERAPY (ART)

Disease Management	Organization	Date	Population	Recommendations	Comments	Source

Human Immunodeficiency Virus (HIV), Antiretroviral Therapy (ART)	HHS	2010	HIV-infected children	1. ART is recommended for all children with symptomatic HIV disease.
				2. Recommends ART for:
				  a. Infants aged < 12 months
				  b. Asymptomatic children with HIV RNA ≥ 100,000 copies/mL
				  c. Children aged 1–5 years with CD4 < 25%
				  d. Children aged ≥ 5 years with CD4 < 350 cells/mm^3
				  e. Children aged ≥ 1 year with acquired immunodeficiency syndrome (AIDS) or symptomatic HIV infection
				3. HIV genotype testing is recommended:
				  a. Prior to initiation of therapy in all treatment-naïve children
				  b. Prior to changing therapy for treatment failure
				4. Recommends evaluating all children 4–8 weeks after initiation of ART for possible side effects and to evaluate response to therapy.
				  a. Reevaluate children every 3–4 months thereafter.
					Specific ART recommendations are beyond the scope of this book.	http://www.guidelines.gov/content.aspx?id=23916

HYPERTENSION: INITIATING TREATMENT
Source: **THE 7TH REPORT OF THE JOINT NATIONAL COMMITTEE ON PREVENTION, DETECTION, EVALUATION, AND TREATMENT OF HIGH BLOOD PRESSURE, 2003**

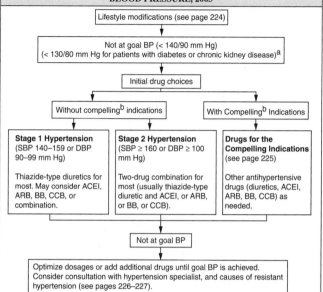

ACEI, ACE inhibitor; ARB, angiotensin receptor blocker; BB, beta-blocker; CCB, calcium channel blocker.

[a]AHA also recommends BP < 130/80 mm Hg for patients with known CHD, carotid artery disease, peripheral arterial disease, abdominal aortic aneurysm, or 10-year Framingham risk score ≥ 10%; and BP < 120/80 for patients with left ventricular dysfunction. (*Circulation*. 2007;115:2761–2788)

[b]Compelling indications: CHF, high CHD risk, diabetes, chronic kidney disease, recurrent stroke prevention, post-MI.

Source: JNC VII, 2003. (*Hypertension*. 2003;42:1206–1252)

Note: Similar recommendations from the Canadian Hypertension Education Program (http://www.hypertension.ca), and the joint European Society of Hypertension and European Society of Cardiology Task Force [*J Hypertension*. 2007;25(9):1751–1762].

Cochrane review (2007): Available evidence does not support use of BB as first-line drugs in treatment of hypertension. BB were inferior to CCB, renin-angiotensin system inhibitors, and thiazide diuretics (although most trials used atenolol). [*Cochrane Database of Systematic Reviews* 2007, Issue 1 (CD002003), http://www.cochrane.org]

LIFESTYLE MODIFICATIONS FOR TREATMENT OF HYPERTENSION[a,b]

Modification	Recommendation	Approximate SBP Reduction (Range)
Weight reduction	Maintain normal body weight (BMI 18.5–24.9 kg/m^2).	5–20 mm Hg per 10-kg weight loss
Adopt DASH eating plan	Consume diet rich in fruits, vegetables, and low-fat dairy products with a reduced content of saturated and total fat.	8–14 mm Hg
Dietary sodium reduction	Reduce dietary sodium intake to less than 100 mmol/day (2.4 g sodium or 6 g sodium chloride).	2–8 mm Hg
Physical activity	Engage in regular aerobic physical activity such as brisk walking (at least 30 min/day, most days of the week).	4–9 mm Hg
Moderation of alcohol consumption	Limit consumption to no more than 2 drinks (1 oz or 30 mL ethanol; eg, 24 oz beer, 10 oz wine, or 3 oz 80-proof whiskey) per day in most men and to no more than 1 drink per day in women and lighter-weight persons.	2–4 mm Hg

[a]For overall cardiovascular risk reduction, stop smoking.
[b]The effects of implementing these modifications are dose-and time dependent and could be greater for some individuals.
DASH = Dietary Approaches to Stop Hypertension
DASH diet found to be effective in lowering SBP in adolescents.
Source: J Pediatr. 2008;152(4):494–501

RECOMMENDED MEDICATIONS FOR COMPELLING INDICATIONS

Compelling Indication[a]	Diuretic	BB	ACEI	ARB	CCB	AldoANT
Heart failure	X	X	X	X		X
Post-MI		X	X			X
High coronary disease risk	X	X	X		X	
Diabetes	X	X	X	X	X	
Chronic kidney disease[b]			X	X		
Recurrent stroke prevention	X		X			

ACEI, ACE inhibitor; ARB, angiotensin receptor blocker;
AldoANT, aldosterone antagonist; BB, beta-blocker; CCB, calcium channel blocker
[a]Compelling indications for antihypertensive drugs are based on benefits from outcome studies or existing clinical guidelines; the compelling indication is managed in parallel with the BP.
[b]ALLHAT: Patients with hypertension and reduced GFR: no difference in renal outcomes (development of ESRD and/or decrement in GFR of $\geq$ 50% from baseline) comparing amlodipine, lisinopril, and chlorthalidone. (*Arch Intern Med.* 2005 Apr 25;165(8):936–946) Data do *not* support preference for CCB, alpha-blockers, or ACEI compared with thiazide diuretics in patients with metabolic syndrome [*Arch Intern Med.* 2008;168(2):207–217].
Note: UCSD Statin Study found modest reduction in SBP and DBP with both simvastatin and pravastatin [*Arch Intern Med.* 2008;168(7):721–727].

HYPERTENSION: CHILDREN AND ADOLESCENTS

Indications for Antihypertensive Drug Therapy in Children and Adolescents

- Symptomatic hypertension
- Secondary hypertension
- Hypertensive target organ damage
- Diabetes (types 1 and 2)
- Persistent hypertension despite nonpharmacologic measures (weight management counseling if overweight; physical activity; diet management)

Sources: Pediatrics. 2004;114:555–576 and *Circulation.* 2006:2710–2738

REFRACTORY HYPERTENSION
Source: **AMERICAN COLLEGE OF CARDIOLOGY/AMERICAN HEART ASSOCIATION/EUROPEAN SOCIETY OF CARDIOLOGY**

Definition:
Failure to reach BP goal (< 140/90 mm Hg, or 130/80 mm Hg in patients with diabetes, heart disease, or chronic kidney disease) using three different antihypertensive drug classes.

Incidence: 20%–30% of HTN patients

Common Causes:
1. Nonadherence to drugs/diet
2. Suboptimal therapy/BP measurement (fluid retention, inadequate dosage)
3. Diet/drug interactions (caffeine, cocaine, alcohol, nicotine, NSAIDs, steroids, BCP, erythropoietin, natural licorice, herbs)
4. Common secondary causes:
   > Obstructive sleep apnea
   > Diabetes
   > Chronic kidney disease
   > Renal artery stenosis
   > Obesity
   > Endocrine disorders (primary hyperaldosteronism, hyperthyroidism, hyperparathyroidism, Cushing's syndrome), pheochromocytoma

Therapy:
- Exclude nonadherence and incorrect BP measurement
- Review drug and diet history
- Screen for secondary causes:

History of sleep disorders/daytime sleepiness/tachycardias/BPs in both arms
Routine labs: sodium, potassium, creatinine, CBC, ECG, urinalysis, blood glucose, cholesterol
Additional evaluation: aldosterone:renin ratio/renal ultrasound with Doppler flow study/serum or urine catecholamine levels/morning cortisol level

- Lifestyle therapy:

Weight loss (10-kg weight loss results in a 5–20 mm Hg decrease in SBP); diet consult for low sodium (2.3 g daily), high fiber, and high potassium (DASH diet results in an 8–14 mm Hg decrease in SBP); exercise aerobic training results in a 4–9 mm Hg decrease in SBP; and restriction of excess alcohol (1 oz in men and 0.5 oz in women) results in a 2–4 mm Hg decrease in SBP

- Pharmacologic therapy:

Consider volume overload
- Switch from HCTZ to chlorthalidone (especially if GFR < 40 mL/min)
- Switch to loop diuretic if GFR < 30 mL/min (e.g., furosemide 40 mg bid)
- Use CCB (amlodipine or nifedipine) + ACE inhibitor or ARB

Consider catecholamine excess
- Switch to vasodilating beta-blocker (carvedilol, labetalol, nebivolol)

Consider aldosterone excess (even with normal serum K + level)
- Spironolactone or eplerenone

Finally, consider hydralazine or minoxidil
   > If already on beta-blocker, clonidine adds little BP benefit

REFRACTORY HYPERTENSION (CONTINUED)
Source: **AMERICAN COLLEGE OF CARDIOLOGY/AMERICAN HEART ASSOCIATION/EUROPEAN SOCIETY OF CARDIOLOGY**

- Nonpharmacologic therapy: still under investigation

  Carotid baroreceptor stimulation (*Hypertension.* 2010;55:1–8)

     May lower BP 33/22 mm Hg

  Renal artery nerve ablation (*N Engl J Med.* 2009;361:932–934)

     May lower BP 32/12 mm Hg with no change in GFR

BP, blood pressure; HTN, hypertension; NSAIDs, nonsteroidal anti-inflammatory drugs; BCP, birth control pill; CBC, complete blood count; ECG, electrocardiogram; SBP, systolic blood pressure; DASH diet, Dietary Approaches to Stop Hypertension diet; HCTZ, hydrochlorothiazide; GFR, glomerular filtration rate; bid, twice a day; CCB, calcium channel blocker; ACE, angiotensin-converting enzyme; ARB, angiotensin receptor blocker.
Sources: AHA Scientific Statement 2008. *Circulation.* 117:e510–e526. JNC VII. *Arch Intern Med.* 2003;289:2560–2572. European 2007 Guidelines. 2007;28:1462–1536.

Disease Management	Organization	Date	Population	Recommendations	Comments	Source
INFLUENZA						

Influenza	IDSA	2009	Adults and children	1. Antiviral treatment is recommended for:
				  a. Lab-confirmed cases of influenza within 48 hours of symptom onset.
				  b. Strongly suspected influenza within 48 hours of symptom onset.
				  c. Hospitalized patients with severe, complicated, or progressive lab-confirmed influenza or influenza-like illness with high likelihood of complications even if >48 hours from symptom onset.
				2. Antiviral options include oseltamivir and zanamivir.
				  a. Oseltamivir for influenza A or B: 75 mg by mouth (PO) twice daily (bid) (adults); 30 mg PO bid (≤ 15 kg); 45 mg PO bid (16–23 kg); 60 mg PO bid (24–40 kg); 75 mg PO bid (> 40 kg or aged ≥ 13 years) × 5 days
				    i. Avoid in children aged < 1 year
				  b. Zanamivir for influenza A or B: 2 puffs bid × 5 days (children aged ≥ 7 years and adults)
				    i. Avoid in asthmatic patients
					1. Consider an influenza nasal swab for diagnosis during influenza season in:
					  a. Persons with acute onset of fever and respiratory illness
					  b. Persons with fever and acute exacerbation of chronic lung disease
					  c. Infants and children with fever of unclear etiology
					  d. Severely ill persons with fever or hypothermia
					2. Rapid influenza antigen tests have a 70%–90% sensitivity in children and a 40%–60% sensitivity in adults.
					3. Direct or indirect fluorescent antibody staining are useful screening tests.
					4. Influenza PCR may be used as a confirmatory test.
						http://www.guidelines.gov/content.aspx?id=14173

Disease Management	Organization	Date	Population	Recommendations	Comments	Source
KIDNEY DISEASE, CHRONIC						

Kidney Disease, Chronic	NICE	2008	Adults	1. Recommends the modification of diet in renal disease (MDRD) equation to estimate GFR.
				 a. Advise patients not to eat any meat in the 12 hours before a blood test for GFR estimation.
				 b. Frequency of GFR testing by chronic kidney disease (CKD) stage:
				    i. Stages 1–2: annually
				    ii. Stage 3: every 6 months
				    iii. Stage 4: every 3 months
				    iv. Stage 5: every 6 weeks
				 2. Recommends urine albumin to creatinine ratio (ACR) to detect low levels of proteinuria.
				 a. Levels $\geq$ 30 mg/mmol are significant
				 3. Recommends checking for urinary tract malignancy for persistent hematuria.
				 4. Recommends a renal ultrasound in CKD and if patient is/has:
				 a. A GFR decline > 5 mL/min/1.73m^2 in 1 year or > 10 mL/min/1.73m^2 in 5 years
				 b. Persistent hematuria
				 c. Symptoms of urinary tract obstruction
				 d. Aged > 20 years and has a family history of polycystic kidney disease
				 e. Stage 4–5 CKD
				 f. Being considered for a renal biopsy
						http://www.nice.org.uk/nicemedia/live/12069/42117/42117.pdf

Disease Management	Organization	Date	Population	Recommendations	Comments	Source
KIDNEY DISEASE, CHRONIC						

Kidney Disease, Chronic (continued)				5. Recommends nephrology referral for:
				  a. Stage 4–5 CKD
				  b. ACR ≥ 70 mg/mmol
				  c. Proteinuria ≥ 1 g/24 h
				  d. Poorly controlled HTN
				  e. Suspected renal artery stenosis
				  f. Rapidly progressive renal impairment
				6. Recommends a check of serum calcium, phosphate, intact parathyroid hormone (iPTH), 25-OH vitamin D, and hemoglobin levels for all stage 4–5 CKD.		

KIDNEY DISEASE, CHRONIC-MINERAL AND BONE DISORDERS (CKD-MBDS)

Disease Management	Organization	Date	Population	Recommendations	Comments	Source

Kidney Disease, Chronic-Mineral and Bone Disorders (CKD-MBDs)	NKF	2009	Adults and children	1. Recommends monitoring serum calcium, phosphorus, iPTH, and alkaline phosphatase levels for:
				  a. Stage 3 CKD (adults)
				  b. Stage 2 CKD (children)
				2. Measure 25-OH vitamin D levels beginning in stage 3 CKD.
				3. Recommends treating all vitamin D deficiency with vitamin D supplementation.
				4. In stages 3–5 CKD, consider a bone biopsy before bisphosphonate therapy if adynamic bone disease is a possibility.
				5. In stages 3–5 CKD, aim to normalize calcium and phosphorus levels.
				6. In Stage 5 CKD, maintain a PTH level of 130–600 pg/mL.
					1. Options for oral phosphate binders:
					  a. Calcium acetate
					  b. Calcium carbonate
					  c. Calcium citrate
					  d. Sevelamer-HCl
					  e. Sevelamer carbonate
					  f. Lanthanum carbonate
						http://www.kdigo.org/guidelines/mbd/index.html

KIDNEY STONES

Disease Management	Organization	Date	Population	Recommendations	Comments	Source

Kidney Stones	EAU	2010	Adults and children with kidney stone disease	1. Recommended imaging study for patients with acute flank pain is a non-contrast CT urogram.
				2. Recommended evaluation for renal colic:
				  a. Urinalysis
				  b. Serum CBC, creatinine, uric acid, calcium, and albumin
				  c. Stone analysis by x-ray crystallography or infrared spectroscopy
				3. Recommends 24-hour urine analysis for complicated calcium stone disease: calcium; oxalate; citrate; creatinine; urate; magnesium; phosphate; sodium; and phosphate.
				4. Recommends a thiazide diuretic for patients with hypercalciuria.
				5. Recommends treatment with an alkaline citrate for hypocitraturia, type 1 renal tubular acidosis (RTA), hypercalciuria, and hyperoxaluria.
				6. Recommends that adults with a history of urinary stones drink sufficient water to maintain a urine output ≥ 2 L/day.
				7. Consider use of an alpha receptor blocker to facilitate spontaneous passage of ureteral stones < 10 mm.
				8. Consider active ureteral stone removal for persistent obstruction, failure of spontaneous passage, or the presence of severe, unremitting colic.
				  a. Options include shockwave lithotripsy or ureteroscopy
					1. Patients at high risk for recurrent stone formation:
					  a. ≥ 3 stones in 3 years
					  b. Infection stones
					  c. Urate stones
					  d. Children and adolescents with stones
					  e. Cystinuria
					  f. Primary hyperoxaluria
					  g. Type 1 RTA
					  h. Cystic fibrosis
					  i. Hyperparathyroidism
					  j. Crohn's disease
					  k. Malabsorption syndromes
					  l. Nephrocalcinosis
					  m. Family history of kidney stone disease
						http://www.uroweb.org/gls/pdf/Urolithiasis%202010.pdf

BACK PAIN, LOW

Disease Management	Organization	Date	Population	Recommendations	Comments	Source

Back Pain, Low	NICE	2009	Adults	1. Educate patients and promote self-management of low back pain.
				2. Recommends offering one of the following treatment options:
				  a. Structure exercise program
				  b. Manual therapy[a]
				  c. Acupuncture
				3. Consider a psychology referral for patients with a high disability and/or who experience significant psychological distress from their low back pain.
				4. Recommends against routine lumbar spine x-rays.
				5. Recommends an MRI scan of lumbar spine only if spinal fusion is under consideration.
				6. Consider a referral for surgery in patients with refractory, severe nonspecific low back pain who have completed the programs above and would consider spinal fusion.
					1. Analgesic ladder for low back pain
					  a. Recommend scheduled acetaminophen
					  b. Add nonsteroidal anti-inflammatory drugs (NSAIDs) and/or weak opioids
					  c. Consider adding a tricyclic antidepressant
					  d. Consider a strong opioid for short-term use for people in severe pain.
					  e. Refer for specialist assessment for people who may require prolonged use of strong opioids
						http://www.nice.org.uk/nicemedia/live/11887/44343/44343.pdf

	ICSI	2010	Adults	See table.		http://www.icsi.org/low_back_pain/adult_low_back_pain__8.html

[a]Manual therapy includes spinal manipulation, spinal mobilization, and massage.

EVALUATION AND MANAGEMENT OF ACUTE LOW BACK PAIN
Source: ICSI, November 2010

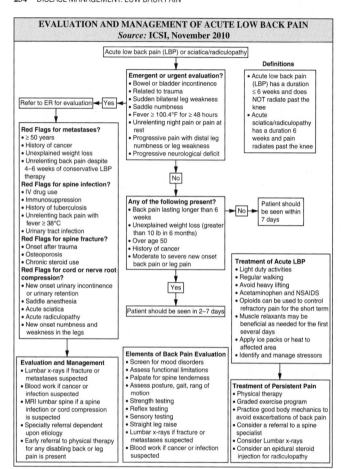

Acute low back pain (LBP) or sciatica/radiculopathy

Emergent or urgent evaluation?
- Bowel or bladder incontinence
- Related to trauma
- Sudden bilateral leg weakness
- Saddle numbness
- Fever ≥ 100.4°F for ≥ 48 hours
- Unrelenting night pain or pain at rest
- Progressive pain with distal leg numbness or leg weakness
- Progressive neurological deficit

Refer to ER for evaluation ◄— Yes

Definitions
- Acute low back pain (LBP) has a duration ≤ 6 weeks and does NOT radiate past the knee
- Acute sciatica/radiculopathy has a duration 6 weeks and pain radiates past the knee

No

Any of the following present?
- Back pain lasting longer than 6 weeks
- Unexplained weight loss (greater than 10 lb in 6 months)
- Over age 50
- History of cancer
- Moderate to severe new onset back pain or leg pain

No ► Patient should be seen within 7 days

Yes

Patient should be seen in 2–7 days

Red Flags for metastases?
- ≥ 50 years
- History of cancer
- Unexplained weight loss
- Unrelenting back pain despite 4–6 weeks of conservative LBP therapy

Red Flags for spine infection?
- IV drug use
- Immunosuppression
- History of tuberculosis
- Unrelenting back pain with fever ≥ 38°C
- Urinary tract infection

Red Flags for spine fracture?
- Onset after trauma
- Osteoporosis
- Chronic steroid use

Red Flags for cord or nerve root compression?
- New onset urinary incontinence or urinary retention
- Saddle anesthesia
- Acute sciatica
- Acute radiculopathy
- New onset numbness and weakness in the legs

Evaluation and Management
- Lumbar x-rays if fracture or metastases suspected
- Blood work if cancer or infection suspected
- MRI lumbar spine if a spine infection or cord compression is suspected
- Specialty referral dependent upon etiology
- Early referral to physical therapy for any disabling back or leg pain is present

Elements of Back Pain Evaluation
- Screen for mood disorders
- Assess functional limitations
- Palpate for spine tenderness
- Assess posture, gait, rang of motion
- Strength testing
- Reflex testing
- Sensory testing
- Straight leg raise
- Lumbar x-rays if fracture or metastases suspected
- Blood work if cancer or infection suspected

Treatment of Acute LBP
- Light duty activities
- Regular walking
- Avoid heavy lifting
- Acetaminophen and NSAIDS
- Opioids can be used to control refractory pain for the short term
- Muscle relaxants may be beneficial as needed for the first several days
- Apply ice packs or heat to affected area
- Identify and manage stressors

Treatment of Persistent Pain
- Physical therapy
- Graded exercise program
- Practice good body mechanics to avoid exacerbations of back pain
- Consider a referral to a spine specialist
- Consider Lumbar x-rays
- Consider an epidural steroid injection for radiculopathy

METABOLIC SYNDROME: IDENTIFICATION & MANAGEMENT
Source: NCEP, ATP III, 2005

Clinical Identification

Risk Factor	Defining Level[a]
Abdominal obesity (waist circumference)[b]	
Men	> 102 cm (> 40 in)
Women	> 88 cm (> 35 in)
Triglycerides	≥ 150 mg/dL
HDL cholesterol	
Men	< 40 mg/dL
Women	< 50 mg/dL
Blood pressure	≥ 135 / ≥ 85 mm Hg
Fasting glucose	≥ 100 mg/dL

Management
- First-line therapy: Lifestyle modification leading to weight reduction and increased physical activity
- Goal: ↓ Body weight by ~ 7%–10% over 6–12 months
- At least 30 minutes of daily moderate-intensity physical activity
- Low intake of saturated fats, trans fats, and cholesterol
- Reduced consumption of simple sugars
- Increased intake of fruits, vegetables, and whole grains
- Avoid extremes in intake of either carbohydrates or fats
- Smoking cessation
- Drug therapy for HTN, elevated LDL cholesterol, and diabetes
- Consider combination therapy with fibrates or nicotinic acid plus a statin
- Low-dose ASA for patients at intermediate and high risk
- Bariatric surgery for BMI > 35 mg/kg^2
- If one component is identified, a systematic search for the others is indicated, together with an active approach to managing all risk factors. (*Eur Heart J.* 2007;28:2375–2414)
- Metabolic syndrome is associated with the presence of subclinical ischemic brain lesions independent of other risk factors. (*Stroke.* 2008;39:1607–1609)
- In patients with atherosclerosis, the presence of metabolic syndrome is associated with an increased risk of cardiovascular event and all-cause mortality, independent of the presence of diabetes. (*Eur Heart J.* 2008;29:213–223)

HDL, high-density lipoprotein; LDL, low-density lipoprotein; ASA, aspirin; BMI, body mass index; HTN, hypertension

[a]NCEP ATP III definition (*Circulation.* 2005;112:2735–2752)—Requires any 3 of the listed components.
[b]Waist circumference can identify persons at greater cardiometabolic risk than are identified by BMI alone. However, further studies are needed to establish waist circumference cutpoints that assess risk not adequately captured by BMI. (*Am J Clin Nutr.* 2007;85:1197–1202)
Note: The World Health Organization (WHO) and International Diabetes Federation (IDF, http://www.idf.org) define metabolic syndrome slightly differently. One study found a 5-fold difference in the prevalence of metabolic syndrome depending on which of seven diagnostic criteria were used [*Metabolism.* 2008;57(3):355–361] There is no official definition of metabolic syndrome in children, but a constellation of conditions confers significant increased risk of coronary heart disease. (*Circulation.* 2007;115:1948–1967)

TREATMENT OF METHICILLIN-RESISTANT *STAPHYLOCOCCUS AUREUS* INFECTIONS (MRSA) IN ADULTS AND CHILDREN

Source: IDSA 2011 Clinical Practice Guideline: *Clin Infect Dis.* 2011;52:1–38

Infection	Primary Therapy	Alternative Therapy	Comments

Abscess associated with extensive involvement; cellulitis; systemic illness; immunosuppression; extremes of age; involvement of face, hands, or genitalia; septic phlebitis; trauma; infected ulcer or burn; or poor response to incision and drainage	1. Incision and drainage
	2. Antibiotics
	  a. Outpatient
	    i. Clindamycin
	    ii. Trimethoprim-sulfamethoxazole (TMP-SMX)
	  b. Inpatient
	    i. Vancomycin
	    ii. Linezolid
	    iii. Daptomycin
		1. Outpatient antibiotics
		  a. Tetracycline
		  b. Linezolid
		2. Inpatient antibiotics
		  a. Telavancin
		  b. Clindamycin
			1. Tetracyclines should not be used in children aged < 8 years.
			2. Vancomycin is recommended for hospitalized children.
			3. Clindamycin and linezolid are alternative choices for children.

Recurrent skin and soft tissue infections (SSTIs)	1. Cover draining wounds.
	2. Maintain good hygiene.
	3. Avoid reusing or sharing personal toiletries.
	4. Use oral antibiotics only for active infections.
		1. Decolonization only if recurrent SSTI despite good hygiene
		  a. Mupirocin per nares bid × 5–10 days
		  b. Chlorhexidine or dilute bleach baths twice weekly (biw) × 1–2 weeks
			Screening cultures prior to decolonization or surveillance cultures after decolonization is not recommended.

Uncomplicated MRSA bacteremia[a]	Vancomycin × 2 weeks	Daptomycin × 2 weeks	Echocardiography is recommended for all MRSA bacteremia

TREATMENT OF METHICILLIN-RESISTANT *STAPHYLOCOCCUS AUREUS* INFECTIONS (MRSA) IN ADULTS AND CHILDREN (CONTINUED)

Source: IDSA 2011 Clinical Practice Guideline: *Clin Infect Dis.* 2011;52:1–38

Infection	Primary Therapy	Alternative Therapy	Comments
MRSA native valve endocarditis	Vancomycin × 6 weeks	Daptomycin × 6 weeks	1. Synergistic gentamicin or rifampin is not indicated for native valve endocarditis. 2. Vancomycin is the drug of choice for children.
MRSA prosthetic valve endocarditis	1. Vancomycin plus rifampin × 6 weeks 2. Gentamicin 1 mg/kg IV q8h × 2 weeks		Recommend early evaluation for valve replacement surgery.
MRSA pneumonia	1. Vancomycin 2. Linezolid	Clindamycin	1. Duration of therapy is 7–21 days 2. Vancomycin for children
MRSA osteomyelitis	1. Surgical débridement 2. Vancomycin 3. Daptomycin 4. Duration of therapy is at least 8 weeks	1. Linezolid 2. TMP-SMX plus rifampin 3. Clindamycin	
MRSA septic arthritis	1. Drain or débride the joint space 2. Vancomycin	Daptomycin	Duration of therapy is 3–4 weeks
MRSA meningitis	1. Vancomycin × 2 weeks	1. Linezolid 2. TMP-SMX	Consider adding rifampin

[a]No endocarditis, no implanted prostheses, defervescence within 72 hours, sterile blood cultures within 72 hours, no evidence of metastatic sites of infection.

MANAGEMENT OF OBESITY IN MATURE ADOLESCENTS AND ADULTS

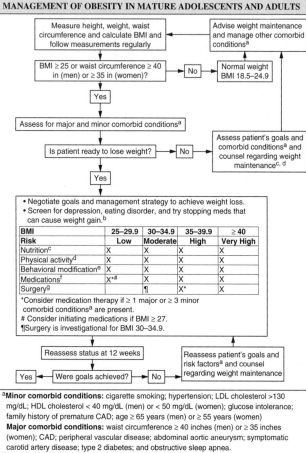

Measure height, weight, waist circumference and calculate BMI and follow measurements regularly

Advise weight maintenance and manage other comorbid conditions[a]

BMI ≥ 25 or waist circumference ≥ 40 in (men) or ≥ 35 in (women)? → No → Normal weight BMI 18.5–24.9

Yes

Assess for major and minor comorbid conditions[a]

Is patient ready to lose weight? → No → Assess patient's goals and comorbid conditions[a] and counsel regarding weight maintenance[c, d]

Yes

- Negotiate goals and management strategy to achieve weight loss.
- Screen for depression, eating disorder, and try stopping meds that can cause weight gain.[b]

BMI	25–29.9	30–34.9	35–39.9	≥ 40
Risk	Low	Moderate	High	Very High
Nutrition[c]	X	X	X	X
Physical activity[d]	X	X	X	X
Behavioral modification[e]	X	X	X	X
Medications[f]	X*#	X	X	X
Surgery[g]		¶	X*	X

*Consider medication therapy if ≥ 1 major or ≥ 3 minor comorbid conditions[a] are present.
Consider initiating medications if BMI ≥ 27.
¶Surgery is investigational for BMI 30–34.9.

Reassess status at 12 weeks

Were goals achieved? → No → Reassess patient's goals and risk factors[a] and counsel regarding weight maintenance

Yes ←

[a]**Minor comorbid conditions:** cigarette smoking; hypertension; LDL cholesterol >130 mg/dL; HDL cholesterol < 40 mg/dL (men) or < 50 mg/dL (women); glucose intolerance; family history of premature CAD; age ≥ 65 years (men) or ≥ 55 years (women)
Major comorbid conditions: waist circumference ≥ 40 inches (men) or ≥ 35 inches (women); CAD; peripheral vascular disease; abdominal aortic aneurysm; symptomatic carotid artery disease; type 2 diabetes; and obstructive sleep apnea.
[b]Sulfonylureas; thiazolidinediones; olanzapine, clozapine; resperidone, quetiapine; lithium; paroxetine, citalopram, sertraline; carbamazepine; pregabalin; corticosteroids; megestrol acetate; cyproheptadine; tricyclic antidepressants; monoamine oxidase inhibitors; mirtazapine; valproic acid; and gabapentin.
[c]Encourage a healthy, balanced diet including daily intake of ≥ 5 servings of fruits/vegetables; 35 g fiber; < 30% calories from fat; eliminate take out, fast food, soda, and desserts; dietician consultation for a calorie reduction between 500–1000 kcal/kg/day to achieve a 1–2 lb weight reduction per week.
[d]Recommend 30–60 minutes of moderate activity at least 5 days a week.

MANAGEMENT OF OBESITY IN MATURE ADOLESCENTS AND ADULTS (CONTINUED)

[e]Identify behaviors that may contribute to weight gain (stress, emotional eating, boredom) and use cognitive behavioral counseling, stimulus control, relapse prevention, and goal setting to decrease caloric intake and increase physical activity.

[f]Medications that are FDA approved for weight loss: phentermine; orlistat; phendimetrazine; diethylpropion; and benzphetamine can be used for up to 3 months as an adjunct for weight loss.

[g]Bariatric surgery is indicated for patients at high risk for complications. They should be motivated, psychologically stable, have no surgical contraindications, and must accept the operative risk involved.

Source: Adapted from the ICSI Guideline on the Prevention and Management of Obesity available at http://www.icsi.org/obesity/obesity_3398.html

Disease Management	Organization	Date	Population	Recommendations	Comments	Source
Osteoporosis	NAMS AACE	2010 2010	Postmenopausal women	1. Recommend maintaining a healthy weight, eating a balanced diet, avoiding excessive alcohol intake, avoiding cigarette smoking, and utilizing measures to avoid falls. 2. Recommend supplemental calcium 1200 mg/day and vitamin D_3 800–1000 international units (IU)/day. 3. Recommend an annual check of height and weight, and assess for chronic back pain. 4. DXA of the hip, femoral neck, and lumbar spine should be measured in women aged ≥ 65 years or postmenopausal women with a risk factor for osteoporosis.[a] 5. Recommend repeat DXA testing every 1–2 years for women taking therapy for osteoporosis and every 2–5 years for untreated postmenopausal women.	1. Options for osteoporosis drug therapy: a. Bisphosphonates i. First-line therapy ii. Options include alendronate, risedronate, or zoledronic acid b. Denosumab i. Consider for women at high fracture risk c. Raloxifene i. Second-line agent in younger women with osteoporosis d. Teriparatide is an option for high fracture risk when bisphosphonates have failed. i. Therapy should not exceed 24 months.	http://www.guidelines.gov/content.aspx?id=15500 http://www.aace.com/pub/pdf/guidelines/OsteoGuidelines2010.pdf

OSTEOPOROSIS

Disease Management	Organization	Date	Population	Recommendations	Comments	Source
OSTEOPOROSIS						

Osteoporosis (continued)				6. Recommend against measurement of biochemical markers of bone turnover.
				7. Recommend drug therapy for osteoporosis for:
				  a. Osteoporotic vertebral or hip fracture
				  b. DXA with T score ≤ −2.5
				  c. DXA with T score ≤ −1 to −2.4 and a 10-year risk of major osteoporotic fracture of ≥ 20% or hip fracture ≥ 3% based on FRAX calculator, available at http://www.shef.ac.uk/FRAX/
				8. Consider the use of hip protectors in women at high risk of falling.
					e. Calcitonin
					  i. Third-line therapy for osteoporosis
					  ii. May be used for bone pain from acute vertebral compression fractures.
					2. Vitamin D therapy should maintain a 25-OH vitamin D level between 30–60 ng/mL.	

ªPrevious fracture after menopause, weight < 127 lb, BMI < 21 kg/m², parent with a history of hip fracture, current smoker, rheumatoid arthritis, or excessive alcohol intake.

OSTEOPOROSIS, GLUCOCORTICOID-INDUCED

Disease Management	Organization	Date	Population	Recommendations	Comments	Source

Osteoporosis, Glucocorticoid-induced	ACR	2010	Glucocorticoid-induced osteoporosis	1. All patients receiving glucocorticoid therapy should receive education and assess risk factors for osteoporosis.
				2. FRAX calculator should be used to place patients at low risk, medium risk, or high risk for major osteoporotic fracture.
				3. If glucocorticoid treatment is expected to last ≥3 months, recommend:
				  a. Weight-bearing activities
				  b. Smoking cessation
				  c. Avoid >2 alcoholic drinks/day
				  d. Calcium 1200–1500 mg/day
				  e. Vitamin D 800–1000 IU/day
				  f. Fall risk assessment
				  g. Baseline DXA test and then every 2 years
				  h. Annual 25-OH vitamin D
				  i. Baseline and annual height measurement
				  j. Assessment of prevalent fragility fractures
				  k. X-rays of spine
				  l. Assessment of degree of osteoporosis medication compliance, if applicable
					1. Clinical factors that may increase the risk of osteoporotic fracture estimated by FRAX calculator:
					  a. BMI < 21 kg/m^2
					  b. Parental history of hip fracture
					  c. Current smoking
					  d. ≥3 alcoholic drinks/day
					  e. Higher glucocorticoid doses or cumulative dose
					  f. IV pulse glucocorticoid use
					  g. Declining central bone mineral density measurement
						http://www.rheumatology.org/practice/clinical/guidelines/ACR_2010_GIOP_Recomm_Clinicians_Guide.pdf

OSTEOPOROSIS, GLUCOCORTICOID-INDUCED						
Disease Management	Organization	Date	Population	Recommendations	Comments	Source

Osteoporosis, Glucocorticoid-induced (continued)				4. For postmenopausal women or men aged > 50 years:
				 a. Low-risk group
				   i. Bisphosphonate if equivalent of prednisone ≥ 7.5 mg/day
				 b. Medium-risk group
				   i. Bisphosphonate if equivalent of prednisolone ≥ 5 mg/day
				 c. High-risk group
				   i. Bisphosphonate for any dose of glucocorticoid
				 5. For premenopausal women or men aged < 50 years with a prevalent fragility (osteoporotic) fracture and glucocorticoid use ≥ 3 months:
				 a. For prednisone ≥ 5 mg/day, use alendronate or risedronate
				 b. For prednisone ≥ 7.5 mg/day, use zoledronic acid
				 c. Consider teriparatide for bisphosphonate failures
					2. Bisphosphonates recommended:
					 a. Low- to Medium-risk patients
					   i. Alendronate
					   ii. Risedronate
					   iii. Zoledronic acid
					 b. High-risk patients
					   i. Same + teriparatide	

OTITIS MEDIA, ACUTE

Disease Management	Organization	Date	Population	Recommendations	Comments	Source

Otitis Media, Acute	ICSI	2008	Children aged 3 months–18 years	1. Diagnosis should be made with pneumatic otoscopy.
				2. Children at low risk[a] should use a wait-and-see approach for 48–72 hours with oral analgesics.
				3. Recommends symptomatic relief with acetaminophen or ibuprofen and warm compresses to the ear.
				4. Educate caregivers about prevention of otitis media: encourage breast-feeding, feed child upright if bottle fed, avoid passive smoke exposure, limit exposure to groups of children, careful handwashing prior to handling child, avoid pacifier use > 10 months, ensure immunizations are up to date.
				5. Amoxicillin is the first-line antibiotic for low-risk children.
				6. Alternative medication if failure to respond to initial treatment; penicillin allergy; presence of a resistant organism found on culture.
					1. Amoxicillin is first-line therapy for low-risk children:
					  a. 40 mg/kg/day if no antibiotics used in last 3 months
					  b. 80 mg/kg/day if child is not low risk
					2. Alternative antibiotics:
					  a. Amoxicillin-clavulanate
					  b. Cefuroxime axetil
					  c. Ceftriaxone
					  d. Cefprozil
					  e. Loracarbef
					  f. Cefdinir
					  g. Cefixime
					  h. Cefpodoxime
					  i. Clarithromycin
					  j. Azithromycin
					  k. Erythromycin
						http://www.icsi.org/ otitis_media/ diagnosis_and_ treatment_of_otitis_ media_in_ children_2304.html

OTITIS MEDIA, ACUTE

Disease Management	Organization	Date	Population	Recommendations	Comments	Source

Otitis Media, Acute (continued)				7. Consider prophylactic antibiotics for recurrent acute otitis media:
				  a. ≥ 3 episodes in 6 months or ≥ 4 episodes in a year
				8. Recommends referral to an ENT specialist for a complication of otitis media: mastoiditis, facial nerve palsy, lateral sinus thrombosis, meningitis, brain abscess, or labyrinthitis.
				9. Recommends against routine recheck at 10–14 days in children feeling well.
				10. Management of otitis media with effusion:
				  a. Educate that effusion will resolve on its own
				  b. Recommends against antihistamines or decongestants
				  c. Recommends a trial of antibiotics for 10–14 days prior to referral for tympanostomy tubes		

[a]Children older than age 2 years without severe disease (temperature > 39ºC and moderate-severe otalgia), otherwise healthy, do not attend daycare, and have had no prior ear infections within the last month.

PALLIATIVE & END-OF-LIFE CARE: PAIN MANAGEMENT	
Principles of Analgesic Use	
By the mouth	The oral route is the preferred route for analgesics, including morphine.
By the clock	Persistent pain requires around-the-clock treatment to prevent further pain. As-needed (prn) dosing is irrational and inhumane; it requires patients to experience pain before becoming eligible for relief. Relief is accomplished with long-acting delayed-release preparations (fentanyl patch, slow-release morphine, or oxycodone).
By the WHO ladder	If a maximum dose of medication fails to adequately relieve pain, move up the ladder, not laterally to a different drug in the same efficiency group. Severe pain requires immediate use of an opioid recommended for controlling severe pain, without progressing sequentially through Steps 1 and 2. When using a long-acting opioid, the dose for breakthrough pain should be 10% of the 24-hour opioid dose (ie, if a patient is on 100 mg/day of an extended-release morphine preparation, their breakthrough dose is 10 mg of morphine or equivalent every 1–2 hours until pain relief is achieved.
Individualize treatment	The right dose of an analgesic is the dose that relieves pain with acceptable side effects for a specific patient.
Monitor	Monitoring is required to ensure the benefits of treatment are maximized while adverse effects are minimized.
Use adjuvant drugs	For example, a nonsteroidal anti-inflammatory drug (NSAID) is almost always needed to help control bone pain. Nonopioid analgesics, such as NSAIDs or acetaminophen, can be used at any step of the ladder. Adjuvant medications also can be used at any step to enhance pain relief or counteract the adverse effects of medications. Neuropathic pain should be treated with gabapentin, nortriptyline, or pregabalin.

Source: Reprinted with permission from the American Academy of Hospice and Palliative Medicine. *Pocket Guide to Hospice/Palliative Medicine.*

ABNORMAL PAP SMEAR ALGORITHM

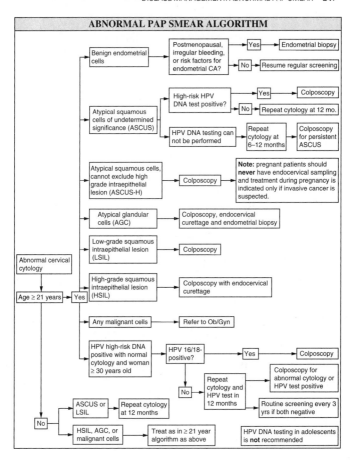

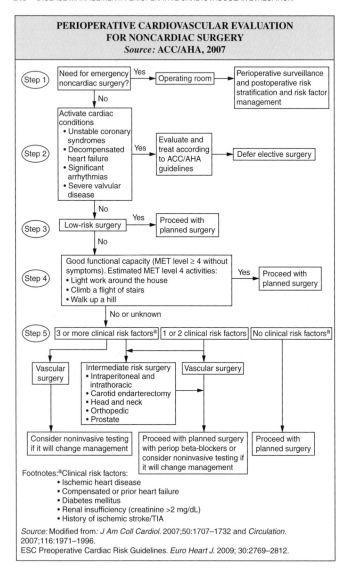

PERIOPERATIVE CARDIOVASCULAR EVALUATION FOR NONCARDIAC SURGERY
Source: ACC/AHA, 2007

Step 1 — Need for emergency noncardiac surgery? → Yes → Operating room → Perioperative surveillance and postoperative risk stratification and risk factor management
↓ No

Step 2 — Activate cardiac conditions
• Unstable coronary syndromes
• Decompensated heart failure
• Significant arrhythmias
• Severe valvular disease
→ Yes → Evaluate and treat according to ACC/AHA guidelines → Defer elective surgery
↓ No

Step 3 — Low-risk surgery → Yes → Proceed with planned surgery
↓ No

Step 4 — Good functional capacity (MET level ≥ 4 without symptoms). Estimated MET level 4 activities:
• Light work around the house
• Climb a flight of stairs
• Walk up a hill
→ Yes → Proceed with planned surgery
↓ No or unknown

Step 5 — 3 or more clinical risk factors[a] | 1 or 2 clinical risk factors | No clinical risk factors[a]

Vascular surgery | Intermediate risk surgery
• Intraperitoneal and intrathoracic
• Carotid endarterectomy
• Head and neck
• Orthopedic
• Prostate | Vascular surgery |

Consider noninvasive testing if it will change management | Proceed with planned surgery with periop beta-blockers or consider noninvasive testing if it will change management | Proceed with planned surgery

Footnotes: [a]Clinical risk factors:
• Ischemic heart disease
• Compensated or prior heart failure
• Diabetes mellitus
• Renal insufficiency (creatinine >2 mg/dL)
• History of ischemic stroke/TIA

Source: Modified from: *J Am Coll Cardiol.* 2007;50:1707–1732 and *Circulation.* 2007;116:1971–1996.
ESC Preoperative Cardiac Risk Guidelines. *Euro Heart J.* 2009; 30:2769–2812.

PERIOPERATIVE CARDIOVASCULAR EVALUATION
Source: ACCF/AHA/ESC, 2009

Perioperative Beta-Blocker Therapy:

- Perioperative beta-blocker recommendations have become more limited.
- Chronic beta-blocker should be continued to prevent rebound HTN, arrhythmias, or myocardial infarction.
- Beta-blockers titrated to heart rate and blood pressure are *probably recommended* for patients undergoing vascular surgery who have CAD or findings of ischemia on preoperative testing.
- Beta-blockers titrated to heart rate and blood pressure are *probably recommended* for patients undergoing intermediate surgery who have CAD or ≥ 1 clinical risk factors.
- Beta-blockers should optimally be started 30 days before surgery, but at least 1 week prior to surgery to allow titrating dose to optimal heart rate and blood pressure.
- Initiation of high-dose beta-blockers should NOT be administered for *potential* benefit due to the observed increased risk of overall death, stroke, and risk of hemodynamic instability. (POISE Trial. *Lancet.* 2008;371:1839–1847)
- A long-acting beta-blocker should be used without intrinsic sympathomimetic activity.
- Beta-blocker therapy should be continued at least 2 months in the postoperative period if there is no other indication for long-term use.

Sources: ACC/AHA 2007 Guidelines. *J Am Coll Cardiol.* 2007;50:1707–1732. 2009 Focused Update on Perioperative Beta Blockade. *J Am Coll Cardiol.* 2009;54(22):2102–2128. European Guidelines. *Euro Heart J.* 2009;30:2769–2812.

PNEUMONIA, COMMUNITY-ACQUIRED: EVALUATION
Source: IDSA, ATS, 2007

Diagnostic Testing	Admission Decision

• CXR or other chest imaging required for diagnosis
• Sputum Gram stain and culture
  • Outpatients: optional
  • Inpatients: if unusual or antibiotic resistance suspected
	• Severity of illness (eg, CURB-65) and prognostic indices (eg, PSI) support decision
	• One must still recognize social and individual factors

CURB-65		Pneumonia Severity Index	
(*Thorax*. 2003;58:337–382)		(*NEJM*. 1997;336:243–250)	

Clinical Factor	Points	Demographic Factor	Points
Confusion	1	Demographic factor	
BUN > 19 mg/dL	1	Men age	Age in years
Respiratory rate ≥ 30 breaths/min	1	Women age	Age in years −10
Systolic BP < 90 mm Hg or Diastolic BP ≤ 60 mm Hg	1	Nursing home resident	+10
Aged > 65 years	1	Coexisting illnesses	
Total points		Neoplastic disease	+30
		Liver disease	+20
• CURB-65 ≥ 2 suggest need for hospitalization		Congestive heart failure	+10
		Cerebrovascular disease	+10
		Renal disease	+10

Score	In-hospital mortality
0	0.7%
1	3.2%
2	3.0%
3	17%
4	42%
5	57%

Physical exam findings	
Altered mental status	+20
Respiratory rate 30 breaths/min	+20
Systolic BP < 90 mm Hg	+20
Temperature < 35°C (95°F)	+15
Temperature > 40°C (104°F)	+15
Pulse > 125 beats/min	+10

Laboratory and radiographic findings	
Arterial blood pH < 7.35	+30
BUN > 30 mg/dL	+20
Sodium level < 130 mmol/L	+20
Glucose level > 250 mg/dL	+10
Hematocrit < 30%	+10
PaO_2 < 60 mm Hg or O_2 sat. < 90%	+10
Pleural effusion	+10

Add up total points to estimate mortality risk

Class	Points	Overall Mortality
I	<51	0.1%
II	51–70	0.6%
III	71–90	0.9%
IV	91–130	9.5%
V	> 130	26.7%

CXR, chest x-ray; CURB-65, confusion, urea nitrogen, respiratory rate, blood pressure, 65 years of age and older; PSI, pneumonia severity index; BP, blood pressure; BUN, blood urea nitrogen
Sources: IDSA and ATS Consensus Guidelines, 2007. (*Clin Infect Diseases*. 2007;44:S27–S72)
Pneumonia Severity Index. (*NEJM*. 1997;336:243)

PNEUMONIA, COMMUNITY-ACQUIRED: SUSPECTED PATHOGENS
Source: IDSA, ATS, 2007

Condition and Risk Factors	Commonly Encountered Pathogens
Alcoholism	*Streptococcus pneumoniae*, oral anaerobes, *Klebsiella pneumoniae*, *Acinetobacter* species, *Mycobacterium tuberculosis*
COPD and/or smoking	*Haemophilus influenzae*, *Pseudomonas aeruginosa*, *Legionella* species, *S. pneumoniae*, *Moraxella catarrhalis*, *Chlamydia pneumoniae*
Aspiration	Gram-negative enteric pathogens, oral anaerobes
Lung abscess	CA-MRSA, oral anaerobes, endemic fungal pneumonia, *M. tuberculosis*, and atypical mycobacteria
Exposure to bat or bird droppings	*Histoplasma capsulatum*
Exposure to birds	*Chlamydophila psittaci* (if poultry: avian influenza)
Exposure to rabbits	*Francisella tularensis*
Exposure to farm animals or parturient cats	*Coxiella burnetii* (Q fever)
HIV infection (early)	*S. pneumoniae*, *H. influenzae*, and *M. tuberculosis*
HIV infection (late)	The pathogens listed for early infection plus *Pneumocystis jiroveci*, *Cryptococcus*, *Histoplasma*, *Aspergillus*, atypical mycobacteria (especially *Mycobacterium kansasii*), *P. aeruginosa*, *H. influenzae*
Hotel or cruise ship stay in previous 2 weeks	*Legionella* species
Travel to or residence in southwestern United States	*Coccidioides* species, *Hantavirus*
Travel to or residence in Southeast and East Asia	*Burkholderia pseudomallei*, avian influenza, SARS
Influenza active in community	Influenza, *S. pneumoniae*, *S. aureus*, *H. influenzae*
Cough ≥ 2 weeks with whoop or posttussive vomiting	*Bordetella pertussis*
Structural lung disease (eg, bronchiectasis)	*P. aeruginosa*, *Burkholderia cepacia*, and *S. aureus*
Injection drug use	*S. aureus*, anaerobes, *M. tuberculosis*, and *S. pneumoniae*
Endobronchial obstruction	Anaerobes, *S. pneumoniae*, *H. influenzae*, *S. aureus*
In context of bioterrorism	*Bacillus anthracis* (anthrax), *Yersinia pestis* (plague), *Francisella tularensis* (tularemia)

CA-MRSA, community-acquired methicillin-resistant *S. aureus*; COPD, chronic obstructive pulmonary disease; SARS, severe acute respiratory syndrome

ROUTINE PRENATAL CARE

Preconception Visit

1. Measure height, weight, blood pressure, and total and HDL cholesterol.
2. Determine rubella, rubeola, and varicella immunity status.
3. Assess all patients for pregnancy risk: substance abuse, domestic violence, sexual abuse, psychiatric disorders, risk factors for preterm labor, exposure to chemicals or infectious agents, hereditary disorders, gestational diabetes, or chronic medical problems.
4. Educate patients about proper nutrition; offer weight reduction strategies for obese patients.
5. Immunize if not current on the following: Tdap, MMR, varicella, or hepatitis B vaccine.
6. Initiate folic acid 400–800 mcg/day; 4 mg/day for a history of a child affected by a neural tube defect.

Initial Prenatal Visit

1. Medical, surgical, social, family, and obstetrical history and do complete exam
2. Pap smear, urine NAAT for gonorrhea and *Chlamydia*, and assess for history of genital herpes.
3. Consider a varicella antibody test if patient unsure about prior varicella infection.
4. Urinalysis for proteinuria and glucosuria, and urine culture for asymptomatic bacteriuria.
5. Order prenatal labs to include a complete blood count, blood type, antibody screen, rubella titer, VDRL, hepatitis B surface antigen, and an HIV test.
6. Order an obstetrical ultrasound for dating if any of the following: beyond 16 weeks gestational age, unsure last menstrual period, size/dates discrepancy on exam, or for inability to hear fetal heart tones by 12 gestational weeks.
7. Discuss fetal aneuploidy screening and counseling regardless of maternal age.
8. Prenatal testing offered for: sickle cell anemia (African descent), thalassemia (African, Mediterranean, Middle Eastern, Southeast Asians), Canavan's disease and Tay-Sachs (Jewish patients), cystic fibrosis (Caucasians and Ashkenazi Jews) and Fragile X syndrome (family history of nonspecified mental retardation).
9. Place a tuberculosis skin test for all medium-to-high risk patients.[a]
10. Consider a 1 hour 50 g glucose tolerance test for certain high-risk groups.[b]
11. Obtain an operative report in all women who have had a prior cesarean section
12. Psychosocial risk assessment for mood disorders, substance abuse, or domestic violence.

Frequency of Visits for Uncomplicated Pregnancies

1. Every 4 weeks until 28 gestational weeks; q2 weeks from 28–36 weeks; weekly > 36 weeks

Routine Checks at Follow-up Prenatal Visits

1. Assess weight, blood pressure, and urine for glucose and protein.
2. Exam: edema, fundal height, and fetal heart tones at all visits; fetal presentation starting at 36 weeks.
3. Ask about regular uterine contractions, leakage of fluid, vaginal bleeding, or decreased fetal movement.
4. Discuss labor precautions.

Antepartum Lab Testing

1. All women should be offered either first trimester, second trimester, or combined testing to screen for fetal aneuploidy; invasive diagnostic testing for fetal aneuploidy should be available to all women regardless of maternal age.
   a. First trimester
   b. Second trimester screening options: amniocentesis at 14 weeks; a Quad Marker Screen at 16–18 weeks; and/or a screening ultrasound with nuchal translucency assessment
2. Consider serial transvaginal sonography of the cervix every 2–3 weeks to assess cervical length for patients at high risk for preterm delivery starting at 16 weeks.

ROUTINE PRENATAL CARE (CONTINUED)

3. No role for routine bacterial vaginosis screening.
4. 1 hour 50 g glucose tolerance test in all women between 24–28 weeks.
5. Rectovaginal swab for group B streptococcal (GBS) testing between 35–37 weeks.
6. Recommend weekly amniotic fluid assessments and twice weekly non-stress testing starting at 41 weeks.

Prenatal Counseling

1. Cessation of smoking, drinking alcohol, or use of any illicit drugs.
2. Avoid cat litter boxes, hot tubs, certain foods (ie, raw fish or unpasteurized cheese)
3. Proper nutrition and expected weight gain: National Academy of Sciences advises weight gain 28–40 lb (pre-pregnancy BMI < 20), 25–35 lb (BMI 20–26), 15–25 lb (BMI 26–29) and 15–20 lb (BMI ≥ 30).
4. Inquire about domestic violence and depression at initial visit, at 28 weeks, and at postpartum visit.
5. Recommend regular mild-moderate exercise 3 or more times a week.
6. Avoid high-altitude activities, scuba diving, and contact sports during pregnancy.
7. Benefits of breast-feeding versus bottle feeding.
8. Discuss postpartum contraceptive options (including tubal sterilization) during third trimester.
9. Discuss analgesia and anesthesia options and offer prenatal classes at 24 weeks.
10. Discuss repeat c-section versus vaginal birth after cesarean (if applicable).
11. Discuss the option of circumcision if a boy is delivered.
12. Avoid air travel and long train or car trips beyond 36 weeks.

Prenatal Interventions

1. Suppressive antiviral medications starting at 36 weeks for women with a history of genital herpes.
2. Cesarean delivery is indicated for women who are HIV-positive or have active genital herpes and are in labor.
3. For patients who report a history of abuse, offer interventions and resources to increase their safety during and after pregnancy.
4. For patients with severe depression, consider treatment with an SSRI (avoid paroxetine if possible).
5. Rh immune globulin 300 mcg IM for all Rh-negative women with negative antibody screens between 26–28 weeks.
6. Refer for nutrition counseling at 10–12 weeks for BMI < 20 kg/m² or at any time during pregnancy for inadequate weight gain.
7. Start prenatal vitamins with iron and folic acid 400–800 mcg/day and 1200 mg elemental calcium/day starting at 4 weeks preconception (or as early as possible during pregnancy) and continued until 6 weeks postpartum.
8. Give inactivated influenza vaccine IM to all pregnant women during influenza season.
9. Consider progesterone therapy IM weekly or intravaginally daily to women at high risk for preterm birth.
10. Recommend an external cephalic version at 37 weeks for all noncephalic presentations.
11. Offer labor induction to women at 41 weeks by good dates.
12. Treat all women with confirmed syphilis with penicillin G during pregnancy.
13. Treat all women with gonorrhea with ceftriaxone; follow treatment with a test of cure.
14. Treat all women with *Chlamydia* with azithromycin; follow treatment with a test of cure.
15. Treat all GBS-positive women with penicillin G when in labor or with spontaneous rupture of membranes.

ROUTINE PRENATAL CARE (CONTINUED)

Postpartum Interventions

1. Treat all infants born to HBV-positive women with hepatitis B immunoglobulin (HBIG) and initiate HBV vaccine series within 12 hours of life.
2. All women with a positive tuberculosis skin test and no evidence of active disease should receive a postpartum chest x-ray; treat with isoniazid 300 mg PO daily for 9 months if chest x-ray is negative.
3. Administer a Tdap booster if tetanus status is unknown or the last Td vaccine has been over 10 years.
4. Administer a MMR vaccine to all rubella nonimmune women.
5. Offer HPV vaccine to all women ≤ 26 weeks who have not been immunized.
6. Initiate contraception.
7. Repeat pap smear at 6 week postpartum check.

[a]Post-gastrectomy, gastric bypass, immunosuppressed (HIV-positive, diabetes, renal failure, chronic steroid/immunosuppressive therapy, head/neck or hematologic malignancies), silicosis, organ transplant recipients, malabsorptive syndromes, alcoholics, intravenous drug users, close contacts of persons with active pulmonary tuberculosis, medically underserved, low socioeconomic class, residents/ employees of long-term care facilities and jails, healthcare workers, and immigrants from endemic areas.

[b]Overweight (BMI ≥ 25 kg/m^2 and an additional risk factor: physical inactivity; first-degree relative with DM; high-risk ethnicity (eg, African-American, Latino, Native American, Asian American, Pacific Islander); history of GDM; prior baby with birthweight > 9 lb; unexplained stillbirth or malformed infant, HTN on therapy or with BP ≥140/90 mmHg; HDL cholesterol level < 35 mg/dL (0.90 mmol/L) and/or a triglyceride level > 250 mg/dL (2.82 mmol/L); polycystic ovary syndrome; history of impaired glucose tolerance with HgbA1c ≥ 5.7%; acanthosis nigicans; cardiovascular disease; or ≥ 2+ glucosuria.

Adapted from ACOG ICSI Guideline on Routine Prenatal Care, July 2010 available at http://www.icsi. org/prenatal_care_4/prenatal_care__routine__full_version__2.html and VA/DoD Clinical Practice Guideline for Management of Pregnancy, 2009 at http://www.guidelines.gov/content.aspx?id=15678

PERINATAL & POSTNATAL GUIDELINES *Source:* AAP, AAFP	
Breast-feeding	Strongly recommends education and counseling to promote breast-feeding
Hemoglobinopathies	Strongly recommends ordering screening tests for hemoglobinopathies in neonates
Hyperbilirubinemia	Perform ongoing systematic assessments during the neonatal period for the risk of an infant developing severe hyperbilirubinemia
Phenylketonuria	Strongly recommends ordering screening tests for phenylketonuria in neonates
Thyroid function abnormalities	Strongly recommends ordering screening tests for thyroid function abnormalities in neonates

Source: Pediatrics. 2004;114:297–316. *Pediatrics.* 2005;115:496–506. (http://www.aafp.org/online/en/home/clinical/exam.html)

Disease Management: Psoriasis, Plaque-type	Organization	Date	Population	Recommendations	Comments	Sources
PSORIASIS, PLAQUE-TYPE						

Psoriasis, Plaque-type	AAD	2009	Adults	Topical Therapies
				1. Topical therapies are most effective for mild–moderate disease.
				2. Topical corticosteroids daily—bid
				  a. Cornerstone of therapy
				  b. Limit Class 1 topical steroids to 4 weeks maximum
				3. Topical agents that have proven efficacy when combined with topical corticosteroids
				  a. Topical vitamin D analogues
				  b. Topical tazarotene
				  c. Topical salicylic acid
				4. Emollients applied 1–3 times daily are a helpful adjunct.
					1. Approximately, 2% of population has psoriasis.
					2. 80% of patients with psoriasis have mild–moderate disease.
					3. Topical steroid toxicity
					  a. Local: skin atrophy, telangiectasia, striae, purpura, or contact dermatitis
					  b. Hypothalamic–pituitary-adrenal axis may be suppressed with prolonged use of medium-high potency steroids
						http://www.aad.org/research/documents/JAADarticle-Section3PsoriasisGuidelines.pdf

	AAD	2009	Adults	Systemic Therapies
				1. Indicated for severe, recalcitrant, or disabling psoriasis
				2. Methotrexate (MTX)
				  a. Dose: 7.5–30 mg PO weekly
				  b. Monitor CBC and liver panel monthly
				3. Cyclosporine
				  a. Initial dose: 2.5–3 mg/kg divided bid
				  b. Monitor for nephrotoxicity, HTN, and hypertrichosis
				4. Acitretin
				  a. Dose: 10–50 mg PO daily
				  b. Monitor: liver panel
					1. MTX contraindications: pregnancy; breast-feeding; alcoholism; chronic liver disease; immunodeficiency syndromes; cytopenias; hypersensitivity reaction
					2. Cyclosporine contraindications: CA; renal impairment; uncontrolled HTN
					3. Acitretin contraindications: pregnancy; chronic liver or renal disease
						http://www.aad.org/research/documents/JAADarticle-Section4PsoriasisGuidelines.pdf

RHEUMATOID ARTHRITIS (RA), BIOLOGIC DISEASE- MODIFYING) ANTIRHEUMATIC DRUGS (DMARDS)

Disease Management	Organization	Date	Population	Recommendations	Comments	Source

Rheumatoid Arthritis (RA), Biologic Disease- modifying Antirheumatic Drugs (DMARDs)	ACR	2008	Adults	1. Anti-(tumor necrosis factor) TNF-α agents
				  a. A tuberculosis (Tb) skin test must be checked before initiating these medications
				  b. Recommended for all patients with high disease activity and presence of poor prognostic features of any duration of disease.
				2. Recommended for patients with disease ≥ 6 months who have failed nonbiologic DMARD therapy and have moderate-high disease activity, especially if poor prognostic features are present
				3. Abatacept has same indications as anti-TNF-α agents.
				4. Rituximab has same indications as anti-TNF-α agents.
				5. Recommends withholding all biologic DMARDs 1 week before or after surgery.
					1. Anti-TNF-α agents, abatacept, and rituximab all contraindicated in:
					  a. Serious bacterial, fungal, and viral infections, or with latent Tb
					  b. Acute viral hepatitis or Child's B or Child's C cirrhosis
					  c. Instances of a lymphoproliferative disorder treated ≤ 5 years ago; decompensated congestive heart failure (CHF); or any demyelinating disorder
						http://www.rheumatology.org/practice/clinical/guidelines/recommendations.pdf

RHEUMATOID ARTHRITIS (RA), NONBIOLOGIC DISEASE-MODIFYING ANTIRHEUMATIC DRUGS (DMARDS) (DMARDs)

Disease Management	Organization	Date	Population	Recommendations	Comments	Source
Rheumatoid Arthritis (RA), Nonbiologic Disease-modifying Antirheumatic Drugs (DMARDs)	ACR	2008	Adults	1. MTX or leflunomide monotherapy may be used for patients with any disease severity or duration. 2. Hydroxychloroquine or minocycline monotherapy recommended if low disease activity and duration ≤ 24 months. 3. Sulfasalazine recommended for all disease durations and without poor prognostic features.[a] 4. MTX plus either hydroxychloroquine or leflunomide recommended for moderate-high disease activity regardless of disease duration. 5. MTX plus sulfasalazine recommended for high disease activity and poor prognostic features.	1. Contraindications to DMARD therapy: a. Serious bacterial, fungal, or viral infections b. Only DMARDs safe with latent Tb are hydroxychloroquine, minocycline, and sulfasalazine. c. Avoid MTX for interstitial pneumonitis and for creatinine clearance < 30 mL/min. d. Avoid MTX and leflunomide for cytopenias, hepatitis, pregnancy, and breast-feeding (also minocycline). e. Avoid all DMARDs in Child's B or Child's C cirrhosis.	http://www.rheumatology.org/practice/clinical/guidelines/recommendations.pdf

[a]Functional limitation, presence of rheumatoid nodules, secondary Sjögren's syndrome, RA vasculitis, Felty's syndrome, and RA lung disease.

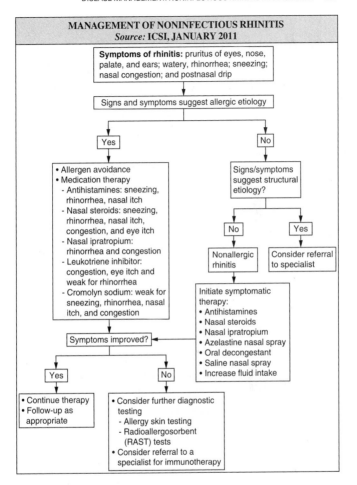

MANAGEMENT OF NONINFECTIOUS RHINITIS
Source: ICSI, JANUARY 2011

Symptoms of rhinitis: pruritus of eyes, nose, palate, and ears; watery, rhinorrhea; sneezing; nasal congestion; and postnasal drip

Signs and symptoms suggest allergic etiology

Yes

No

- Allergen avoidance
- Medication therapy
  - Antihistamines: sneezing, rhinorrhea, nasal itch
  - Nasal steroids: sneezing, rhinorrhea, nasal itch, congestion, and eye itch
  - Nasal ipratropium: rhinorrhea and congestion
  - Leukotriene inhibitor: congestion, eye itch and weak for rhinorrhea
  - Cromolyn sodium: weak for sneezing, rhinorrhea, nasal itch, and congestion

Signs/symptoms suggest structural etiology?

No

Yes

Nonallergic rhinitis

Consider referral to specialist

Initiate symptomatic therapy:
- Antihistamines
- Nasal steroids
- Nasal ipratropium
- Azelastine nasal spray
- Oral decongestant
- Saline nasal spray
- Increase fluid intake

Symptoms improved?

Yes

No

- Continue therapy
- Follow-up as appropriate

- Consider further diagnostic testing
  - Allergy skin testing
  - Radioallergosorbent (RAST) tests
- Consider referral to a specialist for immunotherapy

SEXUALLY TRANSMITTED DISEASES TREATMENT GUIDELINES ADAPTED FROM CDC GUIDELINES, *MMWR.* 2010;59(RR-12):1–116.		
Infection	**Recommended Treatment**	**Alternative Treatment**
Chancroid	• Azithromycin 1 g PO × 1 • Ceftriaxone 250 mg IM × 1	• Ciprofloxacin 500 mg PO bid for 3 days • Erythromycin base 500 mg PO tid for 7 days
First episode of genital HSV	• Acyclovir 400 mg PO tid × 7–10 days[a] • Famciclovir 250 mg PO tid × 7–10 days[a] • Valacyclovir 1 g PO bid × 7–10 days[a]	• Acyclovir 200 mg PO five times a day for 7–10 days[a]
Suppressive therapy for genital HSV	• Acyclovir 400 mg PO bid • Famciclovir 250 mg PO bid	• Valacyclovir 1 g PO daily
Episodic therapy for recurrent genital HSV	• Acyclovir 400 mg PO tid × 5 days • Famciclovir 125 mg PO bid × 5 days • Valacyclovir 500 mg PO bid × 3 days	• Acyclovir 800 mg PO bid × 5 days • Acyclovir 800 mg PO tid × 2 days • Famciclovir 1000 mg PO bid × 1 day • Famciclovir 500 mg PO × 1 then 250 mg bid × 2 days • Valacyclovir 1 g PO daily × 5 days
Suppressive therapy for HIV-positive patients	• Acyclovir 400–800 mg PO bid-tid • Famciclovir 500 mg PO bid • Valacyclovir 500 mg PO bid	
Episodic therapy for recurrent genital HSV in HIV-positive patients	• Acyclovir 400 mg PO tid × 5–10 days • Famciclovir 500 mg PO bid × 5–10 days • Valacyclovir 1 g PO bid × 5–10 days	
Granuloma inguinale (Donovanosis)	• Doxycycline 100 mg PO bid × ≥ 3 weeks and until all lesions have completely healed	• Azithromycin 1 g PO weekly × ≥ 3 weeks • Ciprofloxacin 750 mg PO bid × ≥ 3 weeks • Erythromycin base 500 mg PO qid × ≥ 3 weeks • TMP-SMX one double-strength (160 mg/800 mg) tablet PO bid × ≥ 3 weeks • Continue all of these treatments until all lesions have completely healed
Lymphogranuloma venereum	• Doxycycline 100 mg PO bid for × 21 days	• Erythromycin base 500 mg PO qid × 21 days

SEXUALLY TRANSMITTED DISEASES TREATMENT GUIDELINES (CONTINUED) ADAPTED FROM CDC GUIDELINES, *MMWR.* 2010;59(RR-12):1–116.		
Infection	**Recommended Treatment**	**Alternative Treatment**
Syphilis in adults	• Benzathine penicillin G 2.4 million units IM × 1	
Syphilis in infants and children	• Benzathine penicillin G 50,000 units/kg IM, up to the adult dose of 2.4 million units × 1	
Early latent syphilis in adults	• Benzathine penicillin G 2.4 million units IM × 1	
Early latent syphilis in children	• Benzathine penicillin G 50,000 units/kg IM, up to the adult dose of 2.4 million units × 1	
Late latent syphilis or latent syphilis of unknown duration in adults	• Benzathine penicillin G 2.4 million units IM weekly × 3 doses	
Late latent syphilis or latent syphilis of unknown duration in children	• Benzathine penicillin G 50,000 units/kg, up to the adult dose of 2.4 million units, IM weekly × 3 doses	
Tertiary syphilis	• Benzathine penicillin G 2.4 million units IM weekly × 3 doses	
Neurosyphilis	• Aqueous crystalline penicillin G 3–4 million units IV q4h × 10–14 days	• Procaine penicillin 2.4 million units IM daily × 10–14 days **PLUS** • Probenecid 500 mg PO qid × 10–14 days
Syphilis, pregnant women	• Pregnant women should be treated with the penicillin regimen appropriate for their stage of infection	
Congenital syphilis	• Aqueous crystalline penicillin G 50,000 units/kg/dose IV q12h × 7 days; then q8h × 3 more days	• Procaine penicillin G 50,000 units/kg/dose IM daily × 10 days • Benzathine penicillin G 50,000 units/kg/dose IM × 1
Older children with syphilis	• Aqueous crystalline penicillin G 50,000 units/kg IV q4–6h × 10 days	
Nongonococcal urethritis	• Azithromycin 1 g PO × 1 • Doxycycline 100 mg PO bid × 7 days	• Erythromycin base 500 mg PO qid × 7 days • Erythromycin ethylsuccinate 800 mg PO qid × 7 days • Levofloxacin 500 mg PO daily × 7 days • Ofloxacin 300 mg PO bid × 7 days

SEXUALLY TRANSMITTED DISEASES TREATMENT GUIDELINES (CONTINUED) ADAPTED FROM CDC GUIDELINES, *MMWR*. 2010;59(RR-12):1–116.		
Infection	**Recommended Treatment**	**Alternative Treatment**
Recurrent or persistent urethritis	• Metronidazole 2 g PO × 1 • Tinidazole 2 g PO × 1 • Azithromycin 1 g PO × 1	
Cervicitis[b]	• Azithromycin 1 g PO × 1 • Doxycycline 100 mg PO bid × 7 days	
Chlamydia infections in adolescents, adults[b]	• Azithromycin 1 g PO × 1 • Doxycycline 100 mg PO bid × 7 days	• Erythromycin base 500 mg PO qid × 7 days • Erythromycin ethylsuccinate 800 mg PO qid × 7 days • Levofloxacin 500 mg PO daily × 7 days • Ofloxacin 300 mg PO bid × 7 days
Chlamydia infections in Pregnancy[b]	• Azithromycin 1 g PO × 1 • Amoxicillin 500 mg PO tid × 7 days	• Erythromycin base 500 mg PO qid × 7 days • Erythromycin ethylsuccinate 800 mg PO qid × 7 days
Ophthalmia neonatorum from *Chlamydia*	• Erythromycin base or ethylsuccinate 50 mg/kg/day PO qid × 14 days	
Chlamydia trachomatis pneumonia in infants	• Erythromycin base or ethylsuccinate 50 mg/kg/day PO qid × 14 days	
Chlamydia infections in children < 45 kg	• Erythromycin base or ethylsuccinate 50 mg/kg/day PO qid × 14 days	
Chlamydia infections in children ≥ 45 kg and aged < 8 years	• Azithromycin 1 g PO × 1	
Chlamydia infections in children aged ≥ 8 years	• Azithromycin 1 g PO × 1 • Doxycycline 100 mg PO bid × 7 days	

SEXUALLY TRANSMITTED DISEASES TREATMENT GUIDELINES (CONTINUED) ADAPTED FROM CDC GUIDELINES, *MMWR.* 2010;59(RR-12):1–116.		
Infection	**Recommended Treatment**	**Alternative Treatment**
Uncomplicated gonococcal infections of the cervix, urethra, pharynx, or rectum in adults or children > 45 kg	• Ceftriaxone 250 mg IM × 1 **PLUS** • Azithromycin 1 g PO × 1 **OR** • Doxycycline 100 mg daily × 7 days	
Gonococcal conjunctivitis in adults or children > 45 kg	• Ceftriaxone 1 g IM × 1	
Gonococcal meningitis or endocarditis in adults or children > 45 kg	• Ceftriaxone 1 g IV q12h	
Disseminated gonococcal infection in adults or children > 45 kg	• Ceftriaxone 1 g IV/IM daily	• Cefotaxime 1 g IV q8h • Ceftizoxime 1 g IV q8h
Ophthalmia neonatorum caused by gonococcus	• Ceftriaxone 25–50 mg/kg, not to exceed 125 mg, IV/IM × 1	
Prophylactic treatment of infants born to mothers with gonococcal infection	• Ceftriaxone 25–50 mg/kg, not to exceed 125 mg, IV/IM × 1	
Uncomplicated gonococcal infections of the cervix, urethra, pharynx, or rectum in children ≤ 45 kg	• Ceftriaxone 125 mg IM × 1	
Gonococcal infections with bacteremia or arthritis in children or adults	• Ceftriaxone 50 mg/kg (maximum dose 1 g) IM/IV daily × 7 days	

SEXUALLY TRANSMITTED DISEASES TREATMENT GUIDELINES (CONTINUED) ADAPTED FROM CDC GUIDELINES, *MMWR.* 2010;59(RR-12):1–116.		
Infection	**Recommended Treatment**	**Alternative Treatment**
Ophthalmia neonatorum prophylaxis	• Erythromycin (0.5%) ophthalmic ointment in each eye × 1	
Bacterial vaginosis	• Metronidazole 500 mg PO bid × 7 days[c] • Metronidazole gel 0.75%, one applicator (5 g) IVag daily × 5 days • Clindamycin cream 2%, one applicator (5 g) IVag qhs × 7 days[d]	• Tinidazole 2 g PO daily × 3 days • Clindamycin 300 mg PO bid × 7 days • Clindamycin ovules 100 mg IVag qhs × 3 days
Bacterial vaginosis in pregnancy	• Metronidazole 500 mg PO bid × 7 days • Metronidazole 250 mg PO tid × 7 days • Clindamycin 300 mg PO bid × 7 days	
Trichomoniasis	• Metronidazole 2 g PO × 1[c] • Tinidazole 2 g PO × 1	• Metronidazole 500 mg PO bid × 7 days[c]
Candidal vaginitis	• Butoconazole 2% cream 5 g IVag × 3 days • Clotrimazole 1% cream 5 g IVag × 7–14 days • Clotrimazole 2% cream 5 g IVag × 3 days • Nystatin 100,000-unit vaginal tablet, one tablet IVag × 14 days • Miconazole 2% cream 5 g IVag × 7 days • Miconazole 4% cream 5 g IVag × 3 days • Miconazole 100-mg vaginal suppository, one suppository IVag × 7 days • Miconazole 200-mg vaginal suppository, one suppository IVag × 3 days • Miconazole 1200-mg vaginal suppository, one suppository IVag × 1 • Tioconazole 6.5% ointment 5 g IVag × 1 • Terconazole 0.4% cream 5 g IVag × 7 days • Terconazole 0.8% cream 5 g IVag × 3 days • Terconazole 80-mg vaginal suppository, one suppository IVag × 3 days	• Fluconazole 150 mg oral tablet, one tablet in single dose

SEXUALLY TRANSMITTED DISEASES TREATMENT GUIDELINES (CONTINUED) ADAPTED FROM CDC GUIDELINES, *MMWR.* 2010;59(RR-12):1–116.		
Infection	**Recommended Treatment**	**Alternative Treatment**
Severe pelvic inflammatory disease	• Cefotetan 2 g IV q12h **OR** • Cefoxitin 2 g IV q6h **PLUS** • Doxycycline 100 mg PO/IV bid	• Clindamycin 900 mg IV q8h **PLUS** • Gentamicin loading dose IV or IM (2 mg/kg of body weight), followed by a maintenance dose (1.5 mg/kg) q8h. Single daily dosing (3–5 mg/kg) can be substituted. **OR** • Ampicillin/sulbactam 3 g IV q6h **PLUS** • Doxycycline 100 mg PO/IV bid
Mild-moderate pelvic inflammatory disease	• Ceftriaxone 250 mg IM × 1 **OR** • Cefoxitin 2 g IM × 1 **and** probenecid 1 g PO × 1 **PLUS** • Doxycycline 100 mg PO bid × 14 days +/– metronidazole 500 mg PO bid × 14 days[c]	
Epididymitis	• Ceftriaxone 250 mg IM × 1 **PLUS** • Doxycycline 100 mg PO bid × 10 days	• Levofloxacin 500 mg PO daily × 10 days • Ofloxacin 300 mg PO bid × 10 days
External genital warts	**Provider–Administered:** • Cryotherapy every 1–2 weeks • Podophyllin resin 10%–25% in a compound tincture of benzoin • TCA or BCA 80%–90% • Surgical removal either by tangential scissor excision, tangential shave excision, curettage, or electrosurgery	**Patient-Applied:** • Podofilox 0.5% solution or gel • Imiquimod 5% cream • Sinecatechins 15% ointment
Cervical warts	• Biopsy to exclude high-grade SIL must be performed before treatment is initiated	
Vaginal warts	• TCA or BCA 80%–90% applied only to warts, repeated weekly	
Urethral meatal warts	• Cryotherapy every 1–2 weeks • TCA or BCA 80%–90% applied only to warts, repeated weekly	

SEXUALLY TRANSMITTED DISEASES TREATMENT GUIDELINES (CONTINUED) ADAPTED FROM CDC GUIDELINES, *MMWR*. 2010;59(RR-12):1–116.

Infection	Recommended Treatment	Alternative Treatment
Anal warts	• Cryotherapy every 1–2 weeks • TCA or BCA 80%–90% applied only to warts, repeated weekly	• Surgical removal either by tangential scissor excision, tangential shave excision, curettage, or electrosurgery
Proctitis	• Ceftriaxone 250 mg IM × 1 **PLUS** • Doxycycline 100 mg PO bid × 7 days	
Pediculosis pubis	• Permethrin 1% cream rinse applied to affected areas and washed off after 10 minutes • Pyrethrins with piperonyl butoxide applied to the affected area and washed off after 10 minutes	• Malathion 0.5% lotion applied for 8–12 hours and then washed off • Ivermectin 250 mcg/kg PO, repeated in 2 weeks
Scabies	• Permethrin cream (5%) applied to all areas of the body from the neck down and washed off after 8–14 hours • Ivermectin 200 mcg/kg PO, repeat in 2 weeks	• Lindane (1%) 1 oz of lotion (or 30 g of cream) applied in a thin layer to all areas of the body from the neck down and thoroughly washed off after 8 hours

HSV, herpes simplex virus; PO, by mouth; IM, intramuscular; IVag, intravaginally; bid, twice a day; tid, three times a day; HIV, human immunodeficiency virus; qid, four times a day; TMP-SMX, trimethoprim-sulfamethoxazole; IV, intravenous; q, every; h, hour(s); qhs, at bedtime; TCA, trichloroacetic acid; BCA, bichloracetic acid; SIL, squamous intraepithelial lesion

[a]Treatment can be extended if healing is incomplete after 10 days of therapy.
[b]Consider concomitant treatment of gonorrhea.
[c]Avoid alcohol during treatment and for 24 hours after treatment is completed.
[d]Clindamycin cream may weaken latex condoms and diaphragms during treatment and for 5 days thereafter.

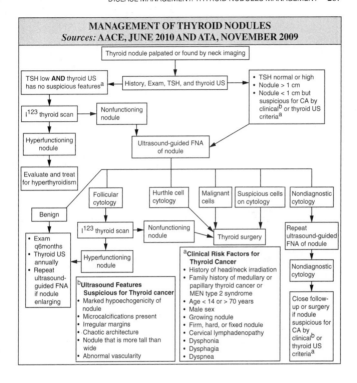

MANAGEMENT OF THYROID NODULES
Sources: AACE, JUNE 2010 AND ATA, NOVEMBER 2009

TOBACCO CESSATION TREATMENT ALGORITHM
Source: U.S. PUBLIC HEALTH SERVICE

Five A's

1. Ask about tobacco use.
2. Advise to quit through clear, personalized messages.
3. Assess willingness to quit.
4. Assist to quit,[a] including referral to Quit Lines (eg, 1-800-NO-BUTTS).
5. Arrange follow-up and support.

[a]Physicians can assist patients to quit by devising a quit plan, providing problem-solving counseling, providing intratreatment social support, helping patients obtain social support from their environment/friends, and recommending pharmacotherapy for appropriate patients. Use caution in recommending pharmacotherapy in patients with medical contraindications, those smoking < 10 cigarettes per day, pregnant/breast-feeding women, and adolescent smokers. As of March 2005, Medicare covers costs for smoking cessation counseling for those who (1) have a smoking-related illness; (2) have an illness complicated by smoking; or (3) take a medication that is made less effective by smoking. (http://www.cms.hhs.gov/mcd/viewdecisionmemo.asp?id=130)
Source: Fiore MC, et al. Treating Tobacco Use and Dependence. Quick Reference Guide for Clinicians. Rockville, MD: U.S. Department of Health and Human Services. Public Health Service, October 2000.

MOTIVATING TOBACCO USERS TO QUIT

Five R's

1. Relevance: personal
2. Risks: acute, long term, environmental
3. Rewards: have patient identify (eg, save money, better food taste)
4. Road blocks: help problem-solve
5. Repetition: at every office visit

TOBACCO CESSATION TREATMENT OPTIONS[a]						
Pharmacotherapy	Precautions/ Contraindications	Side Effects	Dosage	Duration	Availability	Cost/Day[b]
First-Line Pharmacotherapies (approved for use for smoking cessation by the FDA)						
Bupropion SR	History of seizure / History of eating disorder	Insomnia / Dry mouth	150 mg every morning for 3 days, then 150 mg bid. (Begin treatment 1–2 weeks pre-quit.)	7–12 weeks maintenance up to 6 months	Zyban (prescription only)	$5.73
Nicotine gum	—	Mouth soreness / Dyspepsia	1–24 cigarettes/day: 2-mg gum (up to 24 pieces/day) 25+ cigarettes/day: 4-mg gum (up to 24 pieces/day)	Up to 12 weeks	Nicorette, Nicorette Mint (OTC only)	$5.81
Nicotine inhaler	—	Local irritation of mouth and throat	6–16 cartridges/day	Up to 6 months	Nicotrol Inhaler (prescription only)	$6.07
Nicotine nasal spray	—	Nasal irritation	8–40 doses/day	3–6 months	Nicotrol NS (prescription only)	$3.67
Nicotine patch	—	Local skin reaction / Insomnia	21 mg/24 hours / 14 mg/24 hours / 7 mg/24 hours / 15 mg/16 hours	4 weeks Then 2 weeks Then 2 weeks 8 weeks	NicoDerm CQ (OTC only), generic patches (prescription and OTC) Nicotrol (OTC only)	$3.91
Varenicline	Renal impairment	Nausea / Abnormal dreams	0.5 mg QD for 3 days, then 0.5 mg bid for 4 days, then 1.0 mg PO bid	12 weeks or 24 weeks	Chantix (prescription only)	$4.22

TOBACCO CESSATION TREATMENT OPTIONS

TOBACCO CESSATION TREATMENT OPTIONS[a] (CONTINUED)

Pharmacotherapy	Precautions/ Contraindications	Side Effects	Dosage	Duration	Availability	Cost/Day[b]
Second-Line Pharmacotherapies (not approved for use for smoking cessation by the FDA)						
Clonidine	Rebound hypertension	Dry mouth Drowsiness Dizziness Sedation	0.15–0.75 mg/day	3–10 weeks	Oral clonidine–generic, Catapres (prescription only), transdermal Catapres (prescription only)	Clonidine $0.24 for 0.2 mg; Catapres (transdermal) $3.50
Nortriptyline	Risk of arrhythmias	Sedation Dry mouth	75–100 mg/day	12 weeks	Nortriptyline HCL–generic (prescription only)	$0.74 for 75 mg

FDA, Food and Drug Administration; OTC, over-the-counter; QD, every day; bid, twice daily; PO, by mouth
[a]The information contained within this table is not comprehensive. Please see package inserts for additional information.
[b]Prices from Rx for Change, the Regents of the University of California, University of Southern California, and Western University of Health Sciences.
[c]Prices based on retail prices of a national chain pharmacy; 2000.
Source: U.S. Public Health Service.

APPROACH TO ACUTE PHARYNGITIS
Source: ICSI, JANUARY 2011

Symptoms of possible streptococcal pharyngitis: close exposure to strep throat; sudden onset of sore throat; exudative tonsillitis; tender anterior cervical adenopathy; fever; absence of rhinorrhea, cough, or hoarseness; headache and abdominal pain may be present with other symptoms

Obtain a rapid strep test and backup strep culture

Negative and low likelihood of bacterial pharyngitis

Negative and high likelihood of bacterial pharyngitis

Educate and offer home remedies

Send throat strep culture → Positive

Symptoms improved at 1 week?

Negative

Yes → Continue symptomatic therapy

No → Reevaluate and consider testing for mononucleosis

Start penicillin or amoxicillin if positive

Symptoms improved at 48–72 hours?

No → Reevaluate for complications:
- Lemierre's syndrome
- Peritonsillar or retropharyngeal abscess
- Intracranial extension of infection
- Mono testing (if appropriate)

Yes → Complete antibiotic course

URINARY INCONTINENCE, STRESS

Disease Management	Organization	Date	Population	Recommendations	Comments	Source
Urinary Incontinence, Stress	AUA	2009	Adult women	1. Recommends an exam to assess the degree of urethral mobility, pelvic floor relaxation, pelvic organ prolapse, and assess whether any urethral abnormalities exist. 2. Recommends a urinalysis. 3. Assess the post-void residual volume. 4. Surgical options for refractory stress urinary incontinence include: periurethral injections; laparoscopic bladder suspensions; midurethral slings; pubovaginal slings, and retropubic suspensions.		http://www.auanet.org/content/media/stress2009-chapter1.pdf

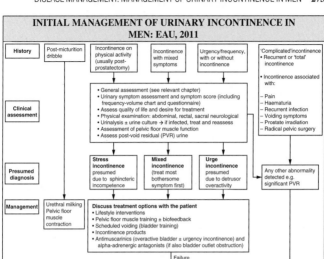

INITIAL MANAGEMENT OF URINARY INCONTINENCE IN MEN: EAU, 2011

History

Post-micturition dribble

Incontinence on physical activity (usually post-prostatectomy)

Incontinence with mixed symptoms

Urgency/frequency, with or without incontinence

'Complicated' incontinence
• Recurrent or 'total' incontinence
• Incontinence associated with:
 – Pain
 – Haematuria
 – Recurrent infection
 – Voiding symptoms
 – Prostate irradiation
 – Radical pelvic surgery

Clinical assessment

• General assessment (see relevant chapter)
• Urinary symptom assessment and symptom score (including frequency-volume chart and questionnaire)
• Assess quality of life and desire for treatment
• Physical examination: abdominal, rectal, sacral neurological
• Urinalysis ± urine culture → if infected, treat and reassess
• Assessment of pelvic floor muscle function
• Assess post-void residual (PVR) urine

Presumed diagnosis

Stress incontinence presumed due to sphincteric incompetence

Mixed incontinence (treat most bothersome symptom first)

Urge incontinence presumed due to detrusor overactivity

Any other abnormality detected e.g. significant PVR

Management

Urethral milking
Pelvic floor muscle contraction

Discuss treatment options with the patient
• Lifestyle interventions
• Pelvic floor muscle training ± biofeedback
• Scheduled voiding (bladder training)
• Incontinence products
• Antimuscarinics (overactive bladder ± urgency incontinence) and alpha-adrenergic antagonists (if also bladder outlet obstruction)

Failure

SPECIALISED MANAGEMENT

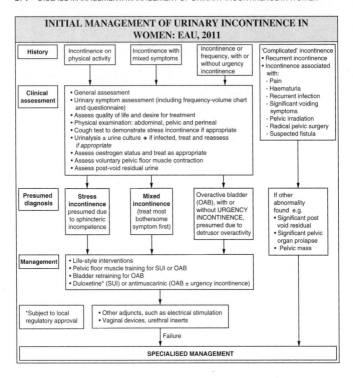

INITIAL MANAGEMENT OF URINARY INCONTINENCE IN WOMEN: EAU, 2011

History

- Incontinence on physical activity
- Incontinence with mixed symptoms
- Incontinence or frequency, with or without urgency incontinence
- 'Complicated' incontinence
  - Recurrent incontinence
  - Incontinence associated with:
    - Pain
    - Haematuria
    - Recurrent infection
    - Significant voiding symptoms
    - Pelvic irradiation
    - Radical pelvic surgery
    - Suspected fistula

Clinical assessment

- General assessment
- Urinary symptom assessment (including frequency-volume chart and questionnaire)
- Assess quality of life and desire for treatment
- Physical examination: abdominal, pelvic and perineal
- Cough test to demonstrate stress incontinence if appropriate
- Urinalysis ± urine culture → if infected, treat and reassess *if appropriate*
- Assess oestrogen status and treat as appropriate
- Assess voluntary pelvic floor muscle contraction
- Assess post-void residual urine

Presumed diagnosis

- **Stress incontinence** presumed due to sphincteric incompetence
- **Mixed incontinence** (treat most bothersome symptom first)
- Overactive bladder (OAB), with or without URGENCY INCONTINENCE, presumed due to detrusor overactivity
- If other abnormality found e.g.
  - Significant post void residual
  - Significant pelvic organ prolapse
  - Pelvic mass

Management

- Life-style interventions
- Pelvic floor muscle training for SUI or OAB
- Bladder retraining for OAB
- Duloxetine* (SUI) or antimuscarinic (OAB ± urgency incontinence)

*Subject to local regulatory approval

- Other adjuncts, such as electrical stimulation
- Vaginal devices, urethral inserts

Failure

SPECIALISED MANAGEMENT

URINARY TRACT INFECTIONS (UTIS)

Disease Management	Organization	Date	Population	Recommendations	Comments	Source

Urinary Tract Infections (UTIs)	ACOG EAU IDSA	2008 2010 2011	Nonpregnant women	1. Screening for and treatment of asymptomatic bacteriuria is not recommended.
				2. Recommend duration of antibiotics:
				  a. Uncomplicated cystitis: 3 days
				    i. Nitrofurantoin requires 5–7 days of therapy
				  b. Uncomplicated pyelonephritis: 7–10 days
				  c. Complicated pyelonephritis or urinary tract infection: 3–5 days after control/elimination of complicating factors and defervescence.
				3. Recommended empiric antibiotics
				For uncomplicated cystitis[a]:
				  a. TMP-SMX
				  b. Fluoroquinolones
				  c. Nitrofurantoin macrocrystals
				  d. Beta-lactam antibiotics are alternative agents[b]
				4. Recommended empiric antibiotics
				For complicated urinary tract infection or uncomplicated pyelonephritis:
				  a. Fluoroquinolones
				  b. Ceftriaxone
				  c. Aminoglycosides
					1. EAU recommends 7 days of antibiotics for men with uncomplicated cystitis.
					2. EAU suggests the following options for antimicrobial prophylaxis of recurrent uncomplicated UTIs in nonpregnant women:
					  a. Nitrofurantoin 50 mg PO daily
					  b. TMP-SMX 40/200 mg/day
					3. EAU suggests the following options for antimicrobial prophylaxis of recurrent uncomplicated UTIs in pregnant women:
					  a. Cephalexin 125 mg PO daily
						http://www.guidelines.gov/content.aspx?id=12628
						
						http://www.uroweb.org/gls/pdf/Urological%20Infections%202010.pdf
						
						http://www.guidelines.gov/content.aspx?id=25652&search=idsa+cystitis+2011

URINARY TRACT INFECTIONS (UTIS)

Disease Management	Organization	Date	Population	Recommendations	Comments	Source

Urinary Tract Infections (UTIs) (continued)				5. Recommended empiric antibiotics for complicated pyelonephritis:
				  a. Fluoroquinolones
				  b. Piperacillin-tazobactam
				  c. Carbapenem
				  d. Aminoglycosides
					4. Once urine culture and sensitivity results are known, antibiotics can be adjusted to the narrowest spectrum antibiotic.	

[a]TMP-SMX only if regional *Escherichia coli* resistance is < 20%; fluoroquinolones include ciprofloxacin, ofloxacin, or levofloxacin.
[b]Amoxicillin–clavulanate, cefdinir, cefaclor, or cefpodoxime–proxetil. Cephalexin may be appropriate in certain settings.

LOWER URINARY TRACT SYMPTOMS (LUTS)

Disease Management	Organization	Date	Population	Recommendations	Comments	Source
Lower Urinary Tract Symptoms (LUTS)	NICE	2010	Adult men	1. All men with LUTS should have a thorough history and exam, including a prostate exam and review of current medications. 2. Recommends supervised bladder training exercises and consider anticholinergic medications for symptoms suggestive of an overactive bladder. 3. Recommends an alpha-blocker for men with moderate-severe LUTS.[a] 4. Consider a 5-alpha reductase inhibitor for men with LUTS with prostate size larger than 30 g. 5. For men with refractory obstructive urinary symptoms despite medical therapy, offer one of three surgeries: transurethral resection, transurethral vaporization, or laser enucleation of the prostate.		http://www.nice.org.uk/nicemedia/live/12984/48557.pdf

[a]Alfuzosin, doxazosin, tamsulosin, or terazosin.

VERTIGO, BENIGN PAROXYSMAL POSITIONAL (BPPV)

Disease Management	Organization	Date	Population	Recommendations	Comments	Source
Vertigo, Benign Paroxysmal Positional (BPPV)	AAO-HNS	2008	Adults	1. Recommends the Dix-Hallpike maneuver to diagnose posterior semicircular canal BPPV. 2. Recommends treatment of posterior semicircular canal BPPV with a particle repositioning maneuver. 3. If the Dix-Hallpike test result is negative, recommends a supine roll test to diagnose lateral semicircular canal BPPV. 4. Recommends offering vestibular rehabilitation exercises for the initial treatment of BPPV. 5. Recommends evaluating patients for an underlying peripheral vestibular or central nervous system disorder if they have an initial treatment failure of presumed BPPV. 6. Recommends against routine radiologic imaging for patients with BPPV. 7. Recommends against routine vestibular testing for patients with BPPV. 8. Recommends against routine use of antihistamines or benzodiazepines for patients with BPPV.	BPPV is the most common vestibular disorder in adults, afflicting 2.4% of adults at some point during their lives.	http://www.entlink.net/Practice/upload/BPPV-guideline-final-journal.pdf

4
Appendices

SCREENING INSTRUMENTS: ALCOHOL ABUSE

SENSITIVITY AND SPECIFICITY OF SCREENING TESTS FOR PROBLEM DRINKING

Instrument Name	Screening Questions/Scoring	Threshold Score	Sensitivity/Specificity (%)	Source
CAGE[a]	See page 257	> 1 > 2 > 3	77/58 53/81 29/92	Am J Psychiatr. 1974;131:1121 J Gen Intern Med. 1998;13:379
AUDIT	See pages 257–258	> 4 > 5 > 6	87/70 77/84 66/90	BMJ. 1997;314:420 J Gen Intern Med. 1998;13:379

[a]The CAGE may be less applicable to binge drinkers (eg, college students), the elderly, and minority populations.

SCREENING INSTRUMENTS: ALCOHOL ABUSE

SCREENING PROCEDURES FOR PROBLEM DRINKING

1. CAGE screening test[a]

Have you ever felt the need to   **C**ut down on drinking?

Have you ever felt   **A**nnoyed by criticism of your drinking?

Have you ever felt   **G**uilty about your drinking?

Have you ever taken a morning   **E**ye opener?

INTERPRETATION: Two "yes" answers are considered a positive screen. One "yes" answer should arouse a suspicion of alcohol abuse.

2. The Alcohol Use Disorder Identification Test (AUDIT)[b] (Scores for response categories are given in parentheses. Scores range from 0–40, with a cut-off score of ≥ 5 indicating hazardous drinking, harmful drinking, or alcohol dependence.)

1) How often do you have a drink containing alcohol?

(0) Never   (1) Monthly or less   (2) Two to four times a month   (3) Two or three times a week   (4) Four or more times a week

2) How many drinks containing alcohol do you have on a typical day when you are drinking?

(0) 1 or 2   (1) 3 or 4   (2) 5 or 6   (3) 7 to 9   (4) 10 or more

3) How often do you have six or more drinks on one occasion?

(0) Never   (1) Less than monthly   (2) Monthly   (3) Weekly   (4) Daily or almost daily

4) How often during the past year have you found that you were not able to stop drinking once you had started?

(0) Never   (1) Less than monthly   (2) Monthly   (3) Weekly   (4) Daily or almost daily

5) How often during the past year have you failed to do what was normally expected of you because of drinking?

(0) Never   (1) Less than monthly   (2) Monthly   (3) Weekly   (4) Daily or almost daily

SCREENING INSTRUMENTS: ALCOHOL ABUSE

SCREENING PROCEDURES FOR PROBLEM DRINKING (CONTINUED)

6) How often during the past year have you needed a first drink in the morning to get yourself going after a heavy drinking session?

(0) Never   (1) Less than monthly   (2) Monthly   (3) Weekly   (4) Daily or almost daily

7) How often during the past year have you had a feeling of guilt or remorse after drinking?

(0) Never   (1) Less than monthly   (2) Monthly   (3) Weekly   (4) Daily or almost daily

8) How often during the past year have you been unable to remember what happened the night before because you had been drinking?

(0) Never   (1) Less than monthly   (2) Monthly   (3) Weekly   (4) Daily or almost daily

9) Have you or has someone else been injured as a result of your drinking?

(0) No   (2) Yes, but not in the past year   (4) Yes, during the past year

10) Has a relative or friend or a doctor or other health worker been concerned about your drinking or suggested you cut down?

(0) No   (2) Yes, but not in the past year   (4) Yes, during the past year

[a]Modified from Mayfield D, McLeod G, and Hall P. The CAGE questionnaire: validation of a new alcoholism screening instrument. *Am J Psychiatr.* 1974;131:1121.
[b]From Piccinelli M, et al. Efficacy of the alcohol use disorders identification test as a screening tool for hazardous alcohol intake and related disorders in primary care: a validity study. *BMJ.* 1997;314:420.

SCREENING INSTRUMENTS: DEPRESSION

SCREENING TESTS FOR DEPRESSION

Instrument Name	Screening Questions/Scoring	Threshold Score	Source
Beck Depression Inventory (short form)	See page 286	0–4: None or minimal depression 5–7: Mild depression 8–15: Moderate depression > 15: Severe depression	*Postgrad Med.* 1972;Dec:81
Geriatric Depression Scale	See page 287	≥ 15: Depression	*J Psychiatr Res.* 1983;17:37
PRIME-MD[b] (mood questions)	1. During the past month, have you often been bothered by feeling down, depressed, or hopeless? 2. During the past month, have you often been bothered by little interest or pleasure in doing things?	"Yes" to either question[a]	*JAMA.* 1994;272:1749 *J Gen Intern Med.* 1997;12:439
Patient Health Questionnaire (PHQ-9)[b]	http://www.pfizer.com/phq-9/ See page 284	*Major depressive syndrome:* if answers to #1a or b and ≥ 5 of #1a–i are at least "More than half the days" (count #1i if present at all) *Other depressive syndrome:* if #1a or b and 2–4 of #1a–i are at least "More than half the days" (count #1i if present at all) 5–9: mild depression 10–14: moderate depression 15–19: moderately severe depression 20–27: severe depression	*JAMA.* 1999;282:1737 *J Gen Intern Med.* 2001;16:606

[a]Sensitivity 86%–96%; specificity 57%–75%.
[b]Pfizer Inc.

\multicolumn{6}{c}{**SCREENING INSTRUMENTS: DEPRESSION**}					

SCREENING INSTRUMENTS: DEPRESSION

PHQ-9 DEPRESSION SCREEN, ENGLISH

Over the last 2 weeks, how often have you been bothered by any of the following problems?

		Not at all	Several days	> Half the days	Nearly every day
a.	Little interest or pleasure in doing things	0	1	2	3
b.	Feeling down, depressed, or hopeless	0	1	2	3
c.	Trouble falling or staying asleep, or sleeping too much	0	1	2	3
d.	Feeling tired or having little energy	0	1	2	3
e.	Poor appetite or overeating	0	1	2	3
f.	Feeling bad about yourself—or that you are a failure or that you have let yourself or your family down	0	1	2	3
g.	Trouble concentrating on things, such as reading the newspaper or watching television	0	1	2	3
h.	Moving or speaking so slowly that other people could have noticed? Or the opposite—being so fidgety or restless that you have been moving around a lot more than usual?	0	1	2	3
i.	Thoughts that you would be better off dead or of hurting yourself in some way	0	1	2	3
	(For office coding: Total Score	—— =	—— +	—— +	——)

Major depressive syndrome: if ≥ 5 items present scored ≥ 2 and one of the items is depressed mood (b) or anhedonia (a). If item "i" is present, then this counts, even if score = 1.
Depressive screen positive: if at least one item ≥ 2 (or item "i" is ≥ 1).

Source: From the Primary Care Evaluation of Mental Disorders Patient Health Questionnaire (PRIME-MD PHQ). The PHQ was developed by Drs. Robert L. et al. For research information, contact Dr. Spitzer at rls8@columbia.edu. PRIME-MD® is a trademark of Pfizer Inc. Copyright © 1999 Pfizer Inc. All rights reserved. Reproduced with permission. FOR OFFICE CODING: Maj Dep Syn if answer to #2a or b and ≥ 5 of #2a–i are at least "More than half the days" (count #2i if present at all). Other Dep Syn if #2a or b and 2, 3, or 4 of #2a–i are at least "More than half the days" (count #2i if present at all).

SCREENING INSTRUMENTS: DEPRESSION				
PHQ-9 DEPRESSION SCREEN, SPANISH				

Durante las últimas 2 semanas, ¿con qué frecuencia le han molestado los siguientes problemas?

		Nunca	Varios dias	> La mitad de los días	Casi todos los días
a.	Tener poco interés o placer en hacer las cosas	0	1	2	3
b.	Sentirse desanimada, deprimida, o sin esperanza	0	1	2	3
c.	Con problemas en dormirse o en mantenerse dormida, o en dormir demasiado	0	1	2	3
d.	Sentirse cansada o tener poca energía	0	1	2	3
e.	Tener poco apetito o comer en exceso	0	1	2	3
f.	Sentir falta de amor propio—o qe sea un fracaso o que decepcionara a sí misma o a su familia	0	1	2	3
g.	Tener dificultad para concentrarse en cosas tales como leer el periódico o mirar la televisión	0	1	2	3
h.	Se mueve o habla tan lentamente que otra gente se podría dar cuenta—o de lo contrario, está tan agitada o inquieta que se mueve mucho más de lo acostumbrado	0	1	2	3
i.	Se le han ocurrido pensamientos de que se haría daño de alguna manera	0	1	2	3
	(For office coding: Total Score	—— =	—— +	—— +	——)

Source: From the Primary Care Evaluation of Mental Disorders Patient Health Questionnaire (PRIME-MD PHQ). The PHQ was developed by Drs Robert L. et al. For research information, contact Dr Spitzer at rls8@columbia.edu. PRIME-MD® is a trademark of Pfizer Inc. Copyright © 1999 Pfizer Inc. All rights reserved. Reproduced with permission. FOR OFFICE CODING: Maj Dep Syn if answer to #2a or b and ≥ 5 of #2a–i are at least "More than half the days" (count #2i if present at all). Other Dep Syn if #2a or b and 2, 3, or 4 of #2a–i are at least "More than half the days" (count #2i if present at all).

SCREENING INSTRUMENTS: DEPRESSION

BECK DEPRESSION INVENTORY, SHORT FORM

Instructions: This is a questionnaire. On the questionnaire are groups of statements. Please read the entire group of statements in each category. Then pick out the one statement in that group that best describes the way you feel today, that is, right now! Circle the number beside the statement you have chosen. If several statements in the group seem to apply equally well, circle each one. Sum all numbers to calculate a score.

Be sure to read all the statements in each group before making your choice.

A. Sadness
3 I am so sad or unhappy that I can't stand it.
2 I am blue or sad all the time and I can't snap out of it.
1 I feel sad or blue.
0 I do not feel sad.

B. Pessimism
3 I feel that the future is hopeless and that things cannot improve.
2 I feel I have nothing to look forward to.
1 I feel discouraged about the future.
0 I am not particularly pessimistic or discouraged about the future.

C. Sense of failure
3 I feel I am a complete failure as a person (parent, husband, wife).
2 As I look back on my life, all I can see is a lot of failures.
1 I feel I have failed more than the average person.
0 I do not feel like a failure.

D. Dissatisfaction
3 I am dissatisfied with everything.
2 I don't get satisfaction out of anything anymore.
1 I don't enjoy things the way I used to.
0 I am not particularly dissatisfied.

E. Guilt
3 I feel as though I am very bad or worthless.
2 I feel quite guilty.
1 I feel bad or unworthy a good part of the time.
0 I don't feel particularly guilty.

F. Self-dislike
3 I hate myself.
2 I am disgusted with myself.
1 I am disappointed in myself.
0 I don't feel disappointed in myself.

G. Self-harm
3 I would kill myself if I had the chance.
2 I have definite plans about committing suicide.
1 I feel I would be better off dead.
0 I don't have any thoughts of harming myself.

H. Social withdrawal
3 I have lost all of my interest in other people and don't care about them at all.
2 I have lost most of my interest in other people and have little feeling for them.
1 I am less interested in other people than I used to be.
0 I have not lost interest in other people.

I. Indecisiveness
3 I can't make any decisions at all anymore.
2 I have great difficulty in making decisions.
1 I try to put off making decisions.
0 I make decisions about as well as ever.

J. Self-image change
3 I feel that I am ugly or repulsive-looking.
2 I feel that there are permanent changes in my appearance and they make me look unattractive.
1 I am worried that I am looking old or unattractive.
0 I don't feel that I look worse than I used to.

K. Work difficulty
3 I can't do any work at all.
2 I have to push myself very hard to do anything.
1 It takes extra effort to get started at doing something.
0 I can work about as well as before.

L. Fatigability
3 I get too tired to do anything.
2 I get tired from doing anything.
1 I get tired more easily than I used to.
0 I don't get any more tired than usual.

M. Anorexia
3 I have no appetite at all anymore.
2 My appetite is much worse now.
1 My appetite is not as good as it used to be.
0 My appetite is no worse than usual.

Source: Reproduced with permission from Beck AT, Beck RW. Screening depressed patients in family practice: a rapid technic. *Postgrad Med.* 1972;52:81.

GERIATRIC DEPRESSION SCALE

Choose the best answer for how you felt over the past week

1. Are you basically satisfied with your life?	yes / no
2. Have you dropped many of your activities and interests?	yes / no
3. Do you feel that your life is empty?	yes / no
4. Do you often get bored?	yes / no
5. Are you hopeful about the future?	yes / no
6. Are you bothered by thoughts you can't get out of your head?	yes / no
7. Are you in good spirits most of the time?	yes / no
8. Are you afraid that something bad is going to happen to you?	yes / no
9. Do you feel happy most of the time?	yes / no
10. Do you often feel helpless?	yes / no
11. Do you often get restless and fidgety?	yes / no
12. Do you prefer to stay at home, rather than going out and doing new things?	yes / no
13. Do you frequently worry about the future?	yes / no
14. Do you feel you have more problems with memory than most?	yes / no
15. Do you think it is wonderful to be alive now?	yes / no
16. Do you often feel downhearted and blue?	yes / no
17. Do you feel pretty worthless the way you are now?	yes / no
18. Do you worry a lot about the past?	yes / no
19. Do you find life very exciting?	yes / no
20. Is it hard for you to get started on new projects?	yes / no
21. Do you feel full of energy?	yes / no
22. Do you feel that your situation is hopeless?	yes / no
23. Do you think that most people are better off than you are?	yes / no
24. Do you frequently get upset over little things?	yes / no
25. Do you frequently feel like crying?	yes / no
26. Do you have trouble concentrating?	yes / no
27. Do you enjoy getting up in the morning?	yes / no
28. Do you prefer to avoid social gatherings?	yes / no
29. Is it easy for you to make decisions?	yes / no
30. Is your mind as clear as it used to be?	yes / no

One point for each response suggestive of depression. (Specifically "no" responses to questions 1, 5, 7, 9, 15, 19, 21, 27, 29, and 30, and "yes" responses to the remaining questions are suggestive of depression.)

A score of ≥ 15 yields a sensitivity of 80% and a specificity of 100%, as a screening test for geriatric depression. *Clin Gerontol*. 1982;1:37.

Source: Reproduced with permission from Yesavage JA, et al. Development and validation of a geriatric depression screening scale: a preliminary report. *J Psychiatr Res*. 1982–83;17:37.

FUNCTIONAL ASSESSMENT SCREENING IN THE ELDERLY			
Target Area	**Assessment Procedure**	**Abnormal Result**	**Suggested Intervention**
Vision	Inquire about vision changes, Snellen chart testing.	Presence of vision changes; inability to read greater than 20/40	Refer to ophthalmologist.
Hearing	Whisper a short, easily answered question such as "What is your name?" in each ear while the examiner's face is out of direct view. Use audioscope set at 40 dB; test using 1000 and 2000 Hz. Brief hearing loss screener	Inability to answer question Inability to hear 1000 or 2000 Hz in both ears or inability to hear frequencies in either ear Brief hearing loss screen score ≥ 3	Examine auditory canals for cerumen and clean if necessary. Repeat test; if still abnormal in either ear, refer for audiometry and possible prosthesis.
Balance and gait	Observe the patient after instructing as follows: "Rise from your chair, walk 10 ft, return, and sit down." Check orthostatic blood pressure and heart rate	Inability to complete task in 15 seconds	Performance-Oriented Mobility Assessment (POMA). Consider referral for physical therapy.
Continence of urine	Ask, "Do you ever lose your urine and get wet?" If yes, then ask, "Have you lost urine on at least 6 separate days?"	"Yes" to both questions	Ascertain frequency and amount. Search for remediable causes, including local irritations, polyuric states, and medications. Consider urologic referral.
Nutrition	Ask, "Without trying, have you lost 10 lb or more in the last 6 months?" Weigh the patient. Measure height.	"Yes" or weight is below acceptable range for height	Do appropriate medical evaluation.
Mental status	Instruct as follows: "I am going to name three objects (pencil, truck, and book). I will ask you to repeat their names now and then again a few minutes from now."	Inability to recall all three objects after 1 minute	Administer Folstein Mini-Mental State Examination. If score is less than 24, search for causes of cognitive impairment. Ascertain onset, duration, and fluctuation of overt symptoms. Review medications. Assess consciousness and affect. Do appropriate laboratory tests.

FUNCTIONAL ASSESSMENT SCREENING IN THE ELDERLY (CONTINUED)			
Target Area	**Assessment Procedure**	**Abnormal Result**	**Suggested Intervention**
Depression	Ask, "Do you often feel sad or depressed?" or "How are your spirits?"	"Yes" or "Not very good, I guess"	Administer Geriatric Depression Scale or PHQ-9. If positive, check for antihypertensive, psychotropic, or other pertinent medications. Consider appropriate pharmacologic or psychiatric treatment.
ADL-IADLª	Ask, "Can you get out of bed yourself?" "Can you dress yourself?" "Can you make your own meals?" "Can you do your own shopping?"	"No" to any question	Corroborate responses with patient's appearance; question family members if accuracy is uncertain. Determine reasons for the inability (motivation compared with physical limitation). Institute appropriate medical, social, or environmental interventions.
Home environment	Ask, "Do you have trouble with stairs inside or outside of your home?" Ask about potential hazards inside the home with bathtubs, rugs, or lighting.	"Yes"	Evaluate home safety and institute appropriate countermeasures.
Social support	Ask, "Who would be able to help you in case of illness or emergency?"	—	List identified persons in the medical record. Become familiar with available resources for the elderly in the community.
Pain	Inquire about pain.	Presence of pain	Pain inventory.
Dentition	Oral examination.	Poor dentition	Dentistry referral.
Falls	Inquire about falls in past year and difficulty with walking or balance.	Presence of falls or gait/balance problems	Falls evaluation (see page 98).

ªActivities of Daily Living–Instrumental Activities of Daily Living.
Source: Modified from Lachs MS, et al. A simple procedure for screening for functional disability in elderly patients. *Ann Intern Med*. 1990;112:699.
Geriatrics At Your Fingertips online edition 2008–2009. (http://www.geriatricsatyourfingertips.org, accessed 10/13/11)

SCREENING AND PREVENTION GUIDELINES IN PERSPECTIVE: PGPC 2011

The following tables highlight areas where differences exist between various organizations' guideline recommendations and areas where a new direction appears to be developing as a result of new or updated guidelines.

1. Areas of significant difference in guideline recommendations

Guidelines	Organization	Recommendations
Adolescent Alcohol Abuse	USPSTF/AAFP	Evidence insufficient
	Bright Futures/ NIAAA	Screen annually
Breast CA Screening, Women aged 40–49 years	UK-NHS	Routine screening not recommended
	ACP	Mammogram and CBE yearly—high-risk patients (> 20% lifetime risk of breast CA) add annual MRI
	USPSTF/AAFP	Mammography ± breast examination every 1–2 years beginning at age 50. In women aged 40–50, counsel regarding risks and benefits
Breast CA Screening, Women aged 50–70 years	UK-NHS	Mammography screening every 3 years
	USPSTF/AAFP	Mammography screening every 1–2 years
	ACS	Annual mammography screening
Cervical CA Screening, Women aged < 50 years	UK-NHS	Begin screening every 3 years after age 25 years
	ACS	Screen 3 years after first sexual intercourse or at age 21, screen annually (or every 2 years if liquid-based Pap smear) until age 30, then every 3 years if consecutive negative Pap smear results
Prostate CA Screening, Men aged > 50 years	USPSTF/AAFP	Evidence insufficient to make recommendation; do not screen men aged > 70 years
	UK-NHS	Informed decision making
	ACS	Offer annual PSA and digital rectal examination, particularly for men who defer to physician's judgment—discuss risks and benefits including treatment options and side effects of treatment
Testicular CA Screening	USPSTF/AAFP	Recommend against screening
	ACS	Perform testicular examination as part of routine CA-related checkup
Depression, Children and Adolescents	USPSTF/AAFP/ CTF/NICE	Insufficient evidence to recommend for or against screening
	Bright Futures	Annual screening for behaviors/emotions that indicate depression or risk of suicide
Family Violence and Abuse, Children and Adolescents	USPSTF/AAFP	Insufficient evidence to recommend for or against screening
	Family Violence Prevention Fund	Assess caregivers/parents and adolescent patients at least annually

SCREENING AND PREVENTION GUIDELINES IN PERSPECTIVE: PGPC 2011 (CONTINUED)

Hearing Loss, Newborns	USPSTF/AAFP	Insufficient evidence to recommend for or against screening during the postpartum hospitalization
	Joint Committee on Infant Hearing	All infants should be screened for neonatal or congenital hearing loss
Thyroid Screening, Adults	USPSTF/AAFP	Evidence insufficient to recommend for or against screening
	ATA	Screen all women aged > 35 years at 5-year intervals
Glaucoma, Adults	USPSTF/AAFP	Evidence insufficient to recommend for or against screening
	AOA	Comprehensive eye examination every 2 years ages 18–60, then every year age > 60
Diabetes Mellitus, Gestational	USPSTF/AAFP	Evidence insufficient to recommend for or against screening asymptomatic pregnant women
	ADA	Risk-assess all women at first prenatal visit

2. New directions resulting from new or updated guidelines

HIV screening: Opt-out screening for practically everyone, actively recommended against written informed consent.

Endocarditis prophylaxis: Now targets those at increased risk of complications from endocarditis, rather than risk of endocarditis.

Perioperative guidelines: New data has emerged on beta blockade that is not reflected in current guidelines. Two randomized trials of perioperative metoprolol found that perioperative metoprolol does not appear to be effective in reducing postoperative death rates among unselected patients.

Osteoporosis:

- WHO Fracture Risk Algorithm (FRAX) developed to calculate the 1-year probability of fracture to guide treatment decisions.
- Screening recommendations for men.
- Recommendation to measure and supplement serum 25-OH vitamin D levels.

Diabetes type 2 prevention: New recommendation to consider metformin for those at very high risk of developing diabetes.

CBE, clinical breast exam; CA, cancer; MRI, magnetic resonance imaging; PSA, prostate-specific antigen; HIV, human immunodeficiency syndrome

95TH PERCENTILE OF BLOOD PRESSURE FOR BOYS

Age (years)	Systolic blood pressure (mm Hg) by percentile of height							Diastolic blood pressure (mm Hg) by percentile of height						
	5%	10%	25%	50%	75%	90%	95%	5%	10%	25%	50%	75%	90%	95%
3	104	105	107	109	110	112	113	63	63	64	65	66	67	67
4	106	107	109	111	112	114	115	66	67	68	69	70	71	71
5	108	109	110	112	114	115	116	69	70	71	72	73	74	74
6	109	110	112	114	115	117	117	72	72	73	74	75	76	76
7	110	111	113	115	117	118	119	74	74	75	76	77	78	78
8	111	112	114	116	118	119	120	75	76	77	78	79	79	80
9	113	114	116	118	119	121	121	76	77	78	79	80	81	81
10	115	116	117	119	121	122	123	77	78	79	80	81	81	82
11	117	118	119	121	123	124	125	78	78	79	80	81	82	82
12	119	120	122	123	125	127	127	78	79	80	81	82	82	83
13	121	122	124	126	128	129	130	79	79	80	81	82	83	83
14	124	125	127	128	130	132	132	80	80	81	82	83	84	84
15	126	127	129	131	133	134	135	81	81	82	83	84	85	85
16	129	130	132	134	135	137	137	82	83	83	84	85	86	87
17	131	132	134	136	138	139	140	84	85	86	87	87	88	89

95TH PERCENTILE OF BLOOD PRESSURE FOR GIRLS

Age (years)	Systolic blood pressure (mm Hg) by percentile of height							Diastolic blood pressure (mm Hg) by percentile of height						
	5%	10%	25%	50%	75%	90%	95%	5%	10%	25%	50%	75%	90%	95%
3	104	104	105	107	108	109	110	65	66	66	67	68	68	69
4	105	106	107	108	110	111	112	68	68	69	70	71	71	72
5	107	107	108	110	111	112	113	70	71	71	72	73	73	74
6	108	109	110	111	113	114	115	72	72	73	74	74	75	76
7	110	111	112	113	115	116	116	73	74	74	75	76	76	77
8	112	112	114	115	116	118	118	75	75	75	76	77	78	78
9	114	114	115	117	118	119	120	76	76	76	77	78	79	79
10	116	116	117	119	120	121	122	77	77	77	78	79	80	80
11	118	118	119	121	122	123	124	78	78	78	79	80	81	81
12	119	120	121	123	124	125	126	79	79	79	80	81	82	82
13	121	122	123	124	126	127	128	80	80	80	81	82	83	83
14	123	123	125	126	127	129	129	81	81	81	82	83	84	84
15	124	125	126	127	129	130	131	82	82	82	83	84	85	85
16	125	126	127	128	130	131	132	82	82	83	84	85	85	86
17	125	126	127	129	130	131	132	82	83	83	84	85	85	86

Source: http://www.nhlbi.nih.gov/guidelines/hypertension/child_tbl.htm, accessed 6/3/08.

BODY MASS INDEX (BMI) CONVERSION TABLE

Height in inches (cm)	BMI 25 kg/m²	BMI 27 kg/m²	BMI 30 kg/m²
	Body weight in pounds (kg)		
58 (147.32)	119 (53.98)	129 (58.51)	143 (64.86)
59 (149.86)	124 (56.25)	133 (60.33)	148 (67.13)
60 (152.40)	128 (58.06)	138 (62.60)	153 (69.40)
61 (154.94)	132 (59.87)	143 (64.86)	158 (71.67)
62 (157.48)	136 (61.69)	147 (66.68)	164 (74.39)
63 (160.02)	141 (63.96)	152 (68.95)	169 (76.66)
64 (162.56)	145 (65.77)	157 (71.22)	174 (78.93)
65 (165.10)	150 (68.04)	162 (73.48)	180 (81.65)
66 (167.64)	155 (70.31)	167 (75.75)	186 (84.37)
67 (170.18)	159 (72.12)	172 (78.02)	191 (86.64)
68 (172.72)	164 (74.39)	177 (80.29)	197 (89.36)
69 (175.26)	169 (76.66)	182 (82.56)	203 (92.08)
70 (177.80)	174 (78.93)	188 (85.28)	207 (93.90)
71 (180.34)	179 (81.19)	193 (87.54)	215 (97.52)
72 (182.88)	184 (83.46)	199 (90.27)	221 (100.25)
73 (185.42)	189 (85.73)	204 (92.53)	227 (102.97)
74 (187.96)	194 (88.00)	210 (95.26)	233 (105.69)
75 (190.50)	200 (90.72)	216 (97.98)	240 (108.86)
76 (193.04)	205 (92.99)	221 (100.25)	246 (111.59)

Metric conversion formula = weight (kg)/ height (m²)

Example of BMI calculation:

A person who weighs 78.93 kg and is 177 cm tall has a BMI of 25:

weight (78.93 kg)/height (1.77 m²) = 25

Nonmetric conversion formula = [weight (pounds)/height (inches²)] × 704.5

Example of BMI calculation:

A person who weighs 164 lb and is 68 in (or 5' 8") tall has a BMI of 25:

[weight (164 lb)/height (68 in²)] × 704.5 = 25

BMI categories:

Underweight = < 18.5

Normal weight = 18.5–24.9

Overweight = 25–29.9

Obesity = ≥ 30

Source: Adapted from NHLBI Obesity Guidelines in Adults: http://www.nhlbi.nih.gov/guidelines/obesity/bmi_tbl.htm, accessed 10/13/11.

BMI on-line calculator: http://www.nhlbisupport.com/bmi/bmicalc.htm, accessed 10/13/11.

ESTIMATE OF 10-YEAR CARDIAC RISK FOR MEN[a]

Age (years)	Points
20–34	–9
35–39	–4
40–44	0
45–49	3
50–54	6
55–59	8
60–64	10
65–69	11
70–74	12
75–79	13

Total Cholesterol	Points				
	Age 20–39	Age 40–49	Age 50–59	Age 60–69	Age 70–79
< 160	0	0	0	0	0
160–199	4	3	2	1	0
200–239	7	5	3	1	0
240–279	9	6	4	2	1
≥ 280	11	8	5	3	1

	Points				
	Age 20–39	Age 40–49	Age 50–59	Age 60–69	Age 70–79
Nonsmoker	0	0	0	0	0
Smoker	8	5	3	1	1

High-Density Lipoprotein (mg/dL)	Points
≥ 60	–1
50–59	0
40–49	1
< 40	2

Systolic Blood Pressure (mm Hg)	If Untreated	If Treated
< 120	0	0
120–129	0	1
130–139	1	2
140–159	1	2
≥ 160	2	3

ESTIMATE OF 10-YEAR CARDIAC RISK FOR MEN[a] (CONTINUED)

Point Total	10-Year Risk %	Point Total	10-Year Risk %	
< 0	< 1	9	5	
0	1	10	6	
1	1	11	8	
2	1	12	10	
3	1	13	12	
4	1	14	16	
5	2	15	20	
6	2	16	25	
7	3	≥ 17	≥ 30	**10-Year Risk ____ %**
8	4			

[a]Framingham point scores.

Source: U.S. Department of Health and Human Services, Public Health Service, National Institutes of Health, National Heart, Lung, and Blood Institute. NIH Publication No. 01-3305, May 2001.
On-line risk calculator: http://hp2010.nhlbihin.net/atpiii/calculator.asp

ESTIMATE OF 10-YEAR CARDIAC RISK FOR WOMEN[a]

Age (years)	Points
20–34	−7
35–39	−3
40–44	0
45–49	3
50–54	6
55–59	8
60–64	10
65–69	12
70–74	14
75–79	16

Total Cholesterol	Points				
	Age 20–39	Age 40–49	Age 50–59	Age 60–69	Age 70–79
< 160	0	0	0	0	0
160–199	4	3	2	1	1
200–239	8	6	4	2	1
240–279	11	8	5	3	2
≥ 280	13	10	7	4	2

	Points				
	Age 20–39	Age 40–49	Age 50–59	Age 60–69	Age 70–79
Nonsmoker	0	0	0	0	0
Smoker	9	7	4	2	1

High-Density Lipoprotein (mg/dL)	Points
≥ 60	−1
50–59	0
40–49	1
< 40	2

Systolic Blood Pressure (mm Hg)	If Untreated	If Treated
< 120	0	0
120–129	1	3
130–139	2	4
140–159	3	5
≥ 160	4	6

ESTIMATE OF 10-YEAR CARDIAC RISK FOR WOMEN[a] (CONTINUED)

Point Total	10-Year Risk %	Point Total	10-Year Risk %	
< 9	< 1	17	5	
9	1	18	6	
10	1	19	8	
11	1	20	11	
12	1	21	14	
13	2	22	17	
14	2	23	22	
15	3	24	27	**10-Year Risk _____ %**
16	4	≥ 25	≥ 30	

[a]Framingham point scores.

Source: U.S. Department of Health and Human Services, Public Health Service, National Institutes of Health, National Heart, Lung, and Blood Institute. NIH Publication No. 01-3305, May 2001. On-line risk calculator: http://hp2010.nhlbihin.net/atpiii/calculator.asp

ESTIMATE OF 10-YEAR STROKE RISK FOR MEN

Age (years)	Points	Untreated Systolic Blood Pressure (mm Hg)	Points
54–56	0	97–105	0
57–59	1	106–115	1
60–62	2	116–125	2
63–65	3	126–135	3
66–68	4	136–145	4
69–72	5	146–155	5
73–75	6	156–165	6
76–78	7	166–175	7
79–81	8	176–185	8
82–84	9	186–195	9
85	10	196–205	10

Treated Systolic Blood Pressure (mm Hg)	Points	History of Diabetes	Points
97–105	0	No	0
106–112	1	Yes	2
113–117	2		
118–123	3		
124–129	4		
130–135	5		
136–142	6		
143–150	7		
151–161	8		
162–176	9		
177–205	10		

Cigarette Smoking	Points	Cardiovascular Disease	Points
No	0	No	0
Yes	3	Yes	4

Atrial Fibrillation	Points	Left Ventricular Hypertrophy on Electrocardiogram	Points
No	0	No	0
Yes	4	Yes	5

ESTIMATE OF 10-YEAR STROKE RISK FOR MEN (CONTINUED)

Point Total	10-Year Risk %	Point Total	10-Year Risk %	
1	3	16	22	
2	3	17	26	
3	4	18	29	
4	4	19	33	
5	5	20	37	
6	5	21	42	
7	6	22	47	
8	7	23	52	
9	8	24	57	
10	10	25	63	
11	11	26	68	
12	13	27	74	
13	15	28	79	
14	17	29	84	10-Year Risk _____ %
15	20	30	88	

Source: Modified Framingham Stroke Risk Profile. *Circulation.* 2006;113:e873–923.

ESTIMATE OF 10-YEAR STROKE RISK FOR WOMEN

Age (years)	Points	Untreated Systolic Blood Pressure (mm Hg)	Points
54–56	0	95–106	1
57–59	1	107–118	2
60–62	2	119–130	3
63–64	3	131–143	4
65–67	4	144–155	5
68–70	5	156–167	6
71–73	6	168–180	7
74–76	7	181–192	8
77–78	8	193–204	9
79–81	9	205–216	10
82–84	10		

ESTIMATE OF 10-YEAR STROKE RISK FOR WOMEN (CONTINUED)

Treated Systolic Blood Pressure (mm Hg)	Points	History of Diabetes	Points
95–106	1	No	0
107–113	2	Yes	3
114–119	3		
120–125	4		
126–131	5		
132–139	6		
140–148	7		
149–160	8		
161–204	9		
205–216	10		

Cigarette Smoking	Points	Cardiovascular Disease	Points
No	0	No	0
Yes	3	Yes	2

Atrial Fibrillation	Points	Left Ventricular Hypertrophy on Electrocardiogram	Points
No	0	No	0
Yes	6	Yes	4

Point Total	10-Year Risk %	Point Total	10-Year Risk %		
1	1	16	19		
2	1	17	23		
3	2	18	27		
4	2	19	32		
5	2	20	37		
6	3	21	43		
7	4	22	50		
8	4	23	57		
9	5	24	64		
10	6	25	71		
11	8	26	78		
12	9	27	84		
13	11	28			
14	13	29		10-Year Risk _____ %	
15	16	30			

Source: Modified Framingham Stroke Risk Profile. *Circulation.* 2006;113:e873–923.

Recommended Immunization Schedule for Persons Aged 0 Through 6 Years—United States • 2011

For those who fall behind or start late, see the catch-up schedule

Vaccine ▼ Age ▶	Birth	1 month	2 months	4 months	6 months	12 months	15 months	18 months	19–23 months	2–3 years	4–6 years
Hepatitis B[1]	HepB	HepB			HepB						
Rotavirus[2]			RV	RV	RV[2]						
Diphtheria, Tetanus, Pertussis[3]			DTaP	DTaP	DTaP		DTaP				DTaP
Haemophilus influenzae type b[4]			Hib	Hib	Hib[4]	Hib					
Pneumococcal[5]			PCV	PCV	PCV	PCV				PPSV	
Inactivated Poliovirus[6]			IPV	IPV		IPV					IPV
Influenza[7]						Influenza (Yearly)					
Measles, Mumps, Rubella[8]						MMR		see footnote[8]			MMR
Varicella[9]						Varicella		see footnote[9]			Varicella
Hepatitis A[10]						HepA (2 doses)				HepA Series	
Meningococcal[11]										MCV4	

Range of recommended ages for all children

Range of recommended ages for certain high-risk groups

This schedule includes recommendations in effect as of December 21, 2010. Any dose not administered at the recommended age should be administered at a subsequent visit, when indicated and feasible. The use of a combination vaccine generally is preferred over separate injections of its equivalent component vaccines. Considerations should include provider assessment, patient preference, and the potential for adverse events. Providers should consult the relevant Advisory Committee on Immunization Practices statement for detailed recommendations: **http://www.cdc.gov/vaccines/pubs/acip-list.htm**. Clinically significant adverse events that follow immunization should be reported to the Vaccine Adverse Event Reporting System (VAERS) at **http://www.vaers.hhs.gov** or by telephone, **800-822-7967**. Use of trade names and commercial sources is for identification only and does not imply endorsement by the U.S. Department of Health and Human Services.

1. Hepatitis B vaccine (HepB). (Minimum age: birth)

At birth:

- Administer monovalent HepB to all newborns before hospital discharge.
- If mother is hepatitis B surface antigen (HBsAg)-positive, administer HepB and 0.5 mL of hepatitis B immune globulin (HBIG) within 12 hours of birth.
- If mother's HBsAg status is unknown, administer HepB within 12 hours of birth. Determine mother's HBsAg status as soon as possible and, if HBsAg-positive, administer HBIG (no later than age 1 week).

Doses following the birth dose:

- The second dose should be administered at age 1 or 2 months. Monovalent HepB should be used for doses administered before age 6 weeks

- Infants born to HBsAg-positive mothers should be tested for HBsAg and antibody to HBsAg 1 to 2 months after completion of at least 3 doses of the HepB series, at age 9 through 18 months (generally at the next well-child visit).
- Administration of 4 doses of HepB to infants is permissible when a combination vaccine containing HepB is administered after the birth dose.
- Infants who did not receive a birth dose should receive 3 doses of HepB on a schedule of 0, 1, and 6 months.
- The final (3rd or 4th) dose in the HepB series should be administered no earlier than age 24 weeks.

2. **Rotavirus vaccine (RV).** (Minimum age: 6 weeks)
   - Administer the first dose at age 6 through 14 weeks (maximum age: 14 weeks 6 days). Vaccination should not be initiated for infants aged 15 weeks 0 days or older.
   - The maximum age for the final dose in the series is 8 months 0 days.
   - If Rotarix is administered at ages 2 and 4 months, a dose at 6 months is not indicated.

3. **Diphtheria and tetanus toxoids and acellular pertussis vaccine (DTaP).** (Minimum age: 6 weeks)
   - The fourth dose may be administered as early as age 12 months, provided at least 6 months have elapsed since the third dose.

4. **Haemophilus influenzae type b conjugate vaccine (Hib).** (Minimum age: 6 weeks)
   - If PRP-OMP (PedvaxHIB or Comvax [Hep-Hib]) is administered at ages 2 and 4 months, a dose at age 6 months is not indicated.
   - Hiberix should not be used for doses at ages 2, 4, or 6 months for the primary series but can be used as the final dose in children aged 12 months through 4 years.

5. **Pneumococcal vaccine.** (Minimum age: 6 weeks for pneumococcal conjugate vaccine [PCV]; 2 years for pneumococcal polysaccharide vaccine [PPSV])
   - PCV is recommended for all children aged younger than 5 years. Administer 1 dose of PCV to all healthy children aged 24 through 59 months who are not completely vaccinated for their age.
   - A PCV series begun with 7-valent PCV (PCV7) should be completed with 13-valent PCV (PCV13).
   - A single supplemental dose of PCV13 is recommended for all children aged 14 through 59 months who have received an age-appropriate series of PCV7.
   - A single supplemental dose of PCV13 is recommended for all children aged 60 through 71 months with underlying medical conditions who have received an age-appropriate series of PCV7.
   - The supplemental dose of PCV13 should be administered at least 8 weeks after the previous dose of PCV7. See *MMWR* 2010;59(No. RR-11).
   - Administer PPSV at least 8 weeks after last dose of PCV to children aged 2 years or older with certain underlying medical conditions, including a cochlear implant.

6. **Inactivated poliovirus vaccine (IPV).** (Minimum age: 6 weeks)
   - If 4 or more doses are administered prior to age 4 years an additional dose should be administered at age 4 through 6 years.
   - The final dose in the series should be administered on or after the fourth birthday and at least 6 months following the previous dose.

7. **Influenza vaccine (seasonal).** (Minimum age: 6 months for trivalent inactivated influenza vaccine [TIV]; 2 years for live, attenuated influenza vaccine [LAIV])
   - For healthy children aged 2 years and older (i.e., those who do not have underlying medical conditions that predispose them to influenza complications), either LAIV or TIV may be used, except LAIV should not be given to children aged 2 through 4 years who have had wheezing in the past 12 months.
   - Administer 2 doses (separated by at least 4 weeks) to children aged 6 months through 8 years who are receiving seasonal influenza vaccine for the first time or who were vaccinated for the first time during the previous influenza season but only received 1 dose.
   - Children aged 6 months through 8 years who received no doses of monovalent 2009 H1N1 vaccine should receive 2 doses of 2010–2011 seasonal influenza vaccine. See *MMWR* 2010;59(No. RR-8):33–34.

8. **Measles, mumps, and rubella vaccine (MMR).** (Minimum age: 12 months)
   - The second dose may be administered before age 4 years, provided at least 4 weeks have elapsed since the first dose.

9. **Varicella vaccine.** (Minimum age: 12 months)
   - The second dose may be administered before age 4 years, provided at least 3 months have elapsed since the first dose.
   - For children aged 12 months through 12 years the recommended minimum interval between doses is 3 months. However, if the second dose was administered at least 4 weeks after the first dose, it can be accepted as valid.

10. **Hepatitis A vaccine (HepA).** (Minimum age: 12 months)
    - Administer 2 doses at least 6 months apart.
    - HepA is recommended for children aged older than 23 months who live in areas where vaccination programs target older children, who are at increased risk for infection, or for whom immunity against hepatitis A is desired.

11. **Meningococcal conjugate vaccine, quadrivalent (MCV4).** (Minimum age: 2 years)
    - Administer 2 doses of MCV4 at least 8 weeks apart to children aged 2 through 10 years with persistent complement component deficiency and anatomic or functional asplenia, and 1 dose every 5 years thereafter.
    - Persons with human immunodeficiency virus (HIV) infection who are vaccinated with MCV4 should receive 2 doses at least 8 weeks apart.
    - Administer 1 dose of MCV4 to children aged 2 through 10 years who travel to countries with highly endemic or epidemic disease and during outbreaks caused by a vaccine serogroup.
    - Administer MCV4 to children at continued risk for meningococcal disease who were previously vaccinated with MCV4 or meningococcal polysaccharide vaccine after 3 years if the first dose was administered at age 2 through 6 years.

The Recommended Immunization Schedules for Persons Aged 0 Through 18 Years are approved by the Advisory Committee on Immunization Practices (**http://www.cdc.gov/vaccines/recs/acip**), the American Academy of Pediatrics (**http://www.aap.org**), and the American Academy of Family Physicians (**http://www.aafp.org**).

The Recommended Immunization Schedules for Persons Aged 0 Through 18 Years are approved by the Advisory Committee on Immunization Practices (**http://www.cdc.gov/vaccines/recs/acip**), the American Academy of Pediatrics (**http://www.aap.org**), and the American Academy of Family Physicians (**http://www.aafp.org**).
Department of Health and Human Services • Centers for Disease Control and Prevention

Recommended Immunization Schedule for Persons Aged 7 Through 18 Years—United States • 2011

For those who fall behind or start late, see the schedule below and the catch-up schedule

This schedule includes recommendations in effect as of December 21, 2010. Any dose not administered at the recommended age should be administered at a subsequent visit, when indicated and feasible. The use of a combination vaccine generally is preferred over separate injections of its equivalent component vaccines. Considerations should include provider assessment, patient preference, and the potential for adverse events. Providers should consult the relevant Advisory Committee on Immunization Practices statement for detailed recommendations: **http://www.cdc.gov/vaccines/recs/acip**. Clinically significant adverse events that follow immunization should be reported to the Vaccine Adverse Event Reporting System (VAERS) at **http://www.vaers.hhs.gov** or by telephone, **800-822-7967**.

1. **Tetanus and diphtheria toxoids and acellular pertussis vaccine (Tdap).** (Minimum age: 10 years for Boostrix and 11 years for Adacel).
   - Persons aged 11 through 18 years who have not received Tdap should receive a dose followed by Td booster doses every 10 years thereafter.
   - Persons aged 7 through 10 years who are not fully immunized against pertussis (including those never vaccinated or with unknown pertussis vaccination status) should receive a single dose of Tdap. Refer to the catch-up schedule if additional doses of tetanus and diphtheria toxoid-containing vaccine are needed.
   - Tdap can be administered regardless of the interval since the last tetanus and diphtheria toxoid-containing vaccine.

2. **Human papillomavirus vaccine (HPV).** (Minimum age: 9 years)
   - Quadrivalent HPV vaccine (HPV4) or bivalent HPV vaccine (HPV2) is recommended for the prevention of cervical precancers and cancers in females.
   - HPV4 is recommended for prevention of cervical precancers, cancers, and genital warts in females.
   - HPV4 may be administered in a 3-dose series to males aged 9 through 18 years to reduce their likelihood of genital warts.
   - Administer the second dose 1 to 2 months after the first dose and the third dose 6 months after the first dose (at least 24 weeks after the first dose).

3. **Meningococcal conjugate vaccine, quadrivalent (MCV4).** (Minimum age: 2 years)
   - Administer MCV4 at age 11 through 12 years with a booster dose at age 16 years.
   - Administer 1 dose at age 13 through 18 years if not previously vaccinated.
   - Persons who received their first dose at age 13 through 15 years should receive a booster dose at age 16 through 18 years.
   - Administer 1 dose to previously unvaccinated college freshmen living in a dormitory.
   - Administer 2 doses at least 8 weeks apart to children aged 2 through 10 years with persistent complement component deficiency and anatomic or functional asplenia, and 1 dose every 5 years thereafter.
   - Persons with HIV infection who are vaccinated with MCV4 should receive 2 doses at least 8 weeks apart.
   - Administer 1 dose of MCV4 to children aged 2 through 10 years who travel to countries with highly endemic or epidemic disease and during outbreaks caused by a vaccine serogroup.
   - Administer MCV4 to children at continued risk for meningococcal disease who were previously vaccinated with MCV4 or meningococcal polysaccharide vaccine after 3 years (if first dose administered at age 2 through 6 years) or after 5 years (if first dose administered at age 7 years or older).

4. **Influenza vaccine (seasonal).**
   - For healthy nonpregnant persons aged 7 through 18 years (i.e., those who do not have underlying medical conditions that predispose them to influenza complications), either LAIV or TIV may be used.
   - Administer 2 doses (separated by at least 4 weeks) to children aged 6 months through 8 years who are receiving seasonal influenza vaccine for the first time or who were not vaccinated for the first time during the previous influenza season but only received 1 dose.
   - Children 6 months through 8 years of age who received no doses of monovalent 2009 H1N1 vaccine should receive 2 doses of 2010-2011 seasonal influenza vaccine. See *MMWR* 2010;59(No. RR-8):33–34.

5. **Pneumococcal vaccines.**
   - A single dose of 13-valent pneumococcal conjugate vaccine (PCV13) may be administered to children aged 6 through 18 years who have functional or anatomic asplenia, HIV infection or other immunocompromising condition, cochlear implant or CSF leak. See *MMWR* 2010;59(No. RR-11).

- The dose of PCV13 should be administered at least 8 weeks after the previous dose of PCV7.
- Administer pneumococcal polysaccharide vaccine at least 8 weeks after the last dose of PCV to children aged 2 years or older with certain underlying medical conditions, including a cochlear implant. A single revaccination should be administered after 5 years to children with functional or anatomic asplenia or an immunocompromising condition.

6. **Hepatitis A vaccine (HepA).**
   - Administer 2 doses at least 6 months apart.
   - HepA is recommended for children aged older than 23 months who live in areas where vaccination programs target older children, or who are at increased risk for infection, or for whom immunity against hepatitis A is desired.

7. **Hepatitis B vaccine (HepB).**
   - Administer the 3-dose series to those not previously vaccinated. For those with incomplete vaccination, follow the catch-up schedule.
   - A 2-dose series (separated by at least 4 months) of adult formulation Recombivax HB is licensed for children aged 11 through 15 years.

8. **Inactivated poliovirus vaccine (IPV).**
   - The final dose in the series should be administered on or after the fourth birthday and at least 6 months following the previous dose.
   - If both OPV and IPV were administered as part of a series, a total of 4 doses should be administered, regardless of the child's current age.

9. **Measles, mumps, and rubella vaccine (MMR).**
   - The minimum interval between the 2 doses of MMR is 4 weeks.

10. **Varicella vaccine.**
    - For persons aged 7 through 18 years without evidence of immunity (see *MMWR* 2007;56[No. RR-4]), administer 2 doses if not previously vaccinated or the second dose if only 1 dose has been administered.
    - For persons aged 7 through 12 years, the recommended minimum interval between doses is 3 months. If the second dose was administered at least 4 weeks after the first dose, it can be accepted as valid.
    - For persons aged 13 years and older, the minimum interval between doses is 4 weeks.

The Recommended Immunization Schedules for Persons Aged 0 Through 18 Years are approved by the Advisory Committee on Immunization Practices (**http://www.cdc.gov/vaccines/recs/acip**), the American Academy of Pediatrics (**http://www.aap.org**), and the American Academy of Family Physicians (**http://www.aafp.org**).
Department of Health and Human Services • Centers for Disease Control and Prevention

Catch-up Immunization Schedule for Persons Aged 4 Months Through 18 Years Who Start Late or Who Are More Than 1 Month Behind—United States • 2011

The table below provides catch-up schedules and minimum intervals between doses for children whose vaccinations have been delayed. A vaccine series does not need to be restarted, regardless of the time that has elapsed between doses. Use the section appropriate for the child's age

Vaccine	Minimum Age for Dose 1	Minimum Interval Between Doses			
		Dose 1 to Dose 2	Dose 2 to Dose 3	Dose 3 to Dose 4	Dose 4 to Dose 5
PERSONS AGED 4 MONTHS THROUGH 6 YEARS					
Hepatitis B[1]	Birth	4 weeks	8 weeks (and at least 16 weeks after first dose)		
Rotavirus[2]	6 wks	4 weeks	4 weeks[2]		
Diphtheria, Tetanus, Pertussis[3]	6 wks	4 weeks	4 weeks	6 months	6 months[3]
Haemophilus influenzae type b[4]	6 wks	4 weeks if first dose administered at younger than age 12 months; 8 weeks (as final dose) if first dose administered at age 12–14 months; No further doses needed if first dose administered at age 15 months or older	4 weeks[4] if current age is younger than 12 months; 8 weeks (as final dose)[4] if current age is 12 months or older and first dose administered at younger than age 12 months and second dose administered at younger than 15 months; No further doses needed if previous dose administered at age 15 months or older	8 weeks (as final dose) This dose only necessary for children aged 12 months through 59 months who received 3 doses before age 12 months	
Pneumococcal[5]	6 wks	4 weeks if first dose administered at younger than age 12 months; 8 weeks (as final dose for healthy children) if first dose administered at age 12 months or older or current age 24 through 59 months; No further doses needed for healthy children if first dose administered at age 24 months or older	4 weeks if current age is younger than 12 months; 8 weeks (as final dose for healthy children) if current age is 12 months or older; No further doses needed for healthy children if previous dose administered at age 24 months or older	8 weeks (as final dose) This dose only necessary for children aged 12 months through 59 months who received 3 doses before age 12 months or for children at high risk who received 3 doses at any age	
Inactivated Poliovirus[6]	6 mos	4 weeks	4 weeks	6 months[6]	
Measles, Mumps, Rubella[7]	12 mos	4 weeks			
Varicella[8]	12 mos	3 months			
Hepatitis A[9]	12 mos	6 months			
PERSONS AGED 7 THROUGH 18 YEARS					
Tetanus, Diphtheria/Tetanus, Diphtheria, Pertussis[10]	7 yrs[10]	4 weeks	4 weeks if first dose administered at younger than age 12 months; 6 months if first dose administered at 12 months or older	6 months if first dose administered at younger than age 12 months	
Human Papillomavirus[11]	9 yrs	Routine dosing intervals are recommended (females)[11]			
Hepatitis A[9]	12 mos	6 months			
Hepatitis B[1]	Birth	4 weeks	8 weeks (and at least 16 weeks after first dose)		
Inactivated Poliovirus[6]	6 wks	4 weeks	4 weeks	6 months[6]	
Measles, Mumps, Rubella[7]	12 mos	4 weeks			
Varicella[8]	12 mos	3 months if person is younger than age 13 years; 4 weeks if person is aged 13 years or older			

1. **Hepatitis B vaccine (HepB).**
   - Administer the 3-dose series to those not previously vaccinated.
   - The minimum age for the third dose of HepB is 24 weeks.
   - A 2-dose series (separated by at least 4 months) of adult formulation Recombivax HB is licensed for children aged 11 through 15 years.

2. **Rotavirus vaccine (RV).**
   - The maximum age for the first dose is 14 weeks 6 days. Vaccination should not be initiated for infants aged 15 weeks 0 days or older.
   - The maximum age for the final dose in the series is 8 months 0 days.
   - If Rotarix was administered for the first and second doses, a third dose is not indicated.

3. **Diphtheria and tetanus toxoids and acellular pertussis vaccine (DTaP).**
   - The fifth dose is not necessary if the fourth dose was administered at age 4 years or older.

4. **Haemophilus influenzae type b conjugate vaccine (Hib).**
   - 1 dose of Hib vaccine should be considered for unvaccinated persons aged 5 years or older who have sickle cell disease, leukemia, or HIV infection, or who have had a splenectomy.
   - If the first 2 doses were PRP-OMP (PedvaxHIB or Comvax), and administered at age 11 months or younger, the third (and final) dose should be administered at age 12 through 15 months and at least 8 weeks after the second dose.
   - If the first dose was administered at age 7 through 11 months, administer the second dose at least 4 weeks later and a final dose at age 12 through 15 months.

5. **Pneumococcal vaccine.**
   - Administer 1 dose of 13-valent pneumococcal conjugate vaccine (PCV13) to all healthy children aged 24 through 59 months with any incomplete PCV schedule (PCV7 or PCV13).
   - For children aged 24 through 71 months with underlying medical conditions, administer 1 dose of PCV13 if 3 doses of PCV were received previously or administer 2 doses of PCV13 at least 8 weeks apart if fewer than 3 doses of PCV were received previously.
   - A single dose of PCV13 is recommended for certain children with underlying medical conditions through 18 years of age. See age-specific schedules for details.
   - Administer pneumococcal polysaccharide vaccine (PPSV) to children aged 2 years or older with certain underlying medical conditions, including a cochlear implant, at least 8 weeks after the last dose of PCV. A single revaccination should be administered after 5 years to children with functional or anatomic asplenia or an immunocompromising condition. See *MMWR* 2010;59(No. RR-11).

6. **Inactivated poliovirus vaccine (IPV).**
   - The final dose in the series should be administered on or after the fourth birthday and at least 6 months following the previous dose.
   - A fourth dose is not necessary if the third dose was administered at age 4 years or older and at least 6 months following the previous dose.
   - In the first 6 months of life, minimum age and minimum intervals are only recommended if the person is at risk for imminent exposure to circulating poliovirus (i.e., travel to a polio-endemic region or during an outbreak).

7. **Measles, mumps, and rubella vaccine (MMR).**
   - Administer the second dose routinely at age 4 through 6 years. The minimum interval between the 2 doses of MMR is 4 weeks.

8. **Varicella vaccine.**
   - Administer the second dose routinely at age 4 through 6 years.
   - If the second dose was administered at least 4 weeks after the first dose, it can be accepted as valid.

9. **Hepatitis A vaccine (HepA).**
   - HepA is recommended for children aged older than age 23 months who live in areas where vaccination programs target older children, or who are at increased risk for infection, or for whom immunity against hepatitis A is desired.

10. **Tetanus and diphtheria toxoids (Td) and tetanus and diphtheria toxoids and acellular pertussis vaccine (Tdap).**
    - Doses of DTaP are counted as part of the Td/Tdap series.
    - Tdap should be substituted for a single dose of Td in the catch-up series for children aged 7 through 10 years or as a booster for children aged 11 through 18 years; use Td for other doses.

11. **Human papillomavirus vaccine (HPV).**
    - Administer the series to females at age 13 through 18 years if not previously vaccinated or have not completed the vaccine series.
    - Quadrivalent HPV vaccine (HPV4) may be administered in a 3-dose series to males 9 through 18 years to reduce their likelihood of genital warts.
    - Use recommended routine dosing intervals for series catch-up (i.e., the second and third doses should be administered at 1 to 2 and 6 months after the first dose). The minimum interval between the first and second doses is 4 weeks. The minimum interval between the second and third doses is 12 weeks, and the third dose should be administered at least 24 weeks after the first dose.

Information about reporting reactions after immunization is available online at http://www.vaers.hhs.gov or by telephone, **800-822-7967**. Suspected cases of vaccine-preventable diseases should be reported to the state or local health department. Additional information, including precautions and contraindications for immunization, is available from the National Center for Immunization and Respiratory Diseases at **800-CDC-INFO** (800-232-4636) or online at http://www.cdc.gov/vaccines or http://www.cdc.gov/vaccines/recs/schedules.

Department of Health and Human Services • Centers for Disease Control and Prevention

Recommended Adult Immunization Schedule
UNITED STATES • 2011

Note: These recommendations *must* be read with the footnotes that follow containing number of doses, intervals between doses, and other important information.

Recommended adult immunization schedule, by vaccine and age group

VACCINE ▼ AGE GROUP ►	19–26 years	27–49 years	50–59 years	60–64 years	≥65 years
Influenza[1],*	1 dose annually				
Tetanus, diphtheria, pertussis (Td/Tdap)[2],*	Substitute 1-time dose of Tdap for Td booster; then boost with Td every 10 yrs			Td booster every 10 yrs	
Varicella[3],*	2 doses				
Human papillomavirus (HPV)[4],*	3 doses (females)				
Zoster[5]				1 dose	
Measles, mumps, rubella (MMR)[6],*	1 or 2 doses		1 dose		
Pneumococcal (polysaccharide)[7,8]	1 or 2 doses				1 dose
Meningococcal[9],*	1 or more doses				
Hepatitis A[10],*	2 doses				
Hepatitis B[11],*	3 doses				

*Covered by the Vaccine Injury Compensation Program.

For all persons in this category who meet the age requirements and who lack evidence of immunity (e.g., lack documentation of vaccination or have no evidence of previous infection)

Recommended if some other risk factor is present (e.g., based on medical, occupational, lifestyle, or other indications)

No recommendation

Report all clinically significant postvaccination reactions to the Vaccine Adverse Event Reporting System (VAERS). Reporting forms and instructions on filing a VAERS report are available at http://www.vaers.hhs.gov or by telephone, 800-822-7967.

Information on how to file a Vaccine Injury Compensation Program claim is available at http://www.hrsa.gov/vaccinecompensation or by telephone, 800-338-2382. Information about filing a claim for vaccine injury is available through the U.S. Court of Federal Claims, 717 Madison Place, N.W., Washington, D.C. 20005; telephone, 202-357-6400.

Additional information about the vaccines in this schedule, extent of available data, and contraindications for vaccination also is available at http://www.cdc.gov/vaccines or from the CDC-INFO Contact Center at 800-CDC-INFO (800-232-4636) in English and Spanish, 24 hours a day, 7 days a week.

Use of trade names and commercial sources is for identification only and does not imply endorsement by the U.S. Department of Health and Human Services.

Vaccines that might be indicated for adults based on medical and other indications

INDICATION ▶ / VACCINE ▼	Pregnancy	Immuno-compromising conditions (excluding human immunodeficiency virus [HIV])3,6,13	HIV infection3,6,12,13 CD4+ T lymphocyte count <200 cells/µL	HIV infection3,6,12,13 CD4+ T lymphocyte count ≥200 cells/µL	Diabetes, heart disease, chronic lung disease, chronic alcoholism	Asplenia12 (including elective splenectomy) and persistent complement component deficiencies	Chronic liver disease	Kidney failure, end-stage renal disease, receipt of hemodialysis	Healthcare personnel
Influenza1,*				1 dose TIV annually					1 dose TIV or LAIV annually
Tetanus, diphtheria, pertussis (Td/Tdap)2,*	Td	Substitute 1-time dose of Tdap for Td booster; then boost with Td every 10 yrs							
Varicella3,*	Contraindicated			2 doses					
Human papillomavirus (HPV)4,*			3 doses through age 26 yrs						
Zoster5	Contraindicated			1 dose					
Measles, mumps, rubella (MMR)6,*	Contraindicated			1 or 2 doses					
Pneumococcal (polysaccharide)7,8		1 or 2 doses							
Meningococcal9,*		1 or more doses							
Hepatitis A10,*		2 doses							
Hepatitis B11,*		3 doses							

*Covered by the Vaccine Injury Compensation Program.

For all persons in this category who meet the age requirements and who lack evidence of immunity (e.g., lack documentation of vaccination or have no evidence of previous infection)

Recommended if some other risk factor is present (e.g., on the basis of medical, occupational, lifestyle, or other indications)

No recommendation

These schedules indicate the recommended age groups and medical indications for which administration of currently licensed vaccines is commonly indicated for adults ages 19 years and older, as of January 1, 2011. For all vaccines being recommended on the adult immunization schedule, a vaccine series does not need to be restarted, regardless of the time that has elapsed between doses. Licensed combination vaccines may be used whenever any components of the combination are indicated and when the vaccine's other components are not contraindicated. For detailed recommendations on all vaccines, including those used primarily for travelers or that are issued during the year, consult the manufacturers' package inserts and the complete statements from the Advisory Committee on Immunization Practices (http://www.cdc.gov/vaccines/pubs/acip-list.htm).

The recommendations in this schedule were approved by the Centers for Disease Control and Prevention's (CDC) Advisory Committee on Immunization Practices (ACIP), the American Academy of Family Physicians (AAFP), the American College of Obstetricians and Gynecologists (ACOG), and the American College of Physicians (ACP).

U.S. DEPARTMENT OF HEALTH AND HUMAN SERVICES
CENTERS FOR DISEASE CONTROL AND PREVENTION

For complete statements by the Advisory Committee on Immunization Practices (ACIP), visit www.cdc.gov/vaccines/pubs/ACIP-list.htm.

1. Influenza vaccination

Annual vaccination against influenza is recommended for all persons aged 6 months and older, including all adults. Healthy, nonpregnant adults aged less than 50 years without high-risk medical conditions can receive either intranasally administered live, attenuated influenza vaccine (FluMist), or inactivated vaccine. Other persons should receive the inactivated vaccine. Adults aged 65 years and older can receive the standard influenza vaccine or the high-dose (Fluzone) influenza vaccine. Additional information about influenza vaccination is available at http://www.cdc.gov/vaccines/vpd-vac/flu/default.htm.

2. Tetanus, diphtheria, and acellular pertussis (Td/Tdap) vaccination

Administer a one-time dose of Tdap to adults aged less than 65 years who have not received Tdap previously or for whom vaccine status is unknown to replace one of the 10-year Td boosters, and as soon as feasible to all 1) postpartum women, 2) close contacts of infants younger than age 12 months (e.g., grandparents and child-care providers), and 3) healthcare personnel with direct patient contact. Adults aged 65 years and older who have not previously received Tdap and who have close contact with an infant aged less than 12 months also should be vaccinated. Other adults aged 65 years and older may receive Tdap. Tdap can be administered regardless of interval since the most recent tetanus or diphtheria-containing vaccine.

Adults with uncertain or incomplete history of completing a 3-dose primary vaccination series with Td-containing vaccines should begin or complete a primary vaccination series. For unvaccinated adults, administer the first 2 doses at least 4 weeks apart and the third dose 6–12 months after the second. If incompletely vaccinated (i.e., less than 3 doses), administer remaining doses. Substitute a one-time dose of Tdap for one of the doses of Td, either in the primary series or for the routine booster, whichever comes first.

If a woman is pregnant and received the most recent Td vaccination 10 or more years previously, administer Td during the second or third trimester. If the woman received the most recent Td vaccination less than 10 years previously, administer Tdap during the immediate postpartum period. At the clinician's discretion, Td may be deferred during pregnancy and Tdap substituted in the immediate postpartum period, or Tdap may be administered instead of Td to a pregnant woman after an informed discussion with the woman.

The ACIP statement for recommendations for administering Td as prophylaxis in wound management is available at http://www.cdc.gov/vaccines/pubs/acip-list.htm.

3. Varicella vaccination

All adults without evidence of immunity to varicella should receive 2 doses of single-antigen varicella vaccine if not previously vaccinated or a second dose if they have received only 1 dose, unless they have a medical contraindication. Special consideration should be given to those who 1) have close contact with persons at high risk for severe disease (e.g., healthcare personnel and family contacts of persons with immunocompromising conditions) or 2) are at high risk for exposure or transmission (e.g., teachers; child-care employees; residents and staff members of institutional settings, including correctional institutions; college students; military personnel; adolescents and adults living in households with children; nonpregnant women of childbearing age; and international travelers).

Evidence of immunity to varicella in adults includes any of the following: 1) documentation of 2 doses of varicella vaccine at least 4 weeks apart; 2) U.S.-born before 1980 (although for healthcare personnel and pregnant women, birth before 1980 should not be considered evidence of immunity); 3) history of varicella based on diagnosis or verification of varicella by a healthcare provider (for a patient reporting a history of or having an atypical case, a mild case, or both, healthcare providers should seek either an epidemiologic link with a typical varicella case or to a laboratory-confirmed case or evidence of laboratory confirmation, if it was performed at the time of acute disease); 4) history of herpes zoster based on diagnosis or verification of herpes zoster by a healthcare provider; or 5) laboratory evidence of immunity or laboratory confirmation of disease.

Pregnant women should be assessed for evidence of varicella immunity. Women who do not have evidence of immunity should receive the first dose of varicella vaccine upon completion or termination of pregnancy and before discharge from the healthcare facility. The second dose should be administered 4–8 weeks after the first dose.

4. Human papillomavirus (HPV) vaccination

HPV vaccination with either quadrivalent (HPV4) vaccine or bivalent vaccine (HPV2) is recommended for females at age 11 or 12 years and catch-up vaccination for females aged 13 through 26 years.

Ideally, vaccine should be administered before potential exposure to HPV through sexual activity; however, females who are sexually active should still be vaccinated consistent with age-based recommendations. Sexually active females who have not been infected with any of the four HPV vaccine types (types 6, 11, 16, and 18, all of which HPV4 prevents) or any of the two HPV vaccine types (types 16 and 18, both of which HPV2 prevents) receive the full benefit of the vaccination. Vaccination is less beneficial for females who have already been infected with one or more of the HPV vaccine types. HPV4 or HPV2 can be administered to persons with a history of genital warts, abnormal Papanicolaou test, or positive HPV DNA test, because these conditions are not evidence of previous infection with all vaccine HPV types.

HPV4 may be administered to males aged 9 through 26 years to reduce their likelihood of genital warts. HPV4 would be most effective when administered before exposure to HPV through sexual contact.

A complete series for either HPV4 or HPV2 consists of 3 doses. The second dose should be administered 1–2 months after the first dose; the third dose should be administered 6 months after the first dose.

Although HPV vaccination is not specifically recommended for persons with the medical indications described in Figure 2, "Vaccines that might be indicated for adults based on medical and other indications," it may be administered to these persons because the HPV vaccine is not a live-virus vaccine. However, the immune response and vaccine efficacy might be less for persons with the medical indications described in Figure 2 than in persons who do not have the medical indications described or who are immunocompetent.

5. Herpes zoster vaccination

A single dose of zoster vaccine is recommended for adults aged 60 years and older regardless of whether they report a previous episode of herpes zoster. Persons with chronic medical conditions may be vaccinated unless their condition constitutes a contraindication.

6. Measles, mumps, rubella (MMR) vaccination

Adults born before 1957 generally are considered immune to measles and mumps. All adults born in 1957 or later should have documentation of 1 or more doses of MMR vaccine unless they have a medical contraindication to the vaccine, laboratory evidence of immunity to each of the three diseases, or documentation of provider-diagnosed measles or mumps disease. For rubella, documentation of provider-diagnosed disease is not considered acceptable evidence of immunity.

Measles component: A second dose of MMR vaccine, administered a minimum of 28 days after the first dose, is recommended for adults who 1) have been recently exposed to measles or are in an outbreak setting; 2) are students in postsecondary educational institutions; 3) work in a healthcare facility; or 4) plan to travel internationally. Persons who received inactivated (killed) measles vaccine or measles vaccine of unknown type during 1963–1967 should be revaccinated with 2 doses of MMR vaccine.

Mumps component: A second dose of MMR vaccine, administered a minimum of 28 days after the first dose, is recommended for adults who 1) live in a community experiencing a mumps outbreak and are in an affected age group; 2) are students in postsecondary educational institutions; 3) work in a healthcare facility; or 4) plan to travel internationally. Persons vaccinated before 1979 with either killed mumps vaccine or mumps vaccine of unknown type who are at high risk for mumps infection (e.g. persons who are working in a healthcare facility) should be revaccinated with 2 doses of MMR vaccine.

Rubella component: For women of childbearing age, regardless of birth year, rubella immunity should be determined. If there is no evidence of immunity, women who are not pregnant should be vaccinated. Pregnant women who do not have evidence of immunity should receive MMR vaccine upon completion or termination of pregnancy and before discharge from the healthcare facility.

Healthcare personnel born before 1957: For unvaccinated healthcare personnel born before 1957 who lack laboratory evidence of measles, mumps, and/or rubella immunity or laboratory confirmation of disease, healthcare facilities should 1) consider routinely vaccinating personnel with 2 doses of MMR vaccine at the appropriate interval (for measles and mumps) and 1 dose of MMR vaccine (for rubella), and 2) recommend 2 doses of MMR vaccine at the appropriate interval during an outbreak of measles or mumps, and 1 dose during an outbreak of rubella. Complete information about evidence of immunity is available at http://www.cdc.gov/vaccines/recs/provisional/default.htm.

7. Pneumococcal polysaccharide (PPSV) vaccination

Vaccinate all persons with the following indications:

Medical: Chronic lung disease (including asthma); chronic cardiovascular diseases; diabetes mellitus; chronic liver diseases; cirrhosis; chronic alcoholism; functional or anatomic asplenia (e.g., sickle cell disease or splenectomy [if elective splenectomy is planned, vaccinate at least 2 weeks before surgery]); immunocompromising conditions (including chronic renal failure or nephrotic syndrome); and cochlear implants and cerebrospinal fluid leaks. Vaccinate as close to HIV diagnosis as possible.

Other: Residents of nursing homes or long-term care facilities and persons who smoke cigarettes. Routine use of PPSV is not recommended for American Indians/Alaska Natives or persons aged less than 65 years unless they have underlying medical conditions that are PPSV indications. However, public health authorities may consider recommending PPSV for American Indians/Alaska Natives and persons aged 50 through 64 years who are living in areas where the risk for invasive pneumococcal disease is increased

8. Revaccination with PPSV

One-time revaccination after 5 years is recommended for persons aged 19 through 64 years with chronic renal failure or nephrotic syndrome; functional or anatomic asplenia (e.g., sickle cell disease or splenectomy); and for persons with immunocompromising conditions. For persons aged 65 years and older, one-time revaccination is recommended if they were vaccinated 5 or more years previously and were aged less than 65 years at the time of primary vaccination.

9. Meningococcal vaccination

Meningococcal vaccine should be administered to persons with the following indications:

Medical: A 2-dose series of meningococcal conjugate vaccine is recommended for adults with anatomic or functional asplenia, or persistent complement component deficiencies. Adults with HIV infection who are vaccinated should also receive a routine 2-dose series. The 2 doses should be administered at 0 and 2 months.

Other: A single dose of meningococcal vaccine is recommended for unvaccinated first-year college students living in dormitories; microbiologists routinely exposed to isolates of Neisseria meningitidis; military recruits; and persons who travel to or live in countries in which meningococcal disease is hyperendemic or epidemic (e.g., the "meningitis belt" of sub-Saharan Africa during the dry season [December through June]), particularly if their contact with local populations will be prolonged. Vaccination is required by the government of Saudi Arabia for all travelers to Mecca during the annual Hajj.

Meningococcal conjugate vaccine, quadrivalent (MCV4) is preferred for adults with any of the preceding indications who are aged 55 years and younger; meningococcal polysaccharide vaccine (MPSV4) is preferred for adults aged 56 years and older. Revaccination with MCV4 every 5 years is recommended for adults previously vaccinated with MCV4 or MPSV4 who remain at increased risk for infection (e.g., adults with anatomic or functional asplenia, or persistent complement component deficiencies).

10. Hepatitis A vaccination

Vaccinate persons with any of the following indications and any person seeking protection from hepatitis A virus (HAV) infection:

Behavioral: Men who have sex with men and persons who use injection drugs.

Occupational: Persons working with HAV-infected primates or with HAV in a research laboratory setting.

Medical: Persons with chronic liver disease and persons who receive clotting factor concentrates.

Other: Persons travelling to or working in countries that have high or intermediate endemicity of hepatitis A (a list of countries is available at http://wwwn.cdc.gov/travel/contentdiseases.aspx).

Unvaccinated persons who anticipate close personal contact (e.g., household or regular babysitting) with an international adoptee during the first 60 days after arrival in the United States from a country with high or intermediate endemicity should be vaccinated. The first dose of the 2-dose hepatitis A vaccine series should be administered as soon as adoption is planned, ideally 2 or more weeks before the arrival of the adoptee.

Single-antigen vaccine formulations should be administered in a 2-dose schedule at either 0 and 6–12 months (Havrix), or 0 and 6–18 months (Vaqta). If the combined hepatitis A and hepatitis B vaccine (Twinrix) is used, administer 3 doses at 0, 1, and 6 months; alternatively, a 4-dose schedule may be used, administered on days 0, 7, and 21–30, followed by a booster dose at month 12.

11. Hepatitis B vaccination

Vaccinate persons with any of the following indications and any person seeking protection from hepatitis B virus (HBV) infection:

Behavioral: Sexually active persons who are not in a long-term, mutually monogamous relationship (e.g., persons with more than one sex partner during the previous 6 months); persons seeking evaluation or treatment for a sexually transmitted disease (STD); current or recent injection-drug users; and men who have sex with men.

Occupational: Healthcare personnel and public-safety workers who are exposed to blood or other potentially infectious body fluids.

Medical: Persons with end-stage renal disease, including patients receiving hemodialysis; persons with HIV infection; and persons with chronic liver disease.

Other: Household contacts and sex partners of persons with chronic HBV infection; clients and staff members of institutions for persons with developmental disabilities; and international travelers to countries with high or intermediate prevalence of chronic HBV infection (a list of countries is available at http://wwwn.cdc.gov/travel/contentdiseases.aspx).

Hepatitis B vaccination is recommended for all adults in the following settings: STD treatment facilities; HIV testing and treatment facilities; facilities providing drug-abuse treatment and prevention services; healthcare settings targeting services to injection-drug users or men who have sex with men; correctional facilities; end-stage renal disease programs and facilities for chronic hemodialysis patients; and institutions and nonresidential day-care facilities for persons with developmental disabilities.

Administer missing doses to complete a 3-dose series of hepatitis B vaccine to those persons not vaccinated or not completely vaccinated. The second dose should be administered 1 month after the first dose; the third dose should be given at least 2 months after the second dose (and at least 4 months after the first dose). If the combined hepatitis A and hepatitis B vaccine (Twinrix) is used, administer 3 doses at 0, 1, and 6 months; alternatively, a 4-dose Twinrix schedule, administered on days 0, 7, and 21 to 30, followed by a booster dose at month 12, may be used.

Adult patients receiving hemodialysis or with other immunocompromising conditions should receive 1 dose of 40 μg/mL (Recombivax HB) administered on a 3-dose schedule or 2 doses of 20 μg/mL (Engerix-B) administered simultaneously on a 4-dose schedule at 0, 1, 2, and 6 months.

12. Selected conditions for which *Haemophilus influenzae* type b (Hib) vaccine may be used

1 dose of Hib vaccine should be considered for persons who have sickle cell disease, leukemia, or HIV infection, or who have had a splenectomy, if they have not previously received Hib vaccine.

13. Immunocompromising conditions

Inactivated vaccines generally are acceptable (e.g., pneumococcal, meningococcal, influenza [inactivated influenza vaccine]) and live vaccines generally are avoided in persons with immune deficiencies or immunocompromising conditions. Information on specific conditions is available at http://www.cdc.gov/vaccines/pubs/acip-list.htm.

PROFESSIONAL SOCIETIES AND GOVERNMENTAL AGENCIES

Abbreviation	Full Name	Internet Address
AACE	American Association of Clinical Endocrinologists	http://www.aace.com
AAD	American Academy of Dermatology	http://www.aad.org
AAFP	American Academy of Family Physicians	http://www.aafp.org
AAHPM	American Academy of Hospice and Palliative Medicine	http://www.aahpm.org
AAN	American Academy of Neurology	http://www.aan.com/professionals
AAO	American Academy of Ophthalmology	http://www.aao.org
AAO-HNS	American Academy of Otolaryngology— Head and Neck Surgery	http://www.entnet.org
AAOS	American Academy of Orthopaedic Surgeons and American Association of Orthopaedic Surgeons	http://www.aaos.org
AAP	American Academy of Pediatrics	http://www.aap.org
ACC	American College of Cardiology	http://www.acc.org
ACCP	American College of Chest Physicians	http://www.chestnet.org
ACIP	Advisory Committee on Immunization Practices	http://www.cdc.gov/vaccines/recs/acip
ACOG	American Congress of Obstetricians and Gynecologists	http://www.acog.com
ACP	American College of Physicians	http://www.acponline.org
ACR	American College of Radiology	http://www.acr.org
ACR	American College of Rheumatology	http://www.rheumatology.org
ACS	American Cancer Society	http://www.cancer.org
ACSM	American College of Sports Medicine	http://www.acsm.org
ADA	American Diabetes Association	http://www.diabetes.org
AGA	American Gastroenterological Association	http://www.gastro.org
AGS	The American Geriatrics Society	http://www.americangeriatrics.org
AHA	American Heart Association	http://www.americanheart.org
ANA	American Nurses Association	http://www.nursingworld.org
AOA	American Optometric Association	http://www.aoa.org
ASA	American Stroke Association	http://www.strokeassociation.org
ASAM	American Society of Addiction Medicine	http://www.asam.org

PROFESSIONAL SOCIETIES AND GOVERNMENTAL AGENCIES (CONTINUED)		
Abbreviation	**Full Name**	**Internet Address**
ASCCP	American Society for Colposcopy and Cervical Pathology	http://www.asccp.org
ASCO	American Society of Clinical Oncology	http://www.asco.org
ASCRS	American Society of Colon and Rectal Surgeons	http://www.fascrs.org
ASGE	American Society for Gastrointestinal Endoscopy	http://asge.org
ASHA	American Speech-Language-Hearing Association	http://www.asha.org
ASN	American Society of Neuroimaging	http://www.asnweb.org
ATA	American Thyroid Association	http://www.thyroid.org
ATS	American Thoracic Society	http://www.thoracic.org
AUA	American Urological Association	http://auanet.org
BASHH	British Association for Sexual Health and HIV	http://www.bashh.org
	Bright Futures	http://brightfutures.org
BGS	British Geriatrics Society	http://www.bgs.org.uk/
BSAC	British Society for Antimicrobial Chemotherapy	http://www.bsac.org.uk
CDC	Centers for Disease Control and Prevention	http://www.cdc.gov
COG	Children's Oncology Group	http://www.childrensoncologygroup.org
CSVS	Canadian Society for Vascular Surgery	http://csvs.vascularweb.org
CTF	Canadian Task Force on Preventive Health Care	http://www.ctfphc.org
EASD	European Association for the Study of Diabetes	http://www.easd.org
EAU	European Association of Urology	http://www.uroweb.org
ERS	European Respiratory Society	http://ersnet.org
ESC	European Society of Cardiology	http://www.escardio.org
ESCDPCP	European and Other Societies on Cardiovascular Disease Prevention in Clinical Practice	http://www.escardio.org
ESH	European Society of Hypertension	http://www.eshonline.org

PROFESSIONAL SOCIETIES AND GOVERNMENTAL AGENCIES (CONTINUED)

Abbreviation	Full Name	Internet Address
IARC	International Agency for Research on Cancer	http://screening.iarc.fr
ICSI	Institute for Clinical Systems Improvement	http://www.icsi.org
IDF	International Diabetes Federation	http://www.idf.org
NAPNAP	National Association of Pediatric Nurse Practitioners	http://www.napnap.org
NCCN	National Comprehensive Cancer Network	http://www.nccn.org/cancer-guidelines.html
NCI	National Cancer Institute	http://www.cancer.gov/cancerinformation
NEI	National Eye Institute	http://www.nei.nih.gov
NGC	National Guideline Clearinghouse	http://www.guidelines.gov
NHLBI	National Heart, Lung, and Blood Institute	http://www.nhlbi.nih.gov
NIAAA	National Institute on Alcohol Abuse and Alcoholism	http://www.niaaa.nih.gov
NICE	National Institute for Health and Clinical Excellence	http://www.nice.org.uk
NIDCR	National Institute of Dental and Craniofacial Research	http://www.nidr.nih.gov
NIHCDC	National Institutes of Health Consensus Development Program	http://www.consensus.nih.gov
NIP	National Immunization Program	http://www.cdc.gov/nip
NKF	National Kidney Foundation	http://www.kidney.org
NOF	National Osteoporosis Foundation	http://www.nof.org
NTSB	National Transportation Safety Board	http://www.ntsb.gov
SCF	Skin Cancer Foundation	http://www.skincancer.org
SGIM	Society of General Internal Medicine	http://www.sgim.org
SKI	Sloan-Kettering Institute	http://www.mskcc.org/mskcc/html/5804.cfm
SVU	Society for Vascular Ultrasound	http://www.svunet.org
UK-NHS	United Kingdom National Health Service	http://www.nhs.uk
USPSTF	United States Preventive Services Task Force	http://www.ahrq.gov/clinic/uspstfix.htm
WHO	World Health Organization	http://www.who.int/en

Index

A

Abdominal aortic aneurysm (AAA), screening for, 2
ABR. *See* Auditory brainstem response
Abuse. *See also* Alcohol abuse and dependence; Drug abuse; Family violence and abuse
DM and, 58–59
Acamprosate, for alcohol abuse, 151
ACEI. *See* Angiotensin-converting enzyme inhibitors
Acetaminophen, for pain management, 246
Acetic acid, for cerumen impaction, 174
Acitretin, for psoriasis, 256
Acne, thyroid cancer and, 44
ACR. *See* Albumin to creatinine ratio
Actinic keratoses, 42
Actinomycin, for cancer, 168
Acute myelocytic leukemia (AML), 166
Acyclovir, for HSV, 260
Addax, for cerumen impaction, 174
Addison's disease, celiac disease and, 45
Adenocarcinoma of gastroesophageal junction, 31
Adenomatous polyps, 25, 26, 100
ADHD. *See* Attention-deficit/ hyperactivity disorder
Adolescents
alcohol abuse and dependence and, 290
with asthma, 154–155
depression in, 290
family violence and abuse and, 290
with HTN, 225
screening for, 74

primary prevention for
for dental caries, 104
for domestic violence, 106
HIV, opportunistic infections, 112
for motor vehicle safety, 128
for obesity, 137
for STDs, 141
with vaccinations, 125
screening of
alcohol abuse and dependence, 3
for cholesterol and lipid disorders, 48
for depression, 55
for HIV, 72, 73
for HSV, 71
for motor vehicle safety, 81
for scoliosis, 87
for smoking, 92
Adrenal cancer, CRC and, 24
Adrenal incidentalomas, management of, 150
AF. *See* Atrial fibrillation
AFP screening
for CRC, 24
for liver cancer, 32
Alanine transaminase (ALT), 68, 215
Albumin to creatinine ratio (ACR), 229
Alcohol abuse and dependence
adolescents and, 290
breast cancer and, 96
CRC and, 99
HTN and, 122
liver cancer and, 101
management for, 151
oral cancer and, 35, 101
pneumonia, community-acquired and, 251

Alcohol abuse and dependence
(*Cont.*):
  screening for, 3
  tools for, 280
Alcohol Use Disorder Identification
  Test (AUDIT), 3, 280–282
Alcoholic cirrhosis, liver cancer and,
  32
Aldehydes, bladder cancer and, 8
Aldosteronism, 150
Alendronate, for osteoporosis, 240
Alkaloids, for cancer, 167
Alkylators, 167, 169
Alopecia, celiac disease and, 45
5-alpha reductase inhibitors, 163, 277
Alpha-1-antitrypsin deficiency, liver
  cancer and, 32
Alpha-blockers, 163, 204
ALT. *See* Alanine transaminase
Amblyopia, 94
Amenorrhea, celiac disease and, 45
Aminoglycosides, for UTIs, 275–276
Aminopenicillin, for COPD, 179
Amiodarone, for AF, 160
AML. *See* Acute myelocytic
  leukemia
Amoxicillin, 244, 262
Ampicillin, for GBS, 111
Anal warts, treatment for, 266
Anastrozole, for breast cancer, 96–97
Androgen deficiency syndrome,
  management of, 152
Anemia, 4, 31
  celiac disease and, 45
Angiotensin receptor blockers
  (ARBs), 133, 225
  for AF, 161
  for DM, 201
  for HTN, 223
  for refractory hypertension, 227
Angiotensin-converting enzyme
  inhibitors (ACEI), 133, 225
  for AF, 161
  for DM, 201

  for HTN, 223
  for refractory hypertension, 227
Anthracycline antibiotics, for cancer,
  166
Antiarrhythmic drug therapy, 160
Antibiotics. *See also specific
    antibiotics*
  for cancer, 166, 168
  for COPD, 179
  for endocarditis, 108
  for GBS, 63, 111
  for MRSA, 236
  for otitis media, 244
Anticholinergic agents, for
  BPH, 163
Anticoagulants, 193, 194
Antiepileptic drugs, migraine and,
  213
Antihistamines, BPPV and, 278
Antihypertensives, for DM, 201
Antioxidants, MI and, 134
Antiphospholipid syndrome, oral
  contraceptives and, 185
Antipsychotic therapy, 153, 195
Antiretroviral regimens (ART),
  220
Antithrombotic therapy, 143,
  158–159
Antiviral therapy, 215, 228
Anxiety, primary prevention for,
  153
ARBs. *See* Angiotensin receptor
  blockers
Aromatase inhibitors, for breast
  cancer, 96
Aromatic amines, bladder cancer and,
  8
Arsenic, bladder cancer and, 9
ART. *See* Antiretroviral regimens
ASA. *See* Aspirin
Aspartate transaminase (AST), for
  CAS, 193
Aspiration, pneumonia, community-
  acquired and, 251

Aspirin (ASA)
for AF, 160
for CAS, 144
for CRC, 99
for metabolic syndrome, 235
for MI, 129, 133, 134
for stroke, 143
AST. *See* Aspartate transaminase
Asthma, management of, 154–155
Atovaquone, 113, 117, 119
for *toxoplasma gondii* encephalitis,
113
Atrial fibrillation (AF)
CAS and, 194
management of
with antithrombotic therapy,
158–159
with HR rate control, 156–157
with rhythm control, 160–162
oral contraceptives and, 186
stroke and, 142
Attention-deficit/hyperactivity
disorder (ADHD), screening
for, 5
Atypical moles, 42
AUDIT. *See* Alcohol Use Disorder
Identification Test
Auditory brainstem response (ABR),
65
Autoimmune hepatitis, celiac disease
and, 45
Autoimmune myocarditis, celiac
disease and, 45
Autosomal dominant polycystic
kidney disease, HTN and, 76
Azithromycin
for cervicitis, 262
for chancroid, 260
for chlamydia, 262
for endocarditis, 108
for MAC, 114, 118
for nongonococcal urethritis, 261
for otitis media, 244
for urethritis, 262

B

Bacille Calmette-Guérin (BCG),
vaccination for, 93
Back pain, low, management of,
233–234
Bacterial vaginosis, 7, 264
Bacteriuria, asymptomatic, screening
for, 5
Bariatric surgery, oral contraceptives
and, 188
Barrett's esophagus, 31
BCG. *See* Bacille Calmette-Guérin
Beck Depression Inventory (BDI),
55, 283, 286
Beclomethasone, for asthma, 180
Benign prostatic hyperplasia (BPD),
78, 163–164
Benzathine penicillin G, for syphilis,
261
Benzene, bladder cancer and, 8
Benzodiazepine, 153, 278
Beta carotene, 101, 134
Beta-agonists, 155, 165
Beta-blockers, 133, 223, 225, 249
migraine and, 213
Bilateral mastectomy, for breast
cancer, 15, 97
Bipolar disorder, celiac disease and,
45
Bisphosphonates, for osteoporosis,
240, 243
Bladder cancer, screening for, 8–9
Bleomycin mitomycin C, for cancer,
166
Blood group O, pancreatic cancer
and, 38
Blood pressure. *See also*
Hypertension
in boys, 292
in girls, 293
Blood-glucose-lowering therapy, 203
BMD. *See* Bone mineral density
Body mass index (BMI), 294. *See
also* Obesity

Bone mineral density (BMD), osteoporosis and, 84

Botulinum toxin, for hoarseness, 217

Boys, blood pressure in, 292

BPD. *See* Benign prostatic hyperplasia

BPPV. *See* Vertigo, benign paroxysmal positional

Brain cancer, CRC and, 24

BRCA1/2
  breast cancer and, 10, 12, 13
  ovarian cancer and, 36, 37
  pancreatic cancer and, 38

Breast cancer
  HRT and, 99
  lifetime risk for, 15
  primary prevention of, 96–97
  screening for, 10–16, 290

Breast self-examination (BSE), 10

Breastfeeding
  cervical cancer and, 98
  HIV and, 221
  oral contraceptives and, 184
  prenatal care and, 255

Bronchitis, management of, 165

Bronchodilators, 154, 179

BSE. *See* Breast self-examination

Budd-Chiari syndrome, oral contraceptives and, 191

Budesonide, for asthma, 180

Bupropion SR, for smoking cessation, 269

Butoconazole, for candidal vaginitis, 264

C

CAD. *See* Coronary artery disease

CAGE, in alcohol abuse screening, 3, 280–282

Calcium acetate, for CKD-MBDs, 231

Calcium carbonate, for CKD-MBDs, 231

Calcium channel blockers, 133, 161, 223, 225
  migraine and, 213

Calcium citrate, for CKD-MBDs, 231

CAM. *See* Confusion Assessment Method

Camptosar, for cancer, 168

Cancer. *See also specific cancers*
  oral contraceptives and, 185
  primary prevention of, 96–103
  survivorship from, management of, 166–170

Candidal vaginitis, treatment for, 264

Capecitabine, for cancer, 168

Carbapenem, for UTIs, 276

Cardiac risk
  for men, 295–296
  oral contraceptives and, 188
  for women, 297–298

Cardiovascular disease (CVD)
  CKD and, 78
  DM and, 202
  from NSAIDs, 99

Carotid artery stenosis (CAS)
  management of, 171
  screening for, 45
  stent therapy for, 193–194
  stroke and, 144–145

Carotid duplex ultrasonography, for CAS, 45

Carotid endarterectomy (CEA), 144, 171

CAS. *See* Carotid artery stenosis

Cataract
  management of, 172–173
  screening for, 94

CBE. *See* Clinical breast exam

CEA. *See* Carotid endarterectomy

Cefazolin, for GBS, 111

Cefdinir, for otitis media, 244

Cefixime, for otitis media, 244

Cefotetan, for pelvic inflammatory disease, 265

Cefoxitin, for pelvic inflammatory disease, 265
Cefpodoxime, for otitis media, 244
Cefprozil, for otitis media, 244
Ceftriaxone
  for chancroid, 260
  for epididymitis, 265
  for gonococcal conjunctivitis, 263
  for gonococcal meningitis, 263
  for ophthalmia neonatorum, 263
  for otitis media, 244
  for pelvic inflammatory disease, 265
  for proctitis, 266
Cefuroxime axetil, for otitis media, 244
Celiac disease, screening for, 46
Cephalexin, for UTIs, 275
Cerebrovascular disease, cholesterol and lipid disorders and, 48
Cerumen impaction, management of, 174
Cerumenex, for cerumen impaction, 174
Cervical cancer
  primary prevention of, 98
  screening for, 17–21, 290
    for ages under 25, 19
    for ages 25-49, 19
    for ages 50-64, 19
    for ages above 65, 19–20
Cervical intraepithelial neoplasia (CIN), 98
Cervical warts, treatment for, 265
Cervicitis, treatment for, 262
Chancroid, 260
CHD. *See* Coronary heart disease
Chemoprophylaxis, for influenza, 126
Chemotherapy. *See also specific chemotherapy agents*
  for cancer, 166–168
  cervical cancer and, 17

Chest x-ray (CXR)
  for asthma, 154
  for lung cancer, 33
  for pneumonia, community-acquired, 250
Children
  alcohol abuse and dependence and, 3
  with asthma, 154–155
  with cerumen impaction, 174
  cholesterol and, 177
  with constipation, 178
  with depression, 290
  with DM, 198–199
  with HIV, 222
  with HTN, 225
    screening for, 74
  with influenza, 228
    chemoprophylaxis for, 126
  lipids and, 177
  primary prevention for
    for CMV, 120
    for dental caries, 104
    for HIV, opportunistic infections, 112
    for MAC, 118
    for malaria, 117
    for motor vehicle safety, 128
    for *Mycobacterium tuberculosis*, 118
    for obesity, 137
    for PCP, 117
    for pressure ulcers, 139
    for *Toxoplasma gondii*, 119
    with vaccinations, 124–125
    for VZV, 119
  screening of
    for ADHD, 5
    for depression, 55
    for DM, 58
    for family violence and abuse, 61
    for growth abnormalities, 64
    for HBV, 68

Children, screening of (*Cont.*):
for lead poisoning, 79–80
for motor vehicle safety, 81
for obesity, 82
for smoking, 92
for speech and language delays, 88
for visual impairment, 94
with syphilis, 261
Chlamydia, 47, 262
Chloroquine, for malaria, 117
Cholecystitis, osteoporotic hip fractures and, 138
Cholesterol. *See also* High-density-lipoprotein cholesterol; Low-density-lipoprotein cholesterol
management of, 175–177
in men, 295
screening for, 48–50
in women, 297
Cholinesterase inhibitor, for dementia, 196
Chronic obstructive pulmonary disease (COPD)
management of, 179–180
pneumonia, community-acquired and, 251
Chronic open angle glaucoma (COAG), 205
CIN. *See* Cervical intraepithelial neoplasia
Cirrhosis, 32, 101, 215
Citalopram, for depression, 197
CKD. *See* Kidney disease, chronic
CKD-MBDs. *See* Kidney disease, chronic-mineral and bone disorders
Clarithromycin
for endocarditis, 108
for MAC, 114, 118
for otitis media, 244
Clindamycin, 111, 236–237, 264, 265
Clinical breast exam (CBE), 10, 14

Clonidine, for smoking cessation, 270
Clotrimazole, for candidal vaginitis, 264
Cluster headache, 209
CMV. *See* Cytomegalovirus
COAG. *See* Chronic open angle glaucoma
Coccidioidomycosis, 114
Colectomy, for CRC, 25
Colonoscopy, for CRC, 22, 23, 25, 26
Colorectal cancer (CRC). *See also* Hereditary nonpolyposis colorectal cancer
adenomatous polyps and, 100
osteoporotic hip fractures and, 138
primary prevention of, 99
screening for, 22–27
vitamin D and, 100
Computed tomography colonography (CTC), 26, 51
Confusion Assessment Method (CAM), 195
Constipation, 45, 178
Contraceptives. *See* Oral contraceptives
COPD. *See* Chronic obstructive pulmonary disease
Coronary artery disease (CAD)
AF and, 160
cholesterol and lipid disorders and, 48
DM and, 202
drugs for, 225
obesity and, 238
osteoporotic hip fractures and, 138
screening for, 51–53
Coronary heart disease (CHD)
cholesterol and, 49, 50, 175
HRT and, 99
HTN and, 121
lipid disorders and, 49, 50
MI and, 129
risk factors for, 54

Corticosteroid, 155, 256
  oral contraceptives and, 189
CRC. *See* Colorectal cancer
CRP, coronary artery disease
    and, 51
Cryptorchid testis, 43
CTC. *See* Computed tomography
    colonography
Cushing's syndrome
  HTN and, 76
  refractory hypertension and, 226
CVD. *See* Cardiovascular disease
CXR. *See* Chest x-ray
Cyclophosphamide, 8, 9
Cyclosporine, for psoriasis, 256
Cypionate, for androgen deficiency
    syndrome, 152
Cystic fibrosis, kidney stones and,
    232
Cystinuria, kidney stones and, 232
Cytarabine, for cancer, 166
Cytomegalovirus (CMV), with HIV,
    in children, 120

D

Dabigatran (Pradaxa), for AF, 159
Dapsone
  for malaria, 117
  for PCP, 113
  for *Toxoplasma gondii*, 113, 119
DAPT. *See* Dual antiplatelet therapy
Daptomycin, for MRSA, 236–237
DBP. *See* Diastolic blood pressure
DCBE. *See* Double-contrast barium
    enema
DDH. *See* Developmental dysplasia
    of the hip
DDP-4. *See* Dipeptidyl peptidase-4
Debrox, for cerumen impaction,
    174
Deep venous thrombosis (DVT)
  oral contraceptives and, 185–186
  ovarian cancer and, 102
Delirium, management of, 195

Dementia
  driving risk with, 106
  management of, 196
  osteoporotic hip fractures
    and, 138
  screening for, 54
Denosumab, for osteoporosis, 240
Dental caries, primary prevention of,
    104
Dental enamel defects, celiac disease
    and, 45
Depot medroxyprogesteone acetate
    (DMPA), 189
Depression
  in adolescents, 290
  celiac disease and, 45
  in children, 290
  in elderly, 287
  management of, 197
  obesity and, 137
  screening for, 55, 290
    tools for, 283–287
Dermatitis herpetiformis, celiac
    disease and, 45
DES. *See* Diethylstilbestrol
Developmental dysplasia of the hip
    (DDH), screening for, 56
Dexamethasone, for cancer, 167
Diabetes
  blood-glucose-lowering therapy
    for, 203
  celiac disease and, 45
  CHD and, 53
  cholesterol and lipid disorders and,
    48
  drugs for, 225
  pancreatic cancer and, 38
  refractory hypertension and, 226
Diabetes mellitus (DM)
  abuse and, 58–59
  CKD and, 78
  liver cancer and, 101
  management of, 198–202
  MI and, 132–133

Diabetes mellitus (DM) (*Cont.*):
  pressure ulcers and, 139
  primary prevention of, 105
Diabetes mellitus, gestational
      (GDM), screening for, 57, 291
Diastolic blood pressure (DBP), 74
Diethylstilbestrol (DES), cervical
      cancer and, 17
Digital rectal exam (DRE), for
      prostate cancer, 39–40
Dipeptidyl peptidase-4 (DDP-4)
      inhibitor, for DM, 200
Disease modifying antirheumatic
      drugs (DMARDs), 257
Diuretics, 133, 201, 225
Divalproex, migraine and, 213
Dix-Hallpike test, for BPPV, 278
DM. *See* Diabetes mellitus
DMARDs. *See* Disease modifying
      antirheumatic drugs
DMPA. *See* Depot medroxyproges-
      teone acetate
DNA tests, for Human papillomavirus
      (HPV), 17
Domestic violence, primary
      prevention of, 106
Double-contrast barium enema
      (DCBE), 26
Down syndrome, celiac disease and,
      45
Doxycycline
  for cervicitis, 262
  for epididymitis, 265
  for granuloma inguinale, 260
  for *Lymphogranuloma venereum*,
      260
  for malaria, 117
  for nongonococcal urethritis, 261
  for pelvic inflammatory disease,
      265
  for proctitis, 266
DRE. *See* Digital rectal exam
Driving risk, primary prevention for,
      107

Dronedarone, 143, 160
Drug abuse
  HCV and, 70
  screening for, 77
Dual antiplatelet therapy (DAPT), for
      CAS, 193
Dual-energy x-ray absorptiometry
      (DXA), 84, 219, 240–241
Dutasteride, for prostate
      cancer, 103
DVT. *See* Deep venous thrombosis
DXA. *See* Dual-energy x-ray
      absorptiometry
Dyslipidemia, cholesterol and lipid
      disorders and, 48

E

Eating disorders, obesity and, 137
ECG. *See* Electrocardiogram
Echocardiography, 51, 160, 236
ED. *See* Erectile dysfunction
EF. *See* Ejection fraction
EIA. *See* Electroimmunoassay
Ejection fraction (EF), 142
Elderly
  depression in, 287
  falls by, primary prevention of,
      109
  screening of
    for falls, 60
    for family violence and abuse,
      61
    for functional assessment,
      288–289
    for visual impairment, 94
Electrocardiogram (ECG), 51, 227
Electroimmunoassay (EIA), for HIV,
      73
Electron-beam CT, for coronary
      artery disease, 51–52
Emergency contraceptive pills, 192
Endocarditis, primary prevention for,
      108
End-of-life, pain management at, 246

Endometrial cancer
  primary prevention of, 100
  screening for, 28–30
Endometrial hyperplasia, oral
      contraceptives and, 189
Engerix-B, 116
Epididymitis, treatment for, 265
Epilepsy, celiac disease and, 45
Epipodophyllotoxins, for cancer, 166
Erectile dysfunction (ED)
  management of, 204
  prostate cancer treatment and, 40,
    102
Eribulin, for cancer, 167
Erythromycin, 111, 244, 264
Esophagogastroduodenoscopy,
      gastric cancer and, 31
Estrogen
  CRC and, 99
  migraine from, 212
  ovarian cancer and, 102
Exenatide, for DM, 200

F
Falls
  by elderly
    primary prevention of, 109
    screening for, 60
  osteoporosis and, 240
Famciclovir, for HSV, 260
Familial adenomatous polyposis
    (FAP), CRC and, 25
Family violence and abuse
  adolescents and, 290
  screening for, 61, 290
FAP. *See* Familial adenomatous
    polyposis
Fecal immunochemical test (FIT), 27
Fecal occult blood test (FOBT), 23,
    25, 27
  for CRC, 22
Finasteride, for prostate cancer, 102
FIT. *See* Fecal immunochemical test
Flecainide, for AF, 160

Flexible sigmoidoscopy (FSIG), for
    CRC, 22, 23, 25, 26
Fluconazole, for coccidioidomycosis,
    114
Fluorescent treponemal antibody
    absorption test (FTA-ABS),
    for syphilis, 89
Fluoride, for dental caries, 104
Fluoroquinolones, for UTIs, 276
Fluoxetine, for depression, 197
FOBT. *See* Fecal occult blood test
Folic acid, 134, 136
Follicular stimulating hormone
    (FSH), androgen deficiency
    syndrome and, 152
Framingham Score, for coronary
    artery disease, 52–53
FRAX, for osteoporosis, 84, 242
FSH. *See* Follicular stimulating
    hormone
FSIG. *See* Flexible sigmoidoscopy
FTA-ABS. *See* Fluorescent
    treponemal antibody
    absorption test
5FU, for cancer, 168

G
Gabapentin
  migraine and, 213
  for pain management, 246
GAD. *See* Generalized anxiety
    disorder
Gastric cancer
  primary prevention of, 100
  screening for, 31
Gastroesophageal reflux disease, 31
GBS. *See* Group B Streptococcal
    disease
GDM. *See* Diabetes mellitus,
    gestational
Gemcitabine, for cancer, 168
Generalized anxiety disorder (GAD),
    153
Genital warts, treatment for, 265

Geriatrics. *See* Elderly
GFR. *See* Glomerular filtration rate
Girls, blood pressure in, 293
Glaucoma
  management of, 205
  screening for, 94, 291
Gleason score, for prostate cancer,
  40, 103
Glomerular filtration rate (GFR), 202
  CKD and, 78, 229
  DM and, 200
  refractory hypertension and, 227
GLP-1. *See* Glucagon-like-peptide-1
Glucagon-like-peptide-1 (GLP-1),
  for DM, 200
Glucocorticoids, osteoporosis and,
  242–243
Gluten, celiac disease and, 45
Gonococcal conjunctivitis, treatment
  for, 263
Gonococcal meningitis, 263
Gonorrhea
  ophthalmia neonatorum, primary
    prevention of, 110
  screening for, 62
Governmental agencies, 303–305
Granuloma inguinale, treatment for,
  260
Group B Streptococcal disease (GBS)
  primary prevention of, 111
  screening for, 63
Growth abnormalities, infant,
  screening for, 64
Gynecomastia, prostate cancer
  treatment and, 102

H
HAART. *See* Highly active
  antiretroviral therapy
Haloperidol, for delirium, 195
HAV. *See* Hepatitis A virus
HBIG. *See* Hepatitis B
  immunoglobulin
HBV. *See* Hepatitis B virus

HCC. *See* Hepatocellular carcinoma
HCTZ. *See* Hydrochlorothiazide
HCV. *See* Hepatitis C virus
HDL. *See* High-density lipoprotein
HDL-C. *See* High-density-
  lipoprotein cholesterol
Headache, 206
  cluster, 209
  menopausal migraine, 211
  menstrual-associated migraine,
    210
  migraine, 207
  perimenopausal migraine, 211
  tension-type, 208
Hearing impairment
  in infants, 291
  screening for, 65, 291
Heart failure (HF)
  AF and, 160
  drugs for, 225
  management of, 214
Heart rate (HR), AF and,
  156–157
Helicobacter pylori, gastric cancer
  and, 31, 100
Hematopoietic cell transplant, for
  cancer, 168
Hematuria, CKD and, 78
Hemochromatosis
  liver cancer and, 32
  screening for, 66
Hemoglobinopathies
  PKU and, 85
  prenatal care and, 255
  screening for, 67
Hepatitis A virus (HAV), 115
Hepatitis B immunoglobulin (HBIG),
  68
Hepatitis B virus (HBV)
  liver cancer and, 101
  management of, 215
  as opportunistic disease, 116
  prenatal care and, 254
  screening for, 68

Hepatitis C virus (HCV)
 liver cancer and, 32
 management of, 216
 screening for, 69–70
Hepatoblastoma, CRC and, 24, 25
Hepatocellular carcinoma (HCC), 32, 101
 HBV and, 215
Hereditary hemochromatosis. *See* Hemochromatosis
Hereditary nonpolyposis colorectal cancer (HNPCC)
 bladder cancer and, 8
 CRC and, 24, 25
 endometrial cancer and, 29, 30
 gastric cancer and, 31
Herpes simplex virus (HSV)
 screening for, 71
 treatment for, 260
HF. *See* Heart failure
HgbA1c, for DM, 200
High-density lipoprotein (HDL), 49
 metabolic syndrome and, 235
 obesity and, 238
High-density-lipoprotein cholesterol (HDL-C), 49, 50
 DM and, 59, 132
Highly active antiretroviral therapy (HAART), 73
High-sensitivity C-reactive protein (hsCRP), 52
Histoplasma capsulatum, 114
HIV. *See* Human immunodeficiency virus
HNPCC. *See* Hereditary nonpolyposis colorectal cancer
Hoarseness, management of, 217
Homocysteine, coronary artery disease and, 51
Hormone replacement therapy (HRT)
 breast cancer and, 96, 99
 CHD and, 99
 HIV and, 219
 MI and, 134

osteoporotic hip fractures and, 138
 ovarian cancer and, 102
 stroke and, 99
HPV. *See* Human papillomavirus
HR. *See* Heart rate
HRT. *See* Hormone replacement therapy
hsCRP. *See* High-sensitivity C-reactive protein
HSV. *See* Herpes simplex virus
HTN. *See* Hypertension
Human immunodeficiency virus (HIV)
 cervical cancer and, 17
 children with, 222
  CMV with, 120
  MAC with, 118
  malaria with, 117
  Mycobacterium tuberculosis with, 118
  PCP with, 117
  Toxoplasma gondii with, 119
  VZV with, 119
 HCV and, 70
 malaria with, 116
 management of, 218–222
 opportunistic infections with, primary prevention of, 112
 pneumonia, community-acquired and, 251
 pregnancy and, 220–221
 screening for, 72–73
 syphilis and, 89
 testicular cancer and, 43
 treatment for, 260
 vaccination and, 119
Human papillomavirus (HPV)
 cervical cancer and, 98
 DNA tests for, 17
 oral cancer and, 35, 101
 prenatal care and, 254
 prostate cancer and, 103
 vaccination for, 17, 18, 98, 101, 115

Hydrochlorothiazide (HCTZ), for refractory hypertension, 227
Hydrogen peroxide, for cerumen impaction, 174
Hydroxychloroquine, 258
Hyperaldosteronism
    HTN and, 76
    refractory hypertension and, 226
Hyperbilirubinemia, prenatal care and, 255
Hypercalcemia, HTN and, 76
Hypercorticalism, 150
Hyperkalemia, HTN and, 76
Hyperlipidemia
    cholesterol and lipid disorders and, 48
    MI and, 131
    stroke and, 146
Hyperparathyroidism, 76, 226, 232
Hypertension (HTN)
    AF and, 160
    CHD and, 53
    cholesterol and, 48, 175
    CKD and, 78
    DM and, 59
    HF and, 214
    initiating treatment for, 223
    lifestyle modifications for, 224
    lipid disorders and, 48
    metabolic syndrome and, 235
    MI and, 131
    obesity and, 238
    OHT, 205
    primary prevention for, 121
        through lifestyle modification, 122
    refractory, 226–227
    screening for
        in adolescents, 74
        in adults, 75–76
        in children, 74
    stroke and, 142
Hypothyroidism, 67, 85, 90
Hysterectomy, Pap smear and, 21

I

IAP. *See* Intrapartum antibiotic prophylaxis
IgA. *See* Immunoglobulin A
IgG. *See* Immunoglobulin G
IGRA. *See* Interferon-gamma release assay
IGT. *See* Impaired glucose tolerance
Immune thrombocytopenic purpura (ITP), celiac disease and, 45
Immunoglobulin A (IgA), celiac disease and, 45
Immunoglobulin G (IgG), 119
Immunosuppression, skin cancer and, 42
Impaired glucose tolerance (IGT), 105
Infants
    with hearing impairment, 291
    with HIV, 220
    primary prevention for
        for gonorrhea, ophthalmia neonatorum, 110
        for motor vehicle safety, 128
        for SIDS, 147
        with vaccinations, 124
    screening of
        for anemia, 4
        for cholesterol and lipid disorders, 48
        for growth abnormalities, 64
        for hearing loss, 65
        for PKU, 85
        for thyroid disease, 90
Inflammatory bowel disease
    CRC and, 25
    oral contraceptives and, 190
Inflammatory disorders, anemia and, 4
Influenza, 114
    chemoprophylaxis for, 126
    management of, 228
    pneumonia, community-acquired and, 251
    vaccination for, 127
INH. *See* Isoniazid

Intact parathyroid hormone (iPTH), CKD and, 230

Interferon-alpha, for HBV, 215

Interferon-gamma release assay (IGRA), for tuberculosis, latent, 93

Intrapartum antibiotic prophylaxis (IAP), for GBS, 111

Intravenous immune globulin (IVIG), 119

iPTH. *See* Intact parathyroid hormone

Iron deficiency, anemia and, 4

Iron dextran, for anemia, 4

Iron sucrose, for anemia, 4

Irritable bowel syndrome, celiac disease and, 45

Isoniazid (INH), for TB, 113, 118

ITP. *See* Immune thrombocytopenic purpura

Itraconazole, for coccidioidomycosis, 114

Ivermectin, for scabies, 266

IVIG. *See* Intravenous immune globulin

Ixabepilone, for cancer, 167

K

Kidney disease, chronic (CKD)
   drugs for, 225
   management of, 229–230
   from NSAIDs, 99
   refractory hypertension and, 226
   screening for, 78

Kidney disease, chronic-mineral and bone disorders (CKD-MBDs), 231

Kidney stones, management of, 232

Klinefelter's syndrome, testicular cancer and, 43

L

Lamivudine, for HBV, 215

Lanthanum carbonate, for CKD-MBDs, 231

Laryngoscopy, for hoarseness, 217

L-asparaginase, for cancer, 168

LDCT. *See* Low-dose CT

LDL-C. *See* Low-density-lipoprotein cholesterol

Lead poisoning, screening for, 79–80

Leflunomide, for RA, 258

Left ventricular hypertrophy (LVH), 160

Leucovorin, 113, 119

Levonorgestrel, 192

LH. *See* Luteinizing hormone

Linezolid, for MRSA, 236–237

Lipid disorders
   management of, 175–177
   screening for, 48–50

Lipoproteins. *See also* High-density lipoprotein; Low-density-lipoprotein cholesterol
   coronary artery disease and, 51
   in men, 295

Liver cancer
   primary prevention of, 101
   screening for, 32

Liver transplantation, alcohol abuse and, 151

Loracarbef, for otitis media, 244

Low-density-lipoprotein cholesterol (LDL-C), 49
   DM and, 132, 202
   metabolic syndrome and, 235
   obesity and, 238

Low-dose CT (LDCT), for lung cancer, 33, 34

Lower urinary tract symptoms (LUTS), 163
   treatment for, 277

Low-grade squamous intraepithelial lesions (LSILs), 18

LSILs. *See* Low-grade squamous intraepithelial lesions

Lung abscess, pneumonia, community-acquired and, 251

Lung cancer
  primary prevention of, 101
  screening for, 33–34
Luteinizing hormone (LH), androgen
  deficiency syndrome and, 152
LUTS. *See* Lower urinary tract
  symptoms
LVH. *See* Left ventricular
  hypertrophy
Lymphogranuloma venereum,
  treatment for, 260
Lymphoma, 12, 45
Lynch syndrome. *See* Hereditary
  nonpolyposis colorectal
  cancer

M

MAC. *See Mycobacterium axiom*
  complex
Macrolide, for COPD, 179
Magnetic resonance imaging (MRI),
  12, 51
  for breast cancer, 11
Malaria, 116
  with HIV, in children, 117
Mammography
  for breast cancer, 12
    ages 20-39, 10
    ages 40-49, 10–12
    ages 50-70, 13
    ages 70-85, 13
    benefits of, 10
  harms of, 16
MAZE, for AF, 160
MDCT. *See* Multidetector computed
  tomography
MDRD. *See* Modification of diet in
  renal disease
Mefloquine, for malaria, 117
Melanoma, 42
Memantine, for dementia, 196
Menopausal migraine, 211
Menstrual-associated migraine, 210
6 mercaptopurine, for cancer, 168

Metabolic bone disease, celiac
  disease and, 45
Metabolic syndrome, management
  of, 235
Metformin, for DM, 105, 200
Methicillin-resistant *Staphylococcus
  aureus* (MRSA), management
  of, 236–237
Methotrexate (MTX)
  for psoriasis, 256
  for RA, 258
Metronidazole
  for bacterial vaginosis, 264
  for pelvic inflammatory disease,
    265
  for trichomoniasis, 264
  for urethritis, 262
MI. *See* Myocardial infarction
Miconazole, for candidal vaginitis,
  264
Microtubular inhibitors, for cancer,
  167
Migraine, 207
  from estrogen, 212
  menopausal, 211
  menstrual-associated, 210
  from oral contraceptives, 212
  perimenopausal, 211
  treatment for, 213
Minocycline, 258
Modification of diet in renal disease
  (MDRD), 229
Moles, 42
Morphine, for pain management,
  246
Motor vehicle safety
  driving risk, 107
  primary prevention with, 128
  screening for, 81
MRI. *See* Magnetic resonance
  imaging
MRSA. *See* Methicillin-resistant
  Staphylococcus aureus
MTX. *See* Methotrexate

Multidetector computed tomography (MDCT), 54
Mycobacterium axiom complex (MAC), 114
  with HIV, in children, 118
Mycobacterium tuberculosis, 113
  with HIV, in children, 118
Myocardial infarction (MI)
  drugs for, 225
  primary prevention for, 129–135
Myocarditis, 45

N

NAAT. *See* Urine nucleic amplification acid test
Naltrexone, for alcohol abuse, 151
National Lung Screening Trial (NLST), 34
Natriuretic-peptide testing, for coronary artery disease, 51
Nephrocalcinosis, kidney stones and, 232
Nephrolithiasis, CKD and, 78
Neural tube defects, primary prevention of, 136
Nicotine, for smoking cessation, 269
Nitrates, ED and, 204
Nitrofurantoin, for UTIs, 275
NLST. *See* National Lung Screening Trial
NNT. *See* Number needed to treat
Nongonococcal urethritis, treatment for, 261
Nonsteroidal anti-inflammatory drugs (NSAIDs)
  for back pain, low, 233
  CKD and, 78
  for CRC, 99
  for pain management, 246
  for refractory hypertension, 227
Norethisterone enanthate, 192
Nortriptyline, 246, 270
NSAIDs. *See* Nonsteroidal anti-inflammatory drugs

Nuclear matrix protein, bladder cancer and, 9
Nucleic acid test, for HCV, 69
Number needed to treat (NNT), 145
Nystatin, for candidal vaginitis, 264

O

OAEs. *See* Otoacoustic emissions
Obesity
  breast cancer and, 96
  CHD and, 53
  cholesterol and lipid disorders and, 48
  CRC and, 99
  DM and, 59
  HTN and, 121
  management of, 238–239
  ovarian cancer and, 102
  primary prevention for, 137
  refractory hypertension and, 226
  screening for, 82–83
Obstructive sleep apnea, refractory hypertension and, 226
Ocular hypertension (OHT), 205
OGTT. *See* Oral glucose tolerance test
OHT. *See* Ocular hypertension
Olanzapine, for delirium, 195
Omega-3 fatty acids, for MI, 134
Omeprazole (Prilosec), for CAS, 193
Ophthalmia neonatorum, treatment for, 263–264
Opioids, for back pain, low, 233
Opportunistic diseases, primary prevention of, 113–116
Oral cancer
  primary prevention of, 101
  screening for, 35
Oral contraceptives
  cervical cancer and, 18, 98
  eligibility criteria for, 184–192
  emergency, 192
  endometrial cancer and, 100
  migraine from, 212

Oral contraceptives (*Cont.*):
  ovarian cancer and, 102
  pregnancy and, 181–183, 192
Oral glucose tolerance test (OGTT),
    for DM, 58
Oropharyngeal squamous cell cancer,
    101
Oseltamivir, for influenza, 126, 228
Osteomas, CRC and, 24
Osteoporosis
  glucocorticoids and, 242–243
  management of, 240–243
  screening for, 84
Osteoporotic hip fractures, primary
    prevention for, 138
Otitis media, management of,
    244–245
Otoacoustic emissions (OAEs), 65
Ovarian cancer
  oral contraceptives and, 186
  primary prevention of, 102
  screening for, 36–37
Oxycodone, for pain management,
    246

P

Pain management, at end-of-life, 246
Pancreatic cancer, screening for, 38
Pancreatitis, alcohol abuse and, 151
Pap smear
  algorithm when abnormal, 247
  for cervical cancer, 17, 18
  for endometrial cancer, 28
  HIV and, 219
  hysterectomy and, 21
  prenatal care and, 254
Patient Health Questionnaire
    (PHQ-9), 283–285
Patient Health Questionnaire for
    Adolescents (PHQ-A), 55
PCP. *See Pneumocystis* pneumonia
PDE5. *See* Phosphodiesterase 5
PE. *See* Pulmonary embolism
Peak expiratory flow (PEF), 154

Pediculosis pubis, treatment for, 266
PEF. *See* Peak expiratory flow
PEG. *See* Polyethylene glycol
Pelvic inflammatory disease,
    treatment for, 265
Pelvic radiation therapy, bladder
    cancer and, 8, 9
Penicillin G
  for GBS, 111
  for syphilis, 261
Pentamidine, 113, 117
Perimenopausal migraine, 211
Perioperative cardiovascular
    evaluation for noncardiac
    surgery, 248
Peripartum cardiomyopathy, oral
    contraceptives and, 188
Peripheral artery disease, cholesterol
    and lipid disorders and, 48
Permethrin, 266
Pernicious anemia, gastric cancer
    and, 31
Pharyngitis, treatment of, 271
Phenylketonuria (PKU), 67, 85, 255
Pheochromocytoma, 76, 150
Phosphodiesterase 5 (PDE5),
    inhibitors of, 204
PHQ-9. *See* Patient Health Question-
    naire
PHQ-A. *See* Patient Health
    Questionnaire for Adolescents
Pioglitazone, for DM, 200
Piperacillin-tazobactam, for UTIs, 276
PKU. *See* Phenylketonuria
PLCO. *See* Prostate, Lung, Colorectal
    and Ovarian Cancer
    Screening Trial
Pneumocystis pneumonia (PCP), 113
  with HIV, in children, 117
Pneumonia, community-acquired,
    management of, 250–251
Polycystic kidney disease, 76
Polyethylene glycol (PEG), for
    constipation, 178

Polyneuropathy, celiac disease and, 45

Postpartum, oral contraceptives and, 184

Potassium, for HTN, 121

PPI. *See* Proton pump inhibitors

Pradaxa. *See* Dabigatran

Prednisolone, for COPD, 179

Prednisone, 167, 242

Pregabalin, for pain management, 246

Pregnancy
  alcohol abuse and dependence and, 3
  bacterial vaginosis and, 264
  chlamydia and, 262
  HIV and, 220–221
  oral contraceptives and, 181–183, 192
  primary prevention for
    for GBS, 111
    for neural tube defects, 136
  screening for
    for anemia, 4
    for bacterial vaginosis, 7
    for bacteriuria, 6
    for DM, 58
    for GBS, 63
    for HCV, 69
    for hepatitis B, 68
    for HIV, 72
    for HSV, 71
    for lead poisoning, 79–80
    for Rh(D) incompatibility, 86
    for smoking, 91
    for syphilis, 89
  syphilis and, 261

Prenatal care, 252–254

Pressure ulcers, primary prevention for, 139–140

Prilosec. *See* Omeprazole

Primary Care Evaluation of Mental Disorders Patient Health Questionnaire (PRIME-MD), 283–285

Proctitis, treatment for, 266

Professional societies, 303–305

Propafenone, for AF, 160

Prostate, Lung, Colorectal and Ovarian Cancer Screening Trial (PLCO), 37

Prostate cancer
  primary prevention of, 102–103
  screening for, 39–41, 290

Prostate-specific antigen (PSA), 39–41

Proteinuria, CKD and, 78, 230

Proton pump inhibitors (PPI), for CAS, 193

PSA. *See* Prostate-specific antigen

Psoriasis, management of, 256

Psychotherapy, for depression, 55

Pulmonary embolism (PE), oral contraceptives and, 185–186

Pulmonary hypertension, oral contraceptives and, 186

Purine agonists, for cancer, 167

Pyrethrins, for pediculosis pubis, 266

Pyrimethamine, 113, 119

R

RA. *See* Rheumatoid arthritis

Radiation therapy, for cancer, 8, 9, 168–169

Radon, lung cancer and, 101

Raloxifene
  for breast cancer, 15
  for osteoporosis, 240

Rapid plasma reagent test (RPR), for syphilis, 89

Refractory hypertension, 226–227

Renal artery stenosis, refractory hypertension and, 226

Renal parenchymal disease, HTN and, 76

Renal tubular acidosis (RTA), kidney stones and, 232

Reynolds Risk Score, for coronary artery disease, 53

Rheumatoid arthritis (RA)
  management of, 257–258
  oral contraceptives and, 189
Rh(D) incompatibility, screening for,
  86
Rhinitis, management of, 259
Rhythm control, for AF, 160–162
Rifampin, for TB, 118
Risedronate, for osteoporosis, 240
Rituximab, for RA, 257
RNA test
  for HCV, 69
  for HIV, 73
RPR. *See* Rapid plasma reagent test
RTA. *See* Renal tubular acidosis

S
Salpingo-oophorectomy, 14
  for breast cancer, 97
  for ovarian cancer, 102
Sarcoidosis, celiac disease and, 45
SASQ, in alcohol abuse screening, 3
SBP. *See* Systolic blood pressure
Scabies, treatment for, 266
Schistosoma haematobium, bladder
  cancer and, 8
Scoliosis, screening for, 87
SCORE Risk System, for coronary
  artery disease, 51
sDNA testing. *See* Stoll DNA
Selective serotonin reuptake
  inhibitors (SSRIs)
  for anxiety, 153
  for depression, 55, 197
Seminoma, testicular cancer and, 43
Sertraline, for anxiety, 153
Serum ferritin, 4
  hemochromatosis and, 66
Sevelamer carbonate, for
  CKD-MBDs, 231
Sevelamer-HCl, for CKD-MBDs, 231
Sexually transmitted diseases
  (STDs), 62. *See also specific
  STDs*

HCV and, 70
HIV and, 72
primary prevention for, 141
treatment guidelines for,
  260–266
Sickle cell disease
  screening for, 67
  stroke and, 146
SIDS. *See* Sudden infant death
  syndrome
Sildenafil, for ED, 204
Sjögren's syndrome, celiac disease
  and, 45
Skin cancer
  CRC and, 24
  screening for, 42
SLE. *See* Systemic lupus
  erythematosus
Smoking
  bladder cancer and, 8, 9
  breast cancer and, 97
  cervical cancer and, 98
  cessation treatment for,
    268–270
  CHD and, 53
  cholesterol and lipid disorders
    and, 48
  CRC and, 99
  HTN and, 122
  lung cancer and, 33, 34, 101
  in men, 295
  metabolic syndrome and, 235
  MI and, 135
  obesity and, 238
  oral cancer and, 35, 101
  osteoporosis and, 242
  pancreatic cancer and, 38
  pneumonia, community-acquired
    and, 251
  primary prevention for,
    148
  screening for, 91–92
  stroke and, 146
  women and, 297

Sodium bicarbonate, for cerumen impaction, 174
Sotalol, for AF, 160
SPARCL Trial, 146
Speech and language delay, screening for, 88
Spiral CT, for lung cancer, 33
SSRIs. *See* Selective serotonin reuptake inhibitors
Statins
    for AF, 161
    breast cancer and, 97
    for DM, 132
    for MI, 135
    for pneumonia, community-acquired, 250
STDs. *See* Sexually transmitted diseases
Sterilization, 192
Steroids, cervical cancer and, 17
Stimulants, for ADHD, 5
Stoll DNA (sDNA testing), for CRC, 27
Strabismus, 94
Streptococcus pneumonia, 114
Stress
    anemia and, 4
    urinary incontinence, 272–274
Stroke
    CAS and, 45
    drugs for, 225
    HRT and, 99
    osteoporotic hip fractures and, 138
    pressure ulcers and, 139
    primary prevention for, 142–146
    risk for
        in men, 299–300
        in women, 301–302
Subacute bacterial endocarditis, oral contraceptives and, 186
Sudden infant death syndrome (SIDS), primary prevention for, 147
Sulfasalazine, 258

Sulfonylurea, for DM, 200
Syphilis
    pregnancy and, 261
    screening for, 89
    treatment for, 261
Systemic lupus erythematosus (SLE), CKD and, 78
Systolic blood pressure (SBP), 74
    in men, 295
    refractory hypertension and, 227
    in women, 297

T
T-ACE, in alcohol abuse screening, 3
Tadalafil, for ED, 204
Tamoxifen
    for breast cancer, 15, 96
    for endometrial cancer, 29
TAT. *See* Triple anticoagulation therapy
Taxanes, for cancer, 167
TB. *See* Tuberculosis
TC. *See* Total cholesterol
TCD. *See* Transcranial Doppler
TEE. *See* Transesophageal echocardiogram
Telavancin, for MRSA, 236
Tension-type headache, 208
Teriparatide, for osteoporosis, 240
Testicular cancer, screening for, 43, 290
Testosterone
    for androgen deficiency syndrome, 152
    for ED, 204
Tetracycline
    for COPD, 179
    for MRSA, 236
Thiazide diuretics, for DM, 201
Thymus gland, thyroid cancer and, 44
Thyroid cancer
    CRC and, 24
    screening for, 44

Thyroid disease
  celiac disease and, 45
  hyperthyroidism, 226
  hypothyroidism, 67, 85, 90
  prenatal care and, 255
  screening for, 90, 291
Thyroid nodules, treatment for, 267
Thyroid-stimulating hormone (TSH), 90
Tinidazole
  for trichomoniasis, 264
  for urethritis, 262
Tioconazole, for candidal vaginitis, 264
Tissue transglutaminase (TTG), celiac disease and, 45
TMP-SMX. *See* Trimethoprim-sulfamethoxazole
TNF-α. *See* Tumor necrosis factor-α
Tobacco. *See* Smoking
Topiramate, migraine and, 213
Topoisomerase I inhibitors, for cancer, 168
Topotecan, for cancer, 168
Total cholesterol (TC), 49, 50
Toxoplasma gondii
  encephalitis, 113
  with HIV, in children, 119
Transcranial Doppler (TCD), 146
Transesophageal echocardiogram (TEE), 160
Transfusions
  anemia and, 4
  for sickle cell disease, 146
Transplantation
  cervical cancer and, 17
  of hematopoietic cells, 168
  of liver, 151
  oral contraceptives and, 190
Transurethral laser ablation, for BPH, 163–164
Transvaginal ultrasound (TVU)
  for endometrial cancer, 28, 29
  for ovarian cancer, 37

Trastuzumab, for cancer, 168
Trichomoniasis, treatment for, 264
Tricyclic antidepressants
  for back pain, low, 233
  migraine and, 213
Triglycerides, 49
  DM and, 59
Trimethoprim-sulfamethoxazole (TMP-SMX)
  for MRSA, 236
  for PCP, 113, 117
  for *Toxoplasma gondii*, 113, 119
  for UTIs, 275
Triple anticoagulation therapy (TAT), for CAS, 193, 194
TSH. *See* Thyroid-stimulating hormone
TST. *See* Tuberculin skin test
TTG. *See* Tissue transglutaminase
Tuberculin skin test (TST), 93
Tuberculosis (TB). *See also* *Mycobacterium tuberculosis*
  latent
    primary prevention of, 113
    screening for, 93
Tumor necrosis factor-α (TNF-α), RA and, 257
Turner's syndrome, celiac disease and, 45
TVU. *See* Transvaginal ultrasound
TWEAK, in alcohol abuse screening, 3

U
Ultrasound. *See also* Transvaginal ultrasound
  for CAS, 45
  for HBV, 215
  for liver cancer, 32
  for thyroid cancer, 44
Upper gastrointestinal bleeding, from NSAIDs, 99
Urethral meatal warts, treatment for, 265